ATLAS of TRAVEL MEDICINE and HEALTH

THIRD EDITION

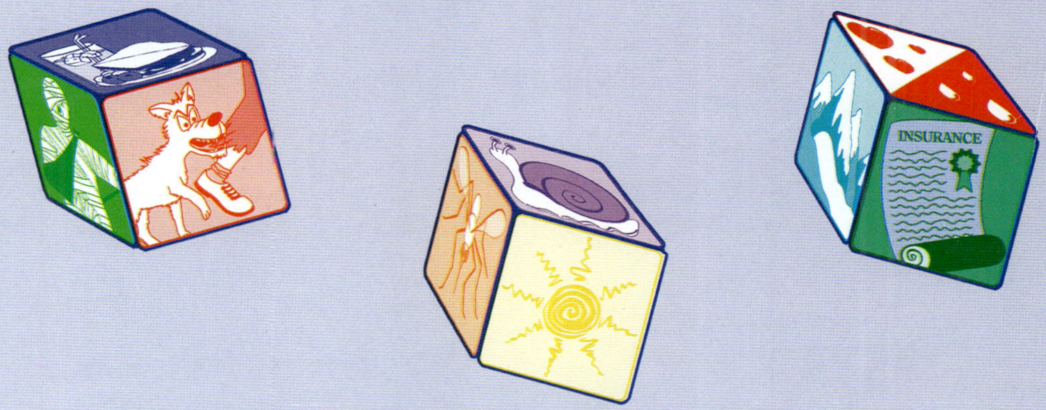

ATLAS of TRAVEL MEDICINE and HEALTH

THIRD EDITION

Jane Chiodini
MSc, RGN, RM,
FFTM RCPS (Glasg)

THE VILLAGE MEDICAL CENTRE
GREAT DENHAM, BEDFORDSHIRE, UK

Lorna Boyne
RGN, MN, DTM (Hon.),
FFTM RCPS (Glasg), PG Cert. Med. Ed.

HEALTH PROTECTION SCOTLAND
GLASGOW, UK

2011
PEOPLE'S MEDICAL PUBLISHING HOUSE–USA
SHELTON, CONNECTICUT

People's Medical Publishing House-USA
2 Enterprise Drive, Suite 509
Shelton, CT 06484
Tel: 203-402-0646; Fax: 203-402-0854
E-mail: info@pmph-usa.com

PMPH-USA

11 12 13 14/PMPH/9 8 7 6 5 4 3 2 1

ISBN-13: 978-1-60795-048-6

ISBN-10: 1-60795-048-0

Printed in China by People's Medical Publishing House
Production/Book design: GYAT, Terrance P. Tor; Staff Editor: Linda Mehta; Cover designer: Mary McKeon

Library of Congress Cataloging-in-Publication Data applied for.

Sales and Distribution

Canada
McGraw-Hill Ryerson Education
Customer Care
300 Water St
Whitby, Ontario L1N 9B6, Canada
Tel: 1-800-565-5758
Fax: 1-800-463-5885
www.mcgrawhill.ca

Foreign Rights
John Scott & Company
International Publisher's Agency
P.O. Box 878
Kimberton, PA 19442, USA
Tel: 610-827-1640
Fax: 610-827-1671

Japan
United Publishers Services Limited
1-32-5 Higashi-Shinagawa
Shinagawa-ku, Tokyo 140-0002, Japan
Tel: 03-5479-7251
Fax: 03-5479-7307
Email: kakimoto@ups.co.jp

United Kingdom, Europe, Middle East, Africa
McGraw Hill Education
Shoppenhangers Road
Maidenhead
Berkshire, SL6 2QL, England
Tel: 44-0-1628-502500
Fax: 44-0-1628-635895
www.mcgraw-hill.co.uk

Singapore, Thailand, Philippines, Indonesia, Vietnam, Pacific Rim, Korea
McGraw-Hill Education
60 Tuas Basin Link
Singapore 638775
Tel: 65-6863-1580
Fax: 65-6862-3354
www.mcgraw-hill.com.sg

Australia, New Zealand, Papua New Guinea, Fiji, Tonga, Solomon Islands, Cook Islands
Woodslane Pty Limited
Unit 7/5 Vuko Place
Warriewood NSW 2102, Australia
Tel: 61-2-9970-5111
Fax: 61-2-9970-5002
www.woodslane.com.au

Brazil
SuperPedido Tecmedd
Beatriz Alves, Foreign Trade Department
R. Sansao Alves dos Santos, 102 | 7th floor
Brooklin Novo
Sao Paolo 04571-090, Brazil
Tel: 55-16-3512-5539
www.superpedidotecmedd.com.br

India, Bangladesh, Pakistan, Sri Lanka, Malaysia
CBS Publishers
4819/X1 Prahlad Street 24
Ansari Road, Darya Ganj, New Delhi-110002
India
Tel: 91-11-23266861/67
Fax: 91-11-23266818
Email: cbspubs@vsnl.com

People's Republic of China
People's Medical Publishing House
International Trade Department
No. 19, Pan Jia Yuan Nan Li, Chaoyang District
Beijing 100021, P.R. China
Tel: 8610-67653342
Fax: 8610-67691034
www.pmph.com/en/

CONTENTS

Section 1: General Advice

Section 2: Travel Related Diseases and Their Global Distribution

Section 3: Country-Specific Advice, Maps, and Weather

Introduction

Many people are unaware of the health risks involved in traveling unprotected to disease risk areas. *The Atlas of Travel Medicine and Health* has been developed to help you improve this situation.

This book should be used a guide by the healthcare professional when discussing travel health. It is assumed a full risk assessment will have been carried out for the traveler before the atlas is referred to. As a result, such information has not been included within this publication but further details can be found in information resources (*see Ref. 2 below*).

The Atlas of Travel Medicine and Health is intended to be used as a reference tool in conjunction with a number of other reference sources. These include:

1. Centers for Disease Control and Prevention. CDC Health Information for International Travel 2010. Atlanta: U.S. Department of Health and Human Services, Public Health Service, 2009 http://wwwnc.cdc.gov/travel/
2. Chiodini J, Boyne L, Grieve S, Jordan A. Royal College of Nursing Competencies: An Integrated Career and Competency Framework for Nurses in Travel Health Medicine. RCN, London: 2007. http://www.rcn.org.uk/__data/assets/pdf_file/0006/78747/003146.pdf
3. Chiodini P, Hill D, Lalloo D, Lea G, Walker E, Whitty C, Bannister B. Guidelines for malaria prevention in travelers from the United Kingdom. London, Health Protection Agency, January 2007 http://www.malaria-reference.co.uk/
4. Department of Health. Immunisation Against Infectious Disease—"the Green Book". The Stationery Office. London, 2006. www.dh.gov.uk/greenbook
5. Field VF, Ford L, Hill DR, eds. Health Information for Overseas Travel. National Travel Health Network and Centre, London, UK: 2010.
6. Fitfortravel online website—this is the public access equivalent of TRAVAX from Health Protection Scotland. www.fitfortravel.nhs.uk
7. Foreign and Commonwealth Office travel advice unit. www.fco.gov.uk/travel
8. National Travel Health Network and Centre (NaTHNaC) online website and database for healthcare professionals and the general public. www.nathnac.org
9. TRAVAX online website for healthcare professionals from Health Protection Scotland. www.travax.nhs.uk
10. World Health Organization. International Travel and Health Geneva: WHO, 2011. www.who.int/ith

ACKNOWLEDGMENTS

The authors wish to thank Michelle White for her significant contribution and original graphics work on the malaria maps and *General Advice* icons. Thanks also go to Tomorrow's Guides Ltd, Hungerford for their permission to use weather statistics from "Weather to Travel" The Travellers' Guide to the World's Weather. Additional thanks to the World Health Organization for permission to use their disease endemicity maps.

How To Use This Atlas

A GUIDE FOR THE HEALTHCARE PROFESSIONAL

The atlas is divided into three main sections.

Sections 1 and 2 contain information for the healthcare professional only. As outlined on the contents page, these sections include key disease information and general advice about: water, food, and personal hygiene; accidents; animal bites, parasitic infection and other hazards; biting insects and bugs; sun and heat; casual sex and blood-borne modes of infection; altitude; and medical coverage, insurance. The disease pages contain information on 19 travel-related diseases considered to be among the most important. The information on these pages is for your reference only and is not intended to be shown to the traveler. You may wish, however, to use the endemicity maps available for some of the diseases if you think this is appropriate in the educational process.

Section 3 is the main part of the atlas. It is intended for use by both the healthcare professional and the traveler, and contains country-specific information for the top holiday destinations, arranged in alphabetical order.

The information provided on each page is as follows:

- ❑ A map of the country showing the capital city and, for some countries, an indication of the malaria risk areas.
- ❑ Vaccination advice (although this should always be used in conjunction with the most up-to-date references in conjunction with your national database for advice if available in the country in which you work).
- ❑ Graphs depicting the average daily sunshine, rainfall, and temperature.
- ❑ Other health considerations depicted by icons illustrating the appropriate advice, as outlined in Section 1, pages 1–8.

For further information on any countries not available in this book, details can be found at www.travax.nhs.uk (membership-only site) or, alternatively, on the public site of this service, valuable for travelers, at www.fitfortravel.nhs.uk.

DISCLAIMER

The material contained within the atlas, including endemicity maps, is designed to be used as a guide only. Information is issued as general information and should not be taken as advice. Country-specific information has been taken from a wide range of sources and may vary according to region. Similarly, the information provided on the annual sunshine, rainfall, and temperature will vary according to region.

While every effort has been made to ensure the accuracy of the information herein supplied, the authors and Health Protection Scotland make no warranty, express or implied, as to the accuracy, completeness, or usefulness of the information, and all liability is excluded, save in respect of any personal injury, caused by their negligence. No responsibility can be accepted for action or inaction as a result of information in this book.

How To Use Malaria Maps

Each country within the *Atlas of Travel Medicine and Health* has a map. Those countries that have a malaria risk will be shaded in one to three risk levels as follows:

Low to no risk antimalarials not usually advised	**Variable risk** antimalarials usually advised	**High risk** antimalarials usually advised	Surrounding countries with malaria risk

- ❑ Low to no malaria risk is shaded in light pink.
- ❑ Variable malaria risk is shaded in mid-pink.
- ❑ High malaria risk is shaded in darker pink.
- ❑ Surrounding areas where malaria is present are in beige.
- ❑ Surrounding areas where malaria is **not** present are in green.
- ❑ Black lines are country borders.
- ❑ A ● denotes the name of town.

These maps are intended only as helpful guides when you are determining whether or not your traveler is entering a malarious area. Remember that mosquitoes which spread malaria do not always respect boundaries, so while every effort has been taken to ensure that information within the maps is correct, they may not be exact. In addition, seasonal variation in malarial risk is not shown. It is essential that a full risk assessment is carried out and healthcare professionals should use another up-to-date reference source to help ascertain your patients' risk and whether or not they should take antimalarial chemoprophylaxis.

SECTION 1 General Advice

Key to General Advice Segments

Information in this section is intended for healthcare professionals. The segments of advice are represented by icons which are used in *Section 3* to illustrate healthcare advised when traveling to specific countries.

WATER, FOOD, AND PERSONAL HYGIENE

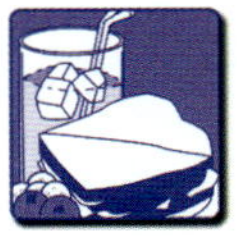

ACCIDENTS

ANIMAL BITES, PARASITIC INFECTION, AND OTHER HAZARDS

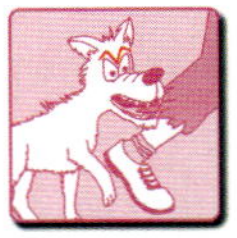

FRESH WATER PARASITES

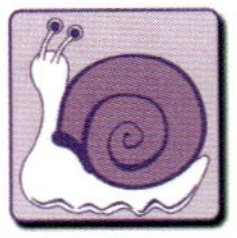

BITING INSECTS AND BUGS

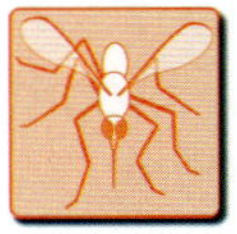

SUN AND HEAT

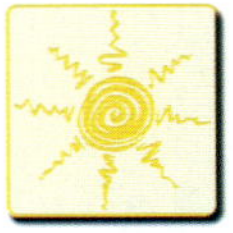

CASUAL SEX AND BLOOD-BORNE MODES OF INFECTION

ALTITUDE

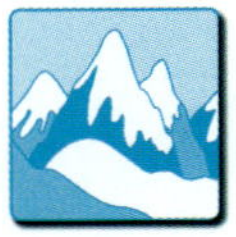

MEDICAL COVERAGE/INSURANCE

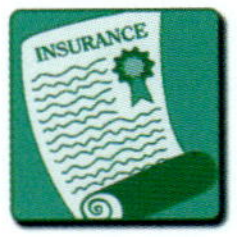

Water, Food, and Personal Hygiene

- ❑ Unless you are sure of the purity of the local water, do not drink it without boiling or sterilizing it first and avoid ice cubes. If unsure, use bottled water in sealed containers. This includes water for cleaning your teeth.
- ❑ Unpasteurized milk should be boiled before use. Caution should be exercised with local dairy produce including ice-cream.
- ❑ Remember that all meats should be cooked thoroughly and eaten hot whenever possible.
- ❑ Avoid leftovers and reheated food.
- ❑ Shellfish is a high risk food, especially when eaten raw. Take local advice, but when in doubt, avoid altogether.
- ❑ Eat only cooked vegetables and avoid salads.
- ❑ Peel all fruit.
- ❑ As a general rule, avoid purchasing food from roadside foodstalls.
- ❑ Always wash your hands thoroughly before eating, handling food, and after using the toilet.

Accidents

Swimming and road traffic accidents are common among travelers. Most accidents are preventable.

Precautions to take include:

- ❑ Avoid alcohol and food before swimming.
- ❑ Do not go swimming alone. Always supervise children.
- ❑ Check the depth of water before diving.
- ❑ Never drink and drive.
- ❑ If renting a vehicle, wherever possible choose a large sturdy one which has been well maintained. Avoid traveling at night.
- ❑ Whether driver or pedestrian, always check on local traffic regulations.
- ❑ Always wear a helmet on a motorbike, moped, or bicycle.
- ❑ Always wear a seat belt in a car.
- ❑ If you are going to take part in potentially hazardous sports such as skiing, canoeing, white water rafting, or para-gliding, follow all relevant safety advice.
- ❑ Know the local emergency facilities.
- ❑ Travelers to resource-poor countries may wish to carry a sterile medical pack with them. For further details, see the section for general advice on casual sex and blood-borne modes of infection.

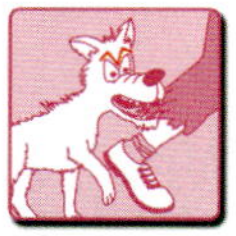

Animal Bites, Parasitic Infection, and Other Hazards

RABIES

Rabies is a viral disease which infects domestic and wild animals. It is transmitted to other animals and humans through close contact with saliva from infected animals, for example bites, scratches, licks on broken skin, and mucous membrane. Dogs are the source of 99% of human rabies deaths. Rabies is present on all continents with the exception of Antarctica, but more than 95% of human deaths occur in Asia and Africa.[1] Once symptoms of the disease develop, rabies is nearly always fatal (see page 27 for disease information). Therefore, prevention of exposure, and/or post exposure prophylaxis in the event of a potential rabies contact, is of immense significance.

Precautions to take include:

- ❑ Do not stroke dogs and cats (even domestic ones) and avoid contact with all wild animals.
- ❑ In rabies-endemic areas, all unprovoked bites or licks should be considered as possible exposure. In that event **immediate** first aid should be administered.
    - The wound should be cleansed thoroughly with soap or detergent and running water for several minutes—the World Health Organization advises 15 minutes duration.[1]
    - Antiseptic should be applied (povidone iodine or, if not available, 40%–70% alcohol will do, for example gin or whisky).
    - Medical assistance should be sought without delay.
    - In the event of possible exposure, attempts should be made to identify the owner of the animal and the animal should be observed for ten days to see if it begins to behave abnormally. The assistance of local officials may be necessary. If the animal is wild or stray, immediate attempts should be made to identify, capture, or even kill the animal involved to determine whether it is rabid.
- ❑ The recommended post-exposure prophylaxis depends on the type of contact with the suspected rabid animal and risk assessment will be required. If there has been contact with broken skin or mucous membranes, prompt post-exposure treatment will be required even if pre-exposure vaccine has been received.
- ❑ As the incubation period for rabies can be prolonged, treatment should still be considered even if the interval from exposure is lengthy. Specialist advice should be sought (contact details in www.dh.gov.uk/greenbook).

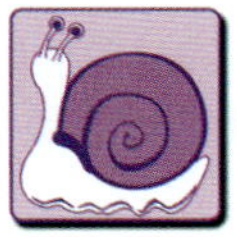

FRESH WATER PARASITES

Swimming and paddling should be avoided in schistosomiasis (bilharzia) endemic areas—for further information see page 29 on schistosomiasis.

OTHER HAZARDS

More adventurous travelers may be exposed to greater risks, e.g., snake bites, scorpion stings, spider bites, marine animals.

General advice includes:[2]

- ❑ ***Snake bite prevention:*** wear boots and long trousers; use a torch and walking stick if outdoors at night; avoid sleeping directly on the ground; avoid collections of rubbish near to a house or campsite and keep grass and foliage cut short.

- ❑ ***Scorpion stings and spider bites:*** avoid bed nets and bed clothes touching the floor for the scorpions and spiders to climb up near the bedding; shake shoes and clothing before putting them on.
- ❑ ***Aquatic species bites or stings:*** Wear plastic shoes in and around water; do not touch coral.

REFERENCES

1. World Health Organization Rabies factsheet no. 99, updated September 2010. Accessed at http://www.who.int/mediacentre/factsheets/fs099/en/.
2. Field VF, Ford L, Hill DR, Eds. Health Information for Overseas Travel. London: National Travel Health Network and Centre; 2010.

Biting Insects and Bugs

In tropical areas, many different mosquitoes, flies, fleas, ticks and bugs can bite, transmitting a variety of diseases. Many of these arthropods bite at night, but some do so during the day. Measures can be taken to prevent these bites.

- ❑ Use insect repellent on exposed skin, preferably one containing DEET; UK guidance suggests up to 50% content DEET for all travelers from 2 months of age, including pregnant and breast feeding women.[1]
- ❑ Wear socks, long trousers or skirts, and long sleeved clothing after sunset. Clothes can be sprayed with repellent or insecticide to give added protection.
- ❑ Air conditioning deters the entry of mosquitoes.
- ❑ If the sleeping area is screened, ensure windows and screens are closed before dusk. Vaporizing mats and knockdown sprays can be used in rooms to kill any mosquitoes that have entered the room during the day. An increased number of devices should be considered in larger rooms.
- ❑ If the room is not air conditioned or screened, sleep under a mosquito net, preferably one that is impregnated with an insecticide (e.g., permethrin).
- ❑ There is no scientific evidence to support the use of garlic, vitamin B, and electric buzzers. They are ineffective.[1]
- ❑ Herbal and homeopathic remedies should not be used.[1]
- ❑ Travelers to areas where there is a risk of tick-borne encephalitis should wear long-sleeved clothing, boots with trousers tucked into socks, and use insect repellent if walking in dense undergrowth in forested areas. Self inspection at the end of each day, to permit prompt removal of attached ticks, is essential.

REFERENCE

1. Chiodini P, et al. Guidelines for malaria prevention in travelers from the United Kingdom. London, Health Protection Agency, Jan 2007 http://www.hpa.org.uk/Topics/InfectiousDiseases/InfectionsAZ/Malaria/Guidelines/.

Sun and Heat

Sunburn and heat exhaustion can both cause great distress to travelers. Sunburn can produce long-term effects, including skin cancer. Both conditions are preventable.

Precautions to take include:

- ❑ Increase exposure to the sun gradually, not more that 20 minutes at a time initially.
- ❑ Use protective creams as appropriate and always reapply after washing or swimming.
- ❑ Wear sensible protective clothing, including hats, and wear sunglasses to filter UV rays.
- ❑ Avoid the sun between 11 AM and 3 PM when its rays are particularly strong, especially at high altitudes, in the snow, or at sea. Remember that you can burn even when swimming and snorkeling.
- ❑ People with pale skin and/or red hair should take special care in the sun.
- ❑ Protect infants and children at all times.
- ❑ Over exposure to sun in a hot and humid climate can lead to heat exhaustion. Avoid strenuous activity during the hottest hours and make sure that you drink plenty of non-alcoholic liquids to balance the loss of body fluids through perspiration. Be aware that alcohol consumption can make you dehydrated.

Casual Sex and Blood-borne Modes of Infection

If the traveler indulges in casual sex, the risk of infection with a sexually transmitted disease is high. Gonorrhea and syphilis may cause long-term disability, especially if treatment is delayed. Hepatitis B and the human immunodeficiency virus (HIV), the cause of AIDS, are spread sexually too, but are also spread by blood transfusion, medical procedures with non-sterile equipment, and the sharing of needles, e.g., tattooing, body piercing, acupuncture, and intravenous (IV) drug use. Hepatitis C is also transmitted via these routes, especially by IV drug use and unscreened blood.

Precautions to take include the following:

- ❑ Casual sexual intercourse is risky. Condoms provide good protection, but not complete protection. (If using condoms, for reliability take products that display evidence that a standard of manufacturing has been met, e.g., the CE Mark which is a requirement for products sold to the European Market). Be aware that hot climates and substances such as suntan oils may perish rubber.
- ❑ Drug taking should be avoided as it might put the traveler in contact with people who have hepatitis B or C or who are HIV-positive. Needle-sharing is very dangerous.

- ❑ Unless you are absolutely certain that the equipment being used is sterile, skin-damaging procedures such as ear/body piercing, tattooing, and acupuncture should be avoided.
- ❑ In many resource-poor countries reuse of medical supplies, including needles and syringes, is common. Travel packs containing sterile equipment for use in an emergency are available from some chemists and travel clinics. A kit should be supplied with a certificate showing contents and the reason for its purchase. This documentation is useful for customs clearance

BLOOD TRANSFUSION

In western Europe, North America, Japan, and Australia all donated blood is now screened for HIV antibodies. However, in most resource-poor countries, there may be only the most basic blood transfusion services and much of the blood donated is unscreened. The risks from blood transfusion in such circumstances are high. Therefore, points to consider are:

- ❑ Accidents are the most common reason for needing a blood transfusion. For further information, see the section for general advice on accident prevention.
- ❑ Blood transfusion should only be accepted when essential:
  - Pregnancy or any other medical condition which may lead to heavy blood loss, should be taken into account before traveling to destinations where good medical facilities will not be available
  - Knowing your blood group in advance may make it easier to find a donor in an emergency

A charitable organization in the United Kingdom called *The Blood Care Foundation* operates a blood care program that is designed to provide screened blood, in an emergency, to its members in any part of the world. The program is also designed to alleviate the shortages of blood that occur in many parts of the resource-poor world. Further information is available from http://www.bloodcare.org.uk.

ALTITUDE

High altitude travel is increasing in popularity. This topic is complex and further reading is required for more detail. Travelers going to extreme altitude should also be seeking specialist advice. A very useful booklet (translated into several different languages) is found at http://medex.org.uk//medex_book/about_book.php.

- ❑ High altitude destinations are considered to be above 2400 meters up to 3658 meters—this would include destinations such as Bogota, Quito, and Cuzco. Very high altitude is from 3658 m to 5500 m in destinations such as La Paz, base camp of Everest. Extreme altitude is from 5500 m to 8848 m—the height of the Mount Everest summit.[1]
- ❑ Altitude illness is a term used to describe a spectrum of illness associated with ascent to altitudes usually higher than 2500 meters. It can be divided into three syndromes: acute mountain sickness (AMS) which is the most common, high-altitude cerebral edema (HACE), and high-altitude pulmonary edema (HAPE).[2]

- Altitude illness can affect any traveler of any age and include those who are physically fit. Risk factors include the altitude gained, rate of ascent, the altitude reached, including the level at which the traveler sleeps and the level of exertion.[1,2]
- Symptoms of AMS include headache, fatigue, loss of appetite, nausea, and sleep disturbance. Mild AMS is usually self-limiting and symptoms can be relieved with analgesia and anti-emetics if required until the traveler has acclimatized.
- AMS progresses in less than 10% of cases to the more severe HACE where travelers experience lethargy, confusion, and ataxia in addition to the symptoms of AMS. HAPE is not necessarily preceded by AMS and symptoms include shortness of breath with exertion, a dry cough initially, becoming productive with blood-stained sputum and shortness of breath at rest. HAPE is frequently accompanied by symptoms of HACE. If a traveler with AMS is not improving then descent should occur by 500 m to 1000 m. However, if a traveler shows signs of HACE or HAPE they must descend completely and immediately. Both these conditions are critical and failure to descend can be life threatening.
- Prevention of altitude illness is not guaranteed, but gradual acclimatization and regular rest are extremely important. Travel to an altitude above 3500 m immediately from sea level should be avoided but if necessary, then several days rest should be taken to acclimatize, thereafter ascending no more than 300–500 m sleeping altitude per day, with a rest day every three days. If symptoms of AMS develop, then no further ascent should be made until recovered.
- Acetazolamide, while unlicensed for the prevention and treatment of AMS in the UK, is sometimes used "off label". Prophylaxis with this agent can speed up acclimatization and relieve symptoms, but it should never be used as an alternative to adequate acclimatization and gradual ascent. It is usually trialed before travel is undertaken to ensure no adverse side effects.

REFERENCES

1. NHS Scotland, Fit for Travel. Basic Information about Mountain Sickness (AMS): http://www.fitfortravel.nhs.uk/advice/advice-for-travelers/acute-mountain-sickness-(ams).aspx.
2. National Travel Health Network and Centre. Health Information Sheet—Altitude Illness: http://www.nathnac.org/pro/factsheets/altitude.htm.

Medical Coverage/Insurance

- Travel insurance covering both injuries and illness when traveling abroad is essential.
- Travelers should be encouraged to buy adequate travel insurance to provide comprehensive cover for cancellation and curtailment, the risks of the trip, and include adequate funds for medical repatriation. The insurance should also include a 24-hour assistance service and ideally, cover for legal services.
- Some credit and charge cards provide health insurance for travelers but this may not provide full travel cover. The policy must be checked to ensure it is adequate.

- When buying insurance any existing medical conditions **must** be declared. It may be necessary to search around for an insurance company to provide adequate protection, and some may charge a premium for this coverage. It is a good idea to carry a physician's letter stating the traveler's medical condition and medication. Having this information translated into the language(s) of the areas to be visited could also be useful.
- Some countries now require proof of adequate health insurance as a condition for entry.
- Some travel insurers require proof of immunizations and/or malaria prophylaxis as a condition of their approval for treatment or repatriation.[1]
- Travelers going on adventure holidays and "gap year" type travelers may find specialist company travel insurance more favorable.
- The group of travelers "Visiting Friends and Relations" (VFRs) should be reminded that travel insurance is an important aspect of their travel arrangements.
- It is good practice to carry a copy of the insurance certificate and contact details of the company together with other travel documents.
- Travelers who receive medical care in other countries may be required to pay in cash or by credit card at the point of service prior to reclaiming costs from their insurance company. Some countries may also have reciprocal agreements for health care which could reduce costs of immediate emergency care; for example the United Kingdom has a European Health Insurance Card (EHIC) for UK residents. This does not replace the need for travel insurance but is an additional option. Further information is available at www.ehic.org.uk.

REFERENCE

1. World Health Organization. International Travel and Health Geneva: WHO, 2011. Accessed at www.who.int/ith.

SECTION 2 Travel-Related Diseases and Their Global Distribution

Nineteen travel-related diseases considered to be among the most important (listed here in alphabetical order with respective page numbers):

*Maps listed with an asterisk denote a WHO map and were accessed May 2011 at www.who.int/ith. The boundaries and names shown and the designations used on the WHO maps do not imply the expression of any opinion whatsoever on the part of the World Health Organization concerning the legal status of any country, territory, city, or area or of its authorities, or concerning the delimination of its frontiers or boundaries. Dotted lines on the maps represent approximate border lines for which there may not yet be full agreement.

CHIKUNGUNYA

COUNTRIES OR AREAS AT RISK

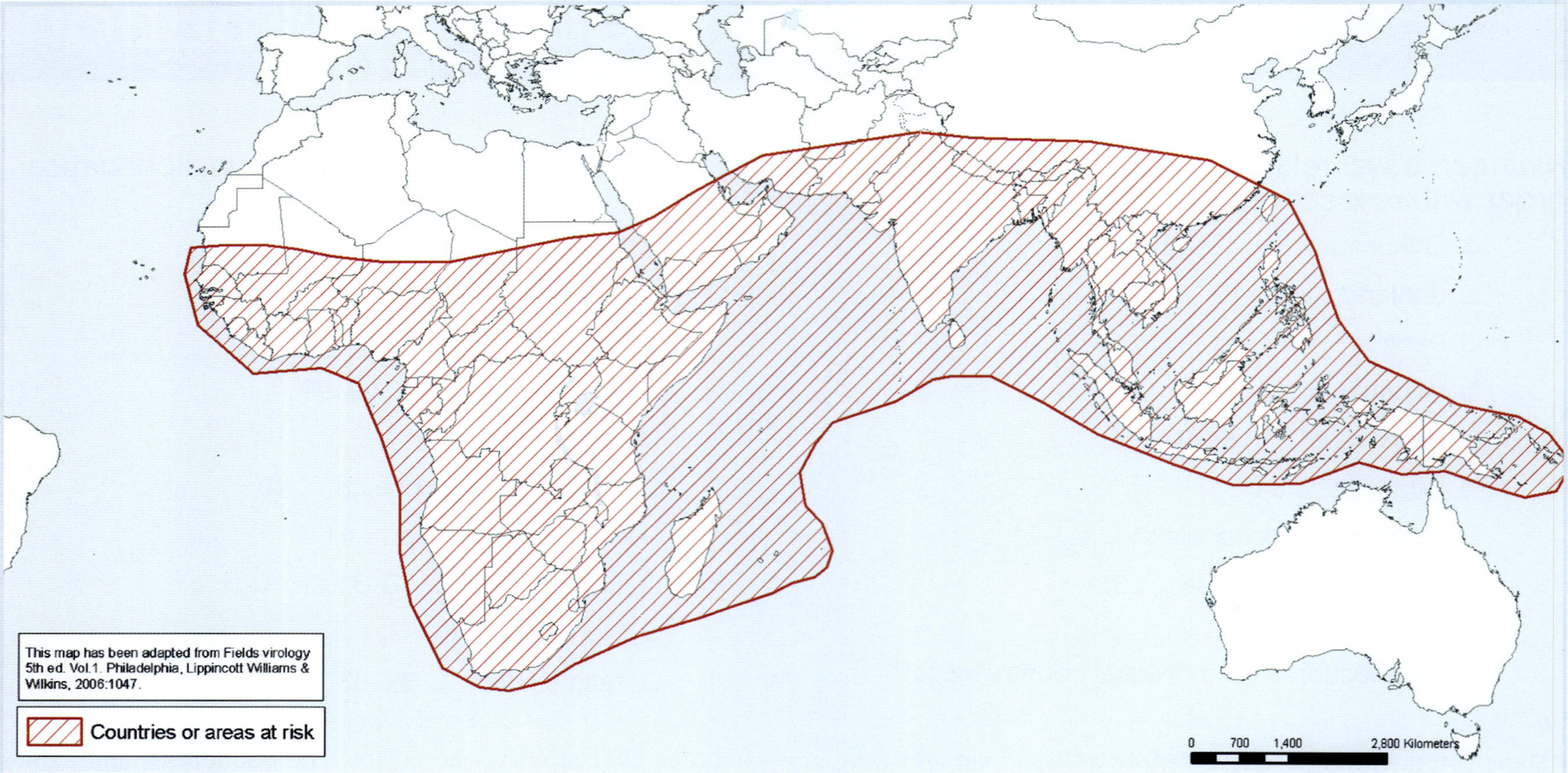

DATA SOURCE: World Health Organization; accessed May 2011. MAP PRODUCTION: Public Health Information and Geographic Information System (GIS) World Health Organization.

CHIKUNGUNYA

- Chikungunya virus (CHIKV) is an RNA arbovirus causing viral infection in humans and nonhuman primates.
- Transmission is mainly by *Aedes aegypti* and *Aedes albopictus*, both day time biting mosquitoes.
- Chikungunya occurs in sub-Saharan Africa, South-East Asia, and tropical areas of the Indian subcontinent, as well as islands in the south-western Indian Ocean.[1]
- Incubation period of CHIKV is usually 4 to 7, up to 12 days.
- Clinical features include a sudden onset of fever, arthralgia, and myalgia.[2] A generalized maculopapular rash may appear after a few days. Unlike dengue, retro orbital pain and thrombocytopenia are both reported to be rare.[3]
- Clinically, chikungunya can be confused with dengue fever but the presence of polyarthralgia is in favor of CHIKV. Blood tests would be required to ascertain the diagnosis (real time PCR for viral RNA and serology for IgM and IgG antibodies are the mainstay of diagnosis).
- There is no specific antiviral therapy so treatment is supportive with fluids, analgesics, anti-inflammatory agents, and rest. Most patients recover well, but up to 10% suffer persistent polyarthralgia, lasting up to 6 months, occasionally longer. Elderly patients with underlying medical conditions are at risk of severe and complicated CHIKV infection.
- Currently, there is no licensed vaccine. Prevention depends entirely on mosquito bite avoidance.

REFERENCES

1. World Health Organization. International Travel and Health Geneva: WHO, 2011. Accessed at www.who.int/ith.
2. Field VF, Ford L, Hill DR (Eds). Health Information for Overseas Travel. London: National Travel Health Network and Centre; 2010.
3. Thiboutout MM, et al. Chikungunya: A Potentially Emerging Epidemic? PLoS Neglected Diseases. 2010; 4: e623.

CHOLERA

AREAS REPORTING OUTBREAKS, 2009–2010

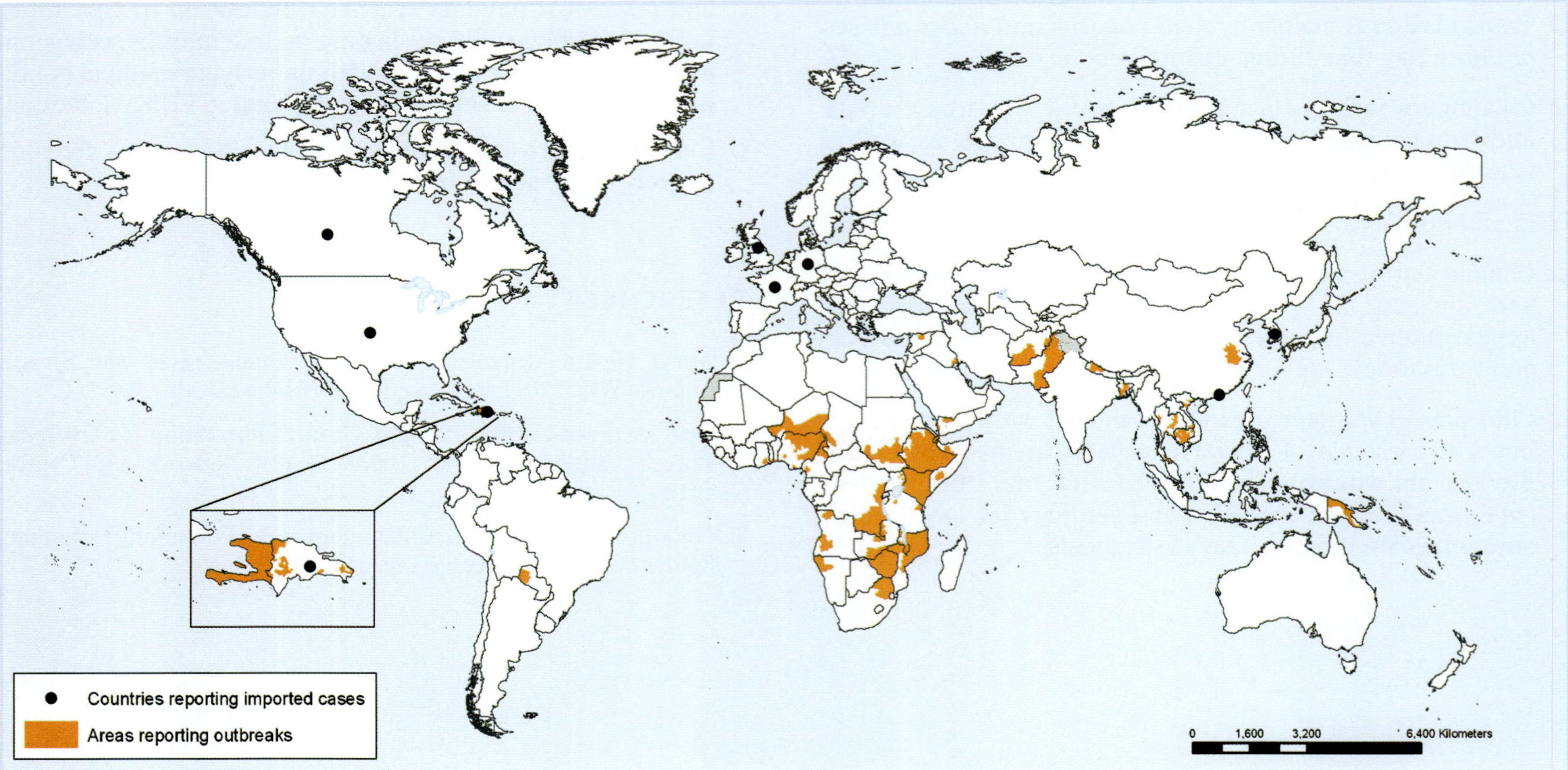

DATA SOURCE: World Health Organization; accessed May 2011. MAP PRODUCTION: Public Health Information and Geographic Information System (GIS) World Health Organization.

CHOLERA

- Cholera is caused by infection with *Vibrio cholerae*, a gram negative bacillus. Of 139 serogroups, only two, O1 and O139, cause cholera. *V. cholerae* O1 exists as two biotypes, classical and El Tor. Each of these biotypes can exist as serotype Ogawa, Inaba or Hikojima.[1] Cholera is a disease of poor sanitation due to ingestion of contaminated water and occasionally food.
- Cholera is predominately a disease of Africa and Asia with most cases occurring in Africa. There are an estimated 3–5 million cholera cases and 100,000–120,000 deaths due to cholera every year.[2]
- Incubation period is usually 2–5 days, but can be as short as 6 hours.
- Clinical features of most infections with *V. cholerae* are mild or inapparent[3] but approximately 11% of classical and 2% of El Tor cases develop severe clinical illness. There is sudden onset of high volume watery diarrhea without tenesmus, often followed by vomiting. Diarrheal volume may be 0.5 to one liter per hour. Severe dehydration with vascular collapse, acidosis, and acute renal tubular necrosis are features of severe cases.
- Diagnosis in an outbreak situation is usually on clinical presentation, but bacterial culture of stool with sero grouping and biotyping of the organism is definitive.
- Treatment includes vigorous fluid replacement and supportive therapy. Antimicrobial therapy shortens the episode of diarrhea by approximately 50% and reduces the length of time for which vibrios are excreted to one or two days from 5 or more days.[4] Tetracycline or doxycycline, macrolides (e.g., erythromycin, azithromycin), ciprofloxacin, and co-trimoxazole can be used, depending on sensitivity tests.
- Good sanitation and good personal hygiene form the basis of prevention. Vaccination is recommended for travelers and aid workers visiting areas where cholera outbreaks due to *V. cholerae* O1 are underway. The inactivated oral vaccine consists of *V. cholerae* O1 Inaba classical and El Tor and O1 Ogaba classical biotypes along with recombinant cholera toxin B,[5] but does not confer protection against O139 strains.

REFERENCES

1. Ward KN, et al. Notes on Medical Microbiology. 2nd Edit. Edinburgh: Churchill Livingstone Elsevier; 2009 (597 pages).
2. World Health Organization. Cholera fact sheet No. 107. Updated June 2010. http://www.who.int/mediacentre/factsheets/fs107/en/index.html.
3. Kaper JB, et al. Cholera. Clinical Microbiology Reviews. 1995;8:48–86.
4. Nelson EJ, et al. Antibiotics for Both Moderate and Severe Cholera. New Engl J Med. December 9, 2010; NEJM.ORG: 1–2.
5. Field VF, Ford L, Hill DR (Eds). Health Information for Overseas Travel. London: National Travel Health Network and Centre; 2010. (http://www.nathnac.org provides purchase information.)

DENGUE

COUNTRIES OR AREAS AT RISK, 2010

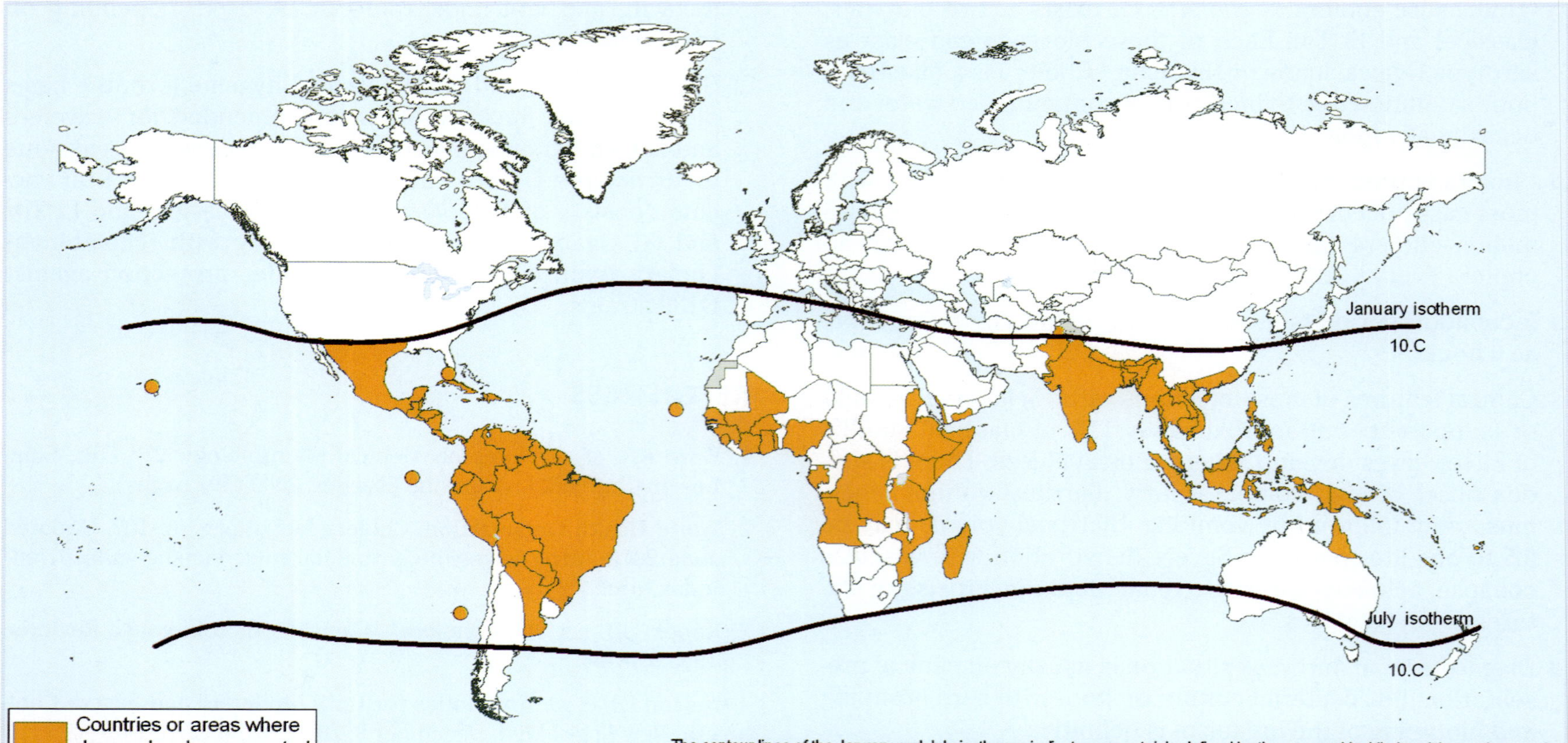

The contour lines of the January and July isotherms indicate areas at risk, defined by the geographical limits of the northern and southern hemispheres for year-round survival of Aedes aegypti, the principal mosquito vector of dengue viruses.

DATA SOURCE: World Health Organization; accessed May 2011. MAP PRODUCTION: Public Health Information and Geographic Information System (GIS) World Health Organization.

DENGUE

- Dengue is an arbovirus infection transmitted by the mosquito *Aedes aegypti*.
- After malaria, dengue is the most common and serious mosquito-borne infection affecting travelers.
- Dengue is widespread in tropical and subtropical regions of central and South America and South and Southeast Asia. It also occurs in Africa and Oceania. The risk is lower at altitudes above 1000 m. The incidence of dengue has grown dramatically around the world in recent decades. Some 2.5 billion people—two fifths of the world's population—are now at risk from dengue. WHO currently estimates there may be 50 million dengue infections worldwide every year.[1] There is a risk for travelers in countries or areas at risk and affected by epidemics.[2]
- The incubation period of dengue is 5 to 8 days.
- Symptoms include high fever, headache, retro orbital pain, severe joint, bone, and muscular pain. A fine maculopapular rash appears around day 4. The illness lasts about one week, but full recovery can take far longer. Dengue fever is also sometimes called "breakbone fever".
- There is no vaccine currently available.
- Prevention of the infection is by stringent mosquito bite prevention methods.
- Mosquitoes that transmit dengue **bite mostly during the daytime.** Avoid mosquito breeding areas, if known.
- A dangerous variant is known as dengue hemorrhagic fever, particularly in Southeast Asia. This disease is thought to be related to previous exposure to a different dengue serotype. The illness can develop to uncontrolled bleeding and shock, requiring intensive care treatment. Fatality rates can be high. Without appropriate hospital care, 40–50% of cases can be fatal; with timely medical care by experienced physicians and nurses the mortality rate can be decreased to 1% or less.[2]

REFERENCES

1. World Health Organization. Dengue and dengue haemorrhagic fever fact sheet No. 117. Updated March, 2009. Accessed at http://www.who.int/mediacentre/factsheets/fs117/en/index.html.
2. World Health Organization. International Travel and Health Geneva: WHO; 2011. Accessed at www.who.int/ith.

HEPATITIS A

COUNTRIES OR AREAS AT RISK

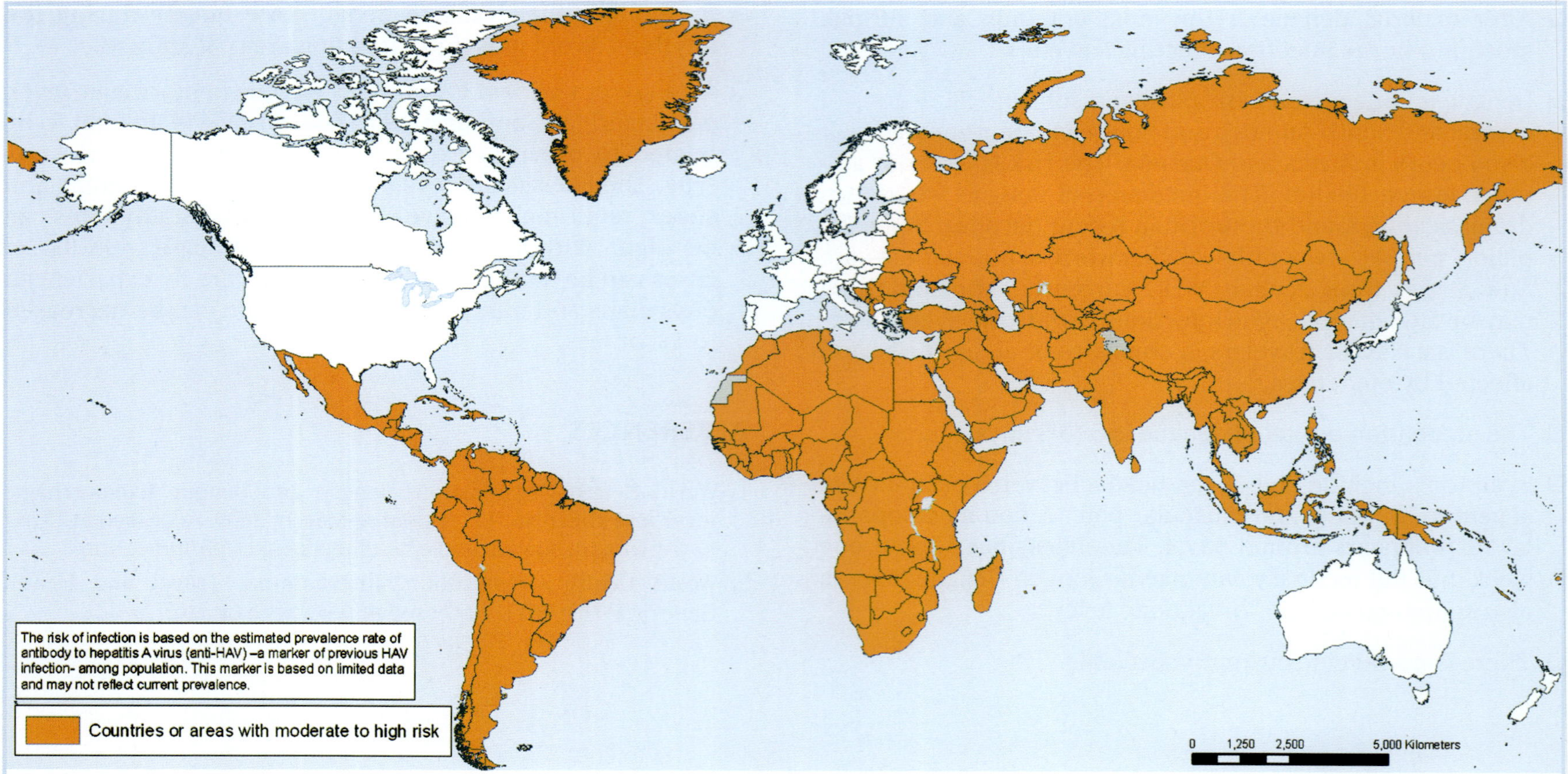

DATA SOURCE: World Health Organization; accessed May 2011. MAP PRODUCTION: Public Health Information and Geographic Information System (GIS) World Health Organization.

HEPATITIS A

- Hepatitis A is a highly infectious disease, caused by a virus (formerly called infectious hepatitis).
- Transmission of hepatitis A is by the fecal-oral route. Person to person spread is the most common method of transmission, although contaminated food and drink is a risk to travelers.
- Hepatitis A is endemic throughout the world and hyperendemic in areas of poor sanitation. Anyone traveling outside northern and western Europe, Scandinavia, North America, Japan, Australia, and New Zealand, should consider being immunized against hepatitis A.
- The highest risk areas for travelers are the Indian subcontinent and the Far East, but the risk extends to Eastern Europe.[1]
- Incubation is usually around 28–30 days, but may sometimes be as short as 15 days and as long as 50 days.[1]
- Symptoms include fever, myalgia, and lassitude. Nausea and vomiting are common, followed later by dark urine, pale stools, and jaundice.
- Asymptomatic or mild disease is common in very young children. However, severity tends to increase with age, with adults being more severely affected and those infected being unable to work for several weeks or months. Case-fatality is greater than 2% for those over 40 years of age and 4% for those over 60.[2]
- Hepatitis A is one of the most common vaccine-preventable infections of travelers.[3]
- Immunization with an inactivated vaccine of 2 doses 6–12 months apart offers prolonged, possibly lifetime, protection following the primary course.[4]
- Travelers should still adhere to food, water, and personal hygiene advice.
- Travelers should be made aware that shellfish are a common source of hepatitis A (they are filter feeders and concentrate the virus from fecally contaminated water).
- Travelers who have suffered hepatitis A infection will have developed lifelong immunity and will not require vaccination. (This should be confirmed with a blood test.)

REFERENCES

1. Department of Health (2006) Immunization Against Infectious Disease—"the Green Book". London: The Stationery Office; 2006. Accessed at and updated online 2009 www.dh.gov.uk/greenbook.
2. World Health Organization. International Travel and Health Geneva: WHO, 2011. Accessed at www.who.int/ith.
3. Centers for Disease Control and Prevention. CDC Health Information for International Travel 2010. Atlanta: U.S. Department of Health and Human Services, Public Health Service; 2009. http://wwwnc.cdc.gov/travel/content/yellowbook/home-2010.aspx.
4. Field VF, Ford L, Hill DR (Eds). Health Information for Overseas Travel. London: National Travel Health Network and Centre; 2010.

HEPATITIS B

COUNTRIES OR AREAS AT RISK

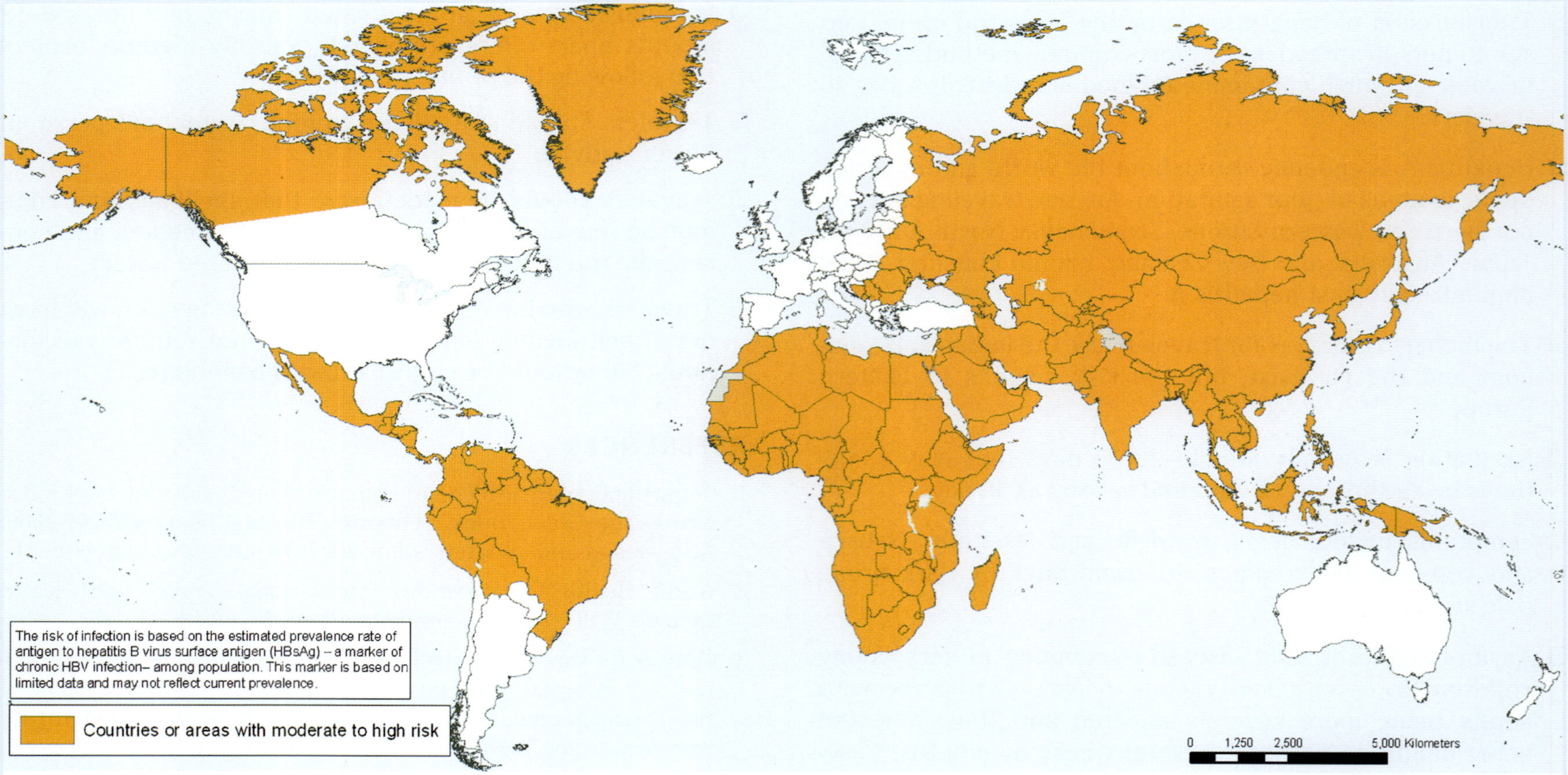

DATA SOURCE: World Health Organization; accessed May 2011. MAP PRODUCTION: Public Health Information and Geographic Information System (GIS) World Health Organization.

HEPATITIS B

- Hepatitis B virus (HBV) is an acute viral infection that attacks the liver and can cause both acute and chronic disease. This chronic liver infection can develop later into cirrhosis of the liver or liver cancer. Chronic infection complications are more common in those infected at a very young age.[1]
- Transmission is through contact with blood or other body fluids of an infected person. For travelers, sexual contact is an important mode of transmission, but infection can also be transmitted by transfusion of contaminated blood or blood products, use of contaminated needles and syringes for injections and other skin-penetrating procedures, including acupuncture, piercing and tattooing. Perinatal transmission from mother to baby is a common mode in resource poor countries.[2] Hepatitis B virus is 50 to 100 times more infectious than human immunodeficiency virus (HIV) and unlike HIV, HBV can survive outside the body for at least 7 days and during that time still cause infection.[1]
- Incubation period ranges from 40 to 160 days, with an average of 60 to 90 days.[2]
- Many HBV infections are asymptomatic or cause mild symptoms which are often unrecognized in adults. Clinical symptoms are similar to hepatitis A, although some cases can progress to acute hepatic necrosis. Among cases requiring hospital admission, the fatality rate is about 1%.[1]
- The prevalence of chronic HBV infection is high (≥8%) in all socioeconomic groups in: all of Africa; Southeast Asia, including China, Korea, Indonesia, and the Philippines; the Middle East, except Israel; South and Western Pacific islands; the interior Amazon River basin; and certain parts of the Caribbean (Haiti and the Dominican Republic). Intermediate risk (2%–7%) is present in South, Central, and Southwest Asia, Israel, Japan, Eastern and Southern Europe, Russia, most areas surrounding the Amazon River basin, Honduras, and Guatemala.[3]
- Hepatitis B is preventable with a safe and effective vaccine.[1] Risk assessment of the traveler and type of trip will help inform the decision to protect including the prevalence of chronic HBV at the destination and the type of activities to be undertaken. The vaccine should be considered for all non-immune individuals traveling to countries or areas with moderate to high risk of infection.[4]
- Immunization is recommended in individuals who are at increased risk of hepatitis B because of their lifestyle, occupation, or other factors such as close contact with a case or carrier.
- Country specific guidance varies on the length of protection hepatitis B vaccination provides. In the UK, travelers are currently advised to have one booster dose of hepatitis B vaccine if at continuing risk of infection, five years after the primary course.[2] Other bodies do not advise a booster and state that a course of immunization provides protection for at least 15 years and, according to current scientific evidence, probably for life.[4]
- It is important that immunization against hepatitis B does not encourage relaxation of good infection-control procedures.

REFERENCES

1. World Health Organization Hepatitis B Fact sheet no. 204 revised August 2008. Accessed at http://www.who.int/mediacentre/factsheets/fs204/en/index.html.
2. Department of Health. Immunization Against Infectious Disease—"the Green Book". London: The Stationery Office. London; 2006. Updated online 2009 http://www.dh.gov.uk/prod_consum_dh/groups/dh_digitalassets/@dh/@en/_documents/digitalasset/dh_108820.pdf .
3. Centers for Disease Control and Prevention. CDC Health Information for International Travel 2010. Atlanta: U.S. Department of Health and Human Services, Public Health Service, 2009
4. World Health Organization. International Travel and Health Geneva: WHO, 2011. Accessed at www.who.int/ith.

JAPANESE B ENCEPHALITIS

COUNTRIES OR AREAS AT RISK, 2008

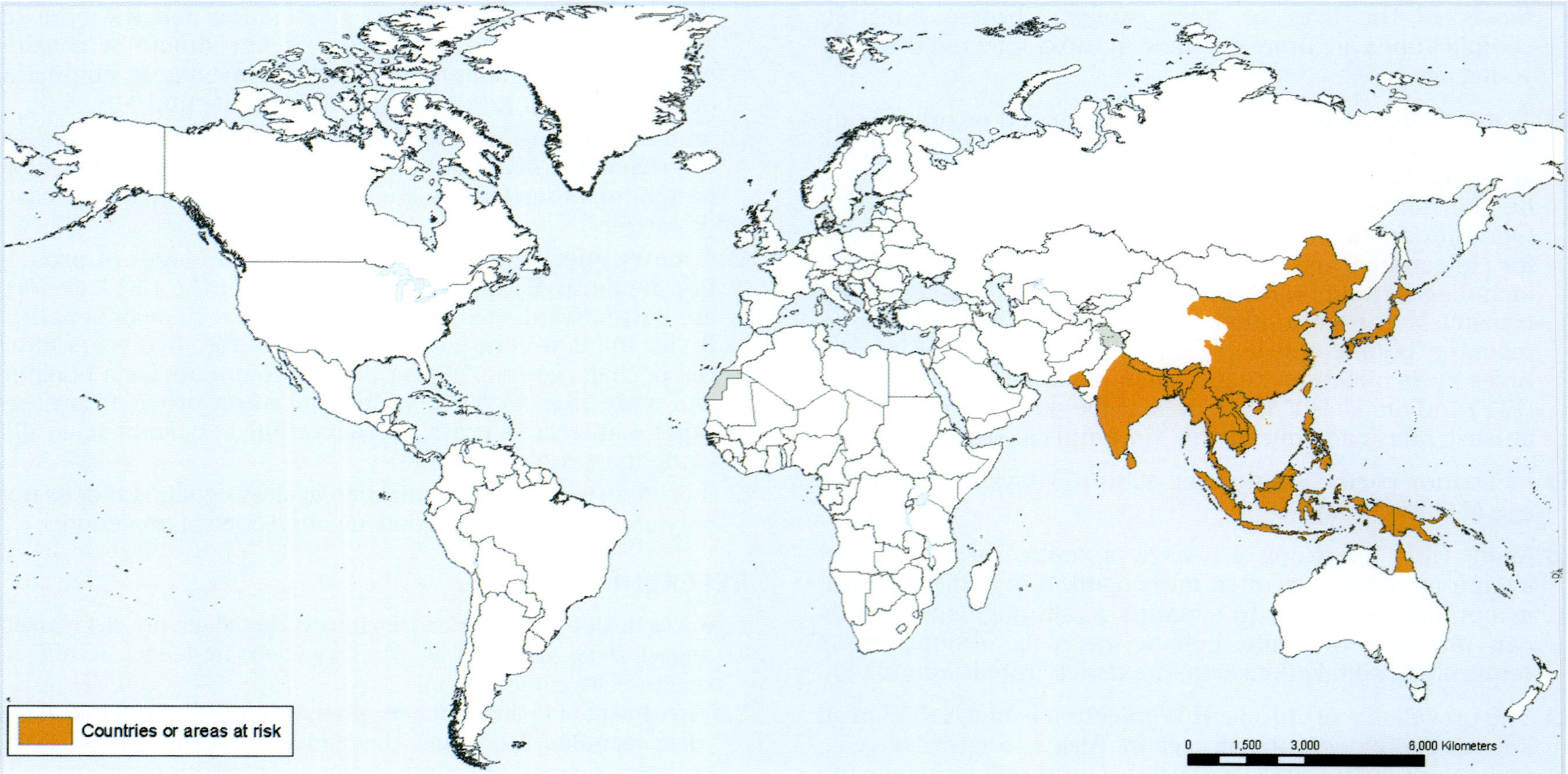

DATA SOURCE: World Health Organization; accessed May 2011. MAP PRODUCTION: Public Health Information and Geographic Information System (GIS) World Health Organization.

JAPANESE ENCEPHALITIS

- ❑ Japanese encephalitis (JE) is a flavivirus transmitted by various species of culicene mosquito from domestic animals (often pigs) and birds to humans. These mosquitoes most commonly breed in rice fields.
- ❑ The disease exists in almost all Asian countries. Largely as a result of immunization, its incidence has been declining in Japan and the Republic of Korea and in some regions of China, but the disease is increasingly reported from Bangladesh, parts of India, Nepal, parts of Pakistan, northern Thailand, and Viet Nam. Transmission occurs principally in rural agricultural locations where flooding irrigation is practized—some of which may be near or within urban centers.[1]
- ❑ Transmission is seasonal and mainly related to the rainy season in Southeast Asia, but year-round transmission occurs, specifically in tropical climate zones. In the temperate regions of China, Japan, the Korean peninsula, and eastern parts of the Russian Federation, transmission occurs mainly during the summer and autumn.[1]
- ❑ Incubation period of JE is 5 to 15 days.[2]
- ❑ JE infection is asymptomatic in the majority of cases; however, if the infection develops into a severe encephalitis, there is a 20% to 30% mortality rate and about 25% to 30% of the survivors are left with neurological sequelae.[3]
- ❑ The disease is extremely rare in travelers, with only two reported cases in UK travelers, in 1982 and 1994. The overall estimated risk is 1 case per 5,000 to 1,000,000 visitors.[3]
- ❑ Risk is increased for long-term travelers, expatriates, and those staying in rural and especially agricultural areas within the endemic zone and in the transmission season.
- ❑ Until recently, the inactivated mouse-brain-derived (IMB) vaccine against Japanese encephalitis was the most widely available commercially, however, a new tissue culture derived vaccine is now available in the UK for use in travelers 18 years and older, but the IMB vaccine is still used for younger travelers. As delayed allergic reactions to the IMB vaccine can occur, the vaccine course should be completed preferably 10 days before travel. Those with history of urticaria or multiple allergies are considered at higher risk of allergic reactions to IMB vaccine. Rare neurological adverse events also occur.[2] Following vaccination, the traveler should be closely observed for 30 minutes within the medical facility.[4]
- ❑ Travelers should be advised to maintain adequate bite prevention measures particularly between dusk and dawn to help prevent JE.

REFERENCES

1. World Health Organization. International Travel and Health Geneva: WHO; 2011. Accessed at www.who.int/ith.
2. Department of Health Immunization Against Infectious Disease—"the Green Book". London: The Stationery Office; 2006, updated online July 2010 http://www.dh.gov.uk/prod_consum_dh/groups/dh_digitalassets/@dh/@en/documents/digitalasset/dh_117991.pdf.
3. Field VF, Ford L, Hill DR (Eds). Health Information for Overseas Travel. London: National Travel Health Network and Centre; 2010.
4. National Travel health Network and Centre. Japanese encephalitis health information. Updated July 2010 http://www.nathnac.org/pro/factsheets/japanese_enc.htm.

MENINGITIS

COUNTRIES OR AREAS AT HIGH RISK, 2009

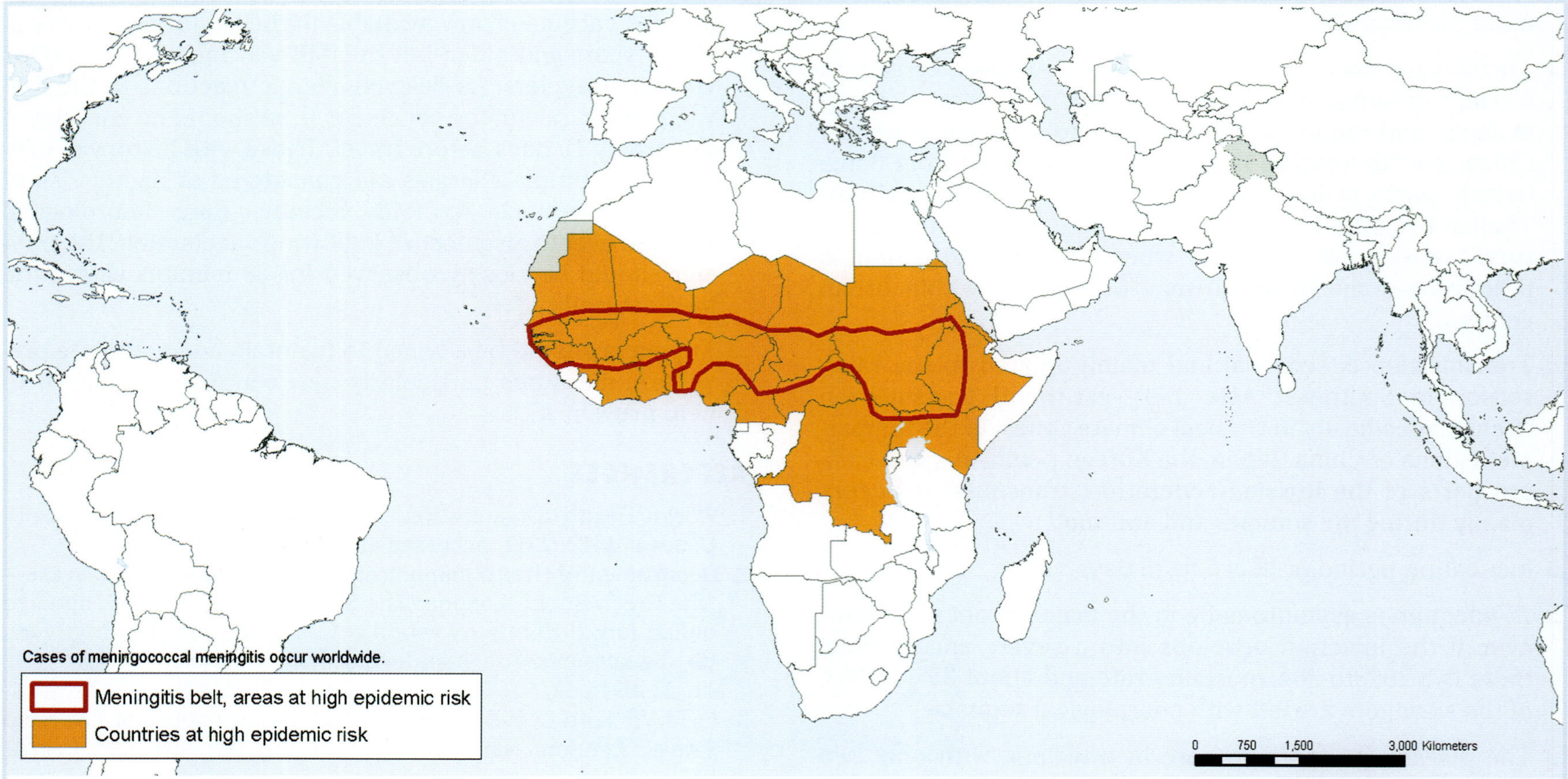

DATA SOURCE: World Health Organization; accessed May 2011. MAP PRODUCTION: Public Health Information and Geographic Information System (GIS) World Health Organization.

MENINGITIS

- Meningitis means inflammation of the membranes covering the brain and spinal cord, caused by many different types of viruses and bacteria. Bacterial meningitis can be rapidly fatal.
- Organisms causing meningitis are transmitted by droplet spread or direct contact from carriers or from individuals in the early stages of the illness; the probable route of invasion is via the nasopharynx.
- Meningococcal meningitis is a systemic bacterial infection caused by the organism *Neisseria meningitidis* which has at least 13 antigenic groups including A, B, C, D, X, Y, Z, W135. Group A organisms cause epidemics, predominantly in sub-Saharan Africa, from Senegal and Gambia in the west to Ethiopia and Somalia in the east and as far south as Zambia, Malawi, and Namibia, particularly in the dry season. Serogroups A and W135, have been responsible for outbreaks in Saudi Arabia in those attending Hajj pilgrimages. Group B meningococci remain the prevalent epidemic organisms of Europe and North America, followed by Group C.
- Incubation period is from 2 to 7 days.[1]
- Symptoms include fever, malaise, vomiting, headache, photophobia, drowsiness or confusion, and joint pains. A typical hemorrhagic rash of meningococcal septicemia may develop. Overall, mortality remains around 10% in the UK with incidence higher in those with septicemia than with those having meningitis alone. In those who survive, approximately 25% may experience a reduced quality of life, with 10–20% developing permanent sequelae.[1] Prompt treatment is essential.
- Immunization (both in conjugate and polysaccharide presentations) is currently available against Groups A, C, W135, and Y providing a minimum of 3 years of protection.[1]
- Travelers visiting areas of risk of meningococcal disease whose planned activities put them at higher risk include healthcare workers, those visiting friends and relatives, and long-term travelers who have close contact with the local population. All are recommended to receive a meningococcal vaccine.[2]
- Travelers attending the Hajj and Umrah pilgrimage in Saudi Arabia are required to receive immunization against groups A, C, W135, and Y to obtain a visa for entry into the country. A certificate of vaccination should be given to the traveler.
- Those with asplenia or splenic dysfunction should be advised to receive the A, C, W135, and Y vaccine if traveling to a country where there is an increased risk of serogroup A, W135, or Y disease. These individuals should receive the Men ACWY conjugate vaccine because of the better immune response, particularly in children and older people.[1]

REFERENCES

1. Department of Health Immunization Against Infectious Disease—"the Green Book". London: The Stationery Office; 2006. Updated on line 2010 www.dh.gov.uk/greenbook; http://www.dh.gov.uk/prod_consum_dh/groups/dh_digitalassets/@dh/@en/documents/digitalasset/dh_122644.pdf.
2. Field VF, Ford L, Hill DR (Eds). Health Information for Overseas Travel. London: National Travel Health Network and Centre; 2010.

POLIO

AFFECTED COUNTRIES FOR WHICH WHO RECOMMENDS POLIO IMMUNIZATION OR BOOSTING TO TRAVELERS*

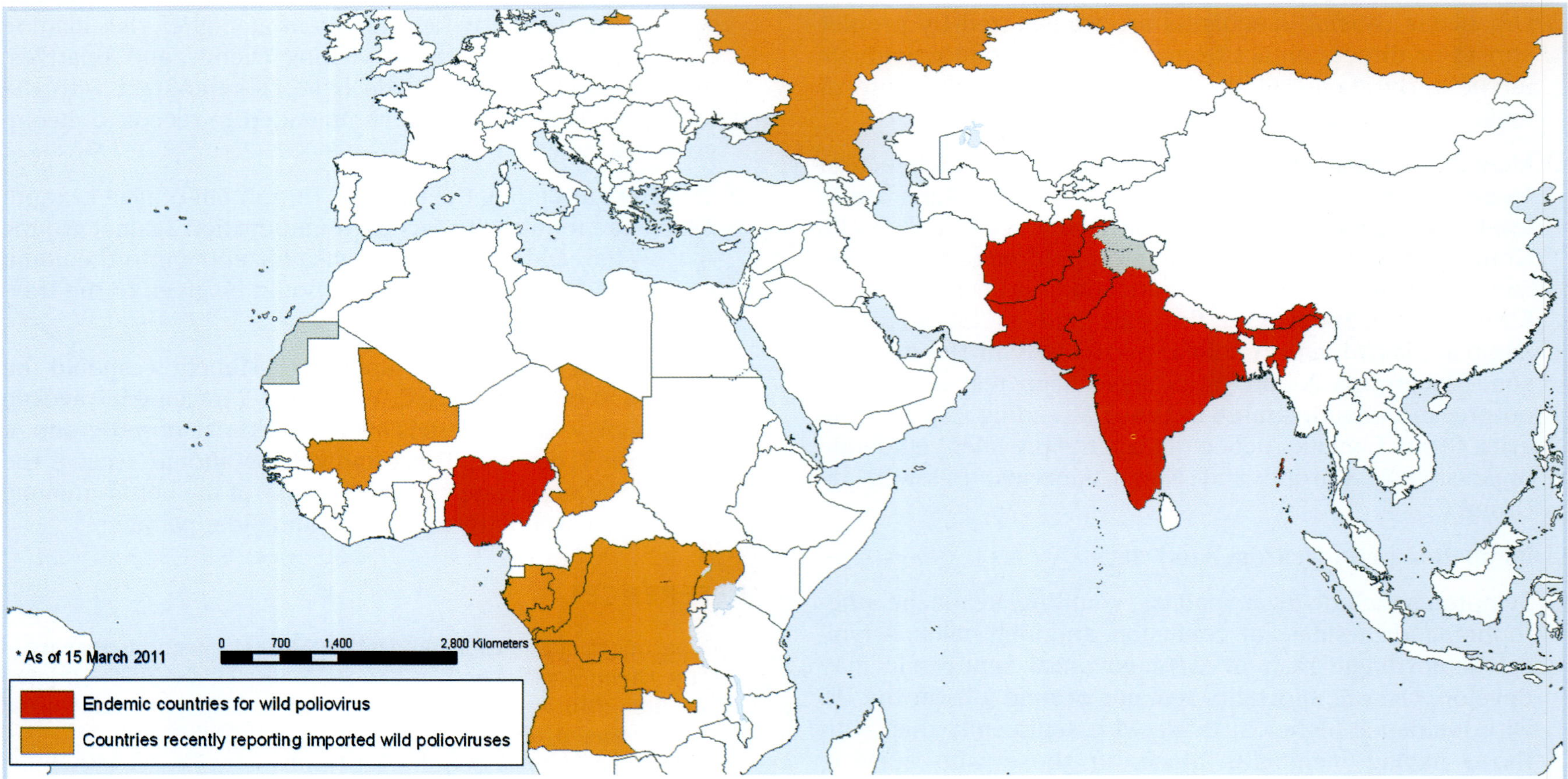

DATA SOURCE: World Health Organization; accessed May 2011. MAP PRODUCTION: Public Health Information and Geographic Information System (GIS) World Health Organization.

POLIO

- Poliomyelitis is an infection caused by one of three types of polio virus. The virus first invades the gastrointestinal tract and a viraemic illness may develop. In some cases the virus invades and destroys the anterior horn cells of the spinal cord. This results in flaccid muscle paralysis, more commonly of the lower limbs. In the most severe cases, the virus attacks the motor neurones of the brain stem causing difficulty in breathing, swallowing, and speaking. In such cases, death can occur unless respiratory support is given.
- Spread is via the fecal oral route, particularly in areas where there is poor food and water hygiene. Transmission is also possible via droplet infection from the nasopharynx of a person in the acute phase, and is more typical in areas where sanitation is good.
- The incubation period ranges from 3 to 21 days.[1]
- Much of the world has been declared polio free and global eradication is anticipated in the future. However, the disease remains endemic in Afghanistan, India, Nigeria, and Pakistan. Exportation of polio from these endemic countries remains a problem with many countries in Asia and Africa being affected.[1] All travelers to and from polio-infected areas should be up to date with polio vaccination according to their national immunization policy; travelers to and from endemic and reinfected countries should be fully protected by vaccination. Updates on countries with ongoing transmission of indigenous and imported wild poliovirus and countries with recent transmission of imported wild poliovirus can be found at www.polioeradication.org/casecount.asp.[2]
- Prevention of spread can be helped by adopting good food, water, and personal hygiene measures. Immunity against polio can be created in two ways: through immunization and after natural infection with polio virus. Short-lived natural immunity is acquired through maternal antibodies for 2 or 3 months after birth. Acquiring poliomyelitis will provide lifelong immunity against the disease, but only against the particular type of virus that caused the illness (type 1, 2, or 3). Infection of one type will not provide protection against the other two polio viruses.
- Inactivated polio vaccine (IPV) will offer immunity against all three types of virus; this is currently the only available vaccine for regular administration in the UK. Oral polio vaccine (OPV) is only stocked for outbreak situations. The current presentation of IPV is combined with other antigens, diphtheria, and tetanus. While 5 doses in the national immunization program provide protection for life within the UK, booster doses at 10 yearly intervals continue to be recommended to travelers at risk, as a routine measure.[3]

REFERENCES

1. Department of Health. Immunization Against Infectious Disease—"the Green Book". London: The Stationery Office; 2006. Accessed at http://www.dh.gov.uk/prod_consum_dh/groups/dh_digitalassets/@dh/@en/documents/digitalasset/dh_108823.pdf.
2. World Health Organization International travel and health Geneva: WHO, 2011. Accessed at www.who.int/ith.
3. Field VF, Ford L, Hill DR (Eds). Health Information for Overseas Travel. London: National Travel Health Network and Centre; 2010.

RABIES

COUNTRIES OR AREAS AT RISK, 2008

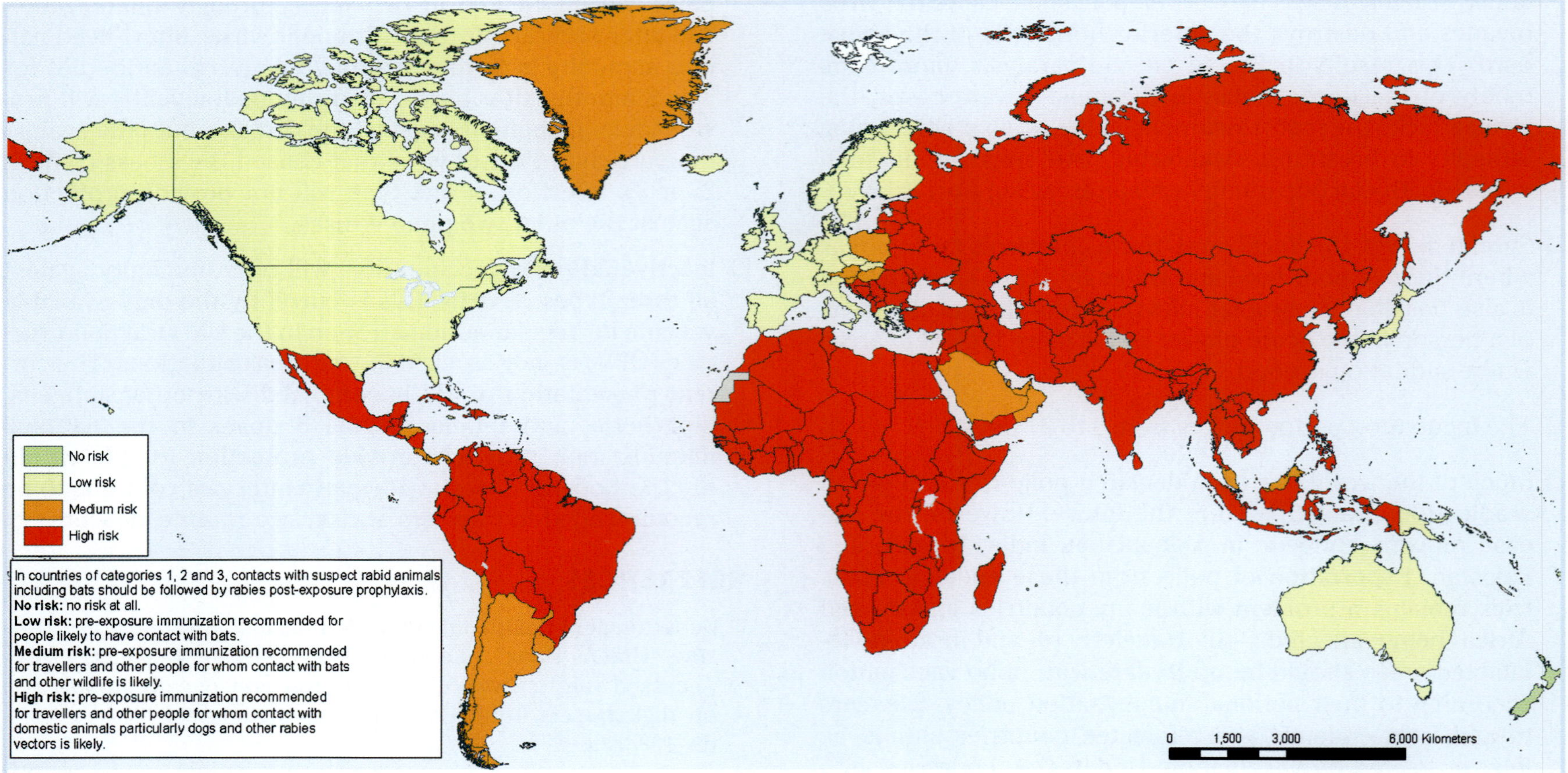

DATA SOURCE: World Health Organization; accessed May 2011. MAP PRODUCTION: Public Health Information and Geographic Information System (GIS) World Health Organization.

RABIES

- Rabies is a viral disease which infects domestic and wild animals. It is transmitted to other animals and humans through close contact with saliva from infected animals, for example bites, scratches, licks on broken skin, and mucous membrane. Dogs are the source of 99% of human rabies deaths.[1]
- Rabies is present on all continents with the exception of Antarctica, but more than 95% of human deaths occur in Asia and Africa. Once symptoms of the disease develop, rabies is nearly always fatal.[1]
- Worldwide, more than 55,000 people die of rabies every year and 40% of people who are bitten by suspect rabid animals are children under 15 years of age. Every year, more than 15 million people worldwide receive a post-exposure preventive regimen to avert the disease.[1]
- The incubation period for rabies is typically 1 to 3 months, but may vary from less than 1 week to more than a year.[1]
- The first symptoms of rabies are usually nonspecific and suggest involvement of the respiratory, gastrointestinal, and/or central nervous systems. Presentation may include parasthesiae around the site of the wound, fever, headache, and malaise. In the acute stage, the disease may present with spasms, hydrophobia, hallucinations, and maniacal behavior progressing to paralysis and coma resulting in death, usually from respiratory failure.
- Pre-exposure vaccination is advised to travelers with extensive outdoor exposure in rural areas—such as might occur while running, bicycling, hiking, camping, backpacking—as they may be at risk, even if the duration of travel is short; for children living in or visiting rabies-endemic areas, where they are an easy target for rabid animals; for persons traveling to isolated areas or to areas where immediate access to appropriate medical care is limited or to countries where human rabies immunoglobulin (HRIG) particularly but also rabies vaccine itself are in short supply and locally available rabies vaccines might be unsafe and/or ineffective.[2]
- A primary course of pre-exposure vaccination consists of three doses of 1.0 ml of rabies vaccine given by intramuscular administration. There are currently two rabies vaccines licensed for use in the UK: human diploid cell vaccine (HDCV) and purified chick embryo cell rabies vaccine (PCEC).[3]
- Follow general advice for animal bites, parasitic infection and other hazards in *Section 1, page 3* if exposure to rabies infection is suspected.
- It is essential to advise **all** travelers to seek immediate medical help for post-exposure prophylaxis if infection is suspected. This would consist of rabies vaccine and possibly anti-rabies immunoglobulin, depending on the extent of the wound and availability of HRIG. Post-exposure prophylaxis must be administered as soon as possible.

REFERENCES

1. World Health Organization Rabies factsheet no 99 updated September 2010 http://www.who.int/mediacentre/factsheets/fs099/en/ .
2. World Health Organization International Travel and Health Geneva: WHO, 2011. www.who.int/ith.
3. Department of Health. Immunization Against Infectious Disease—"the Green Book". The Stationery Office. London, 2006. http://www.dh.gov.uk/prod_consum_dh/groups/dh_digitalassets/@dh/@en/documents/digitalasset/dh_063658.pdf.

SCHISTOSOMIASIS

COUNTRIES OR AREAS AT HIGH RISK, 2008

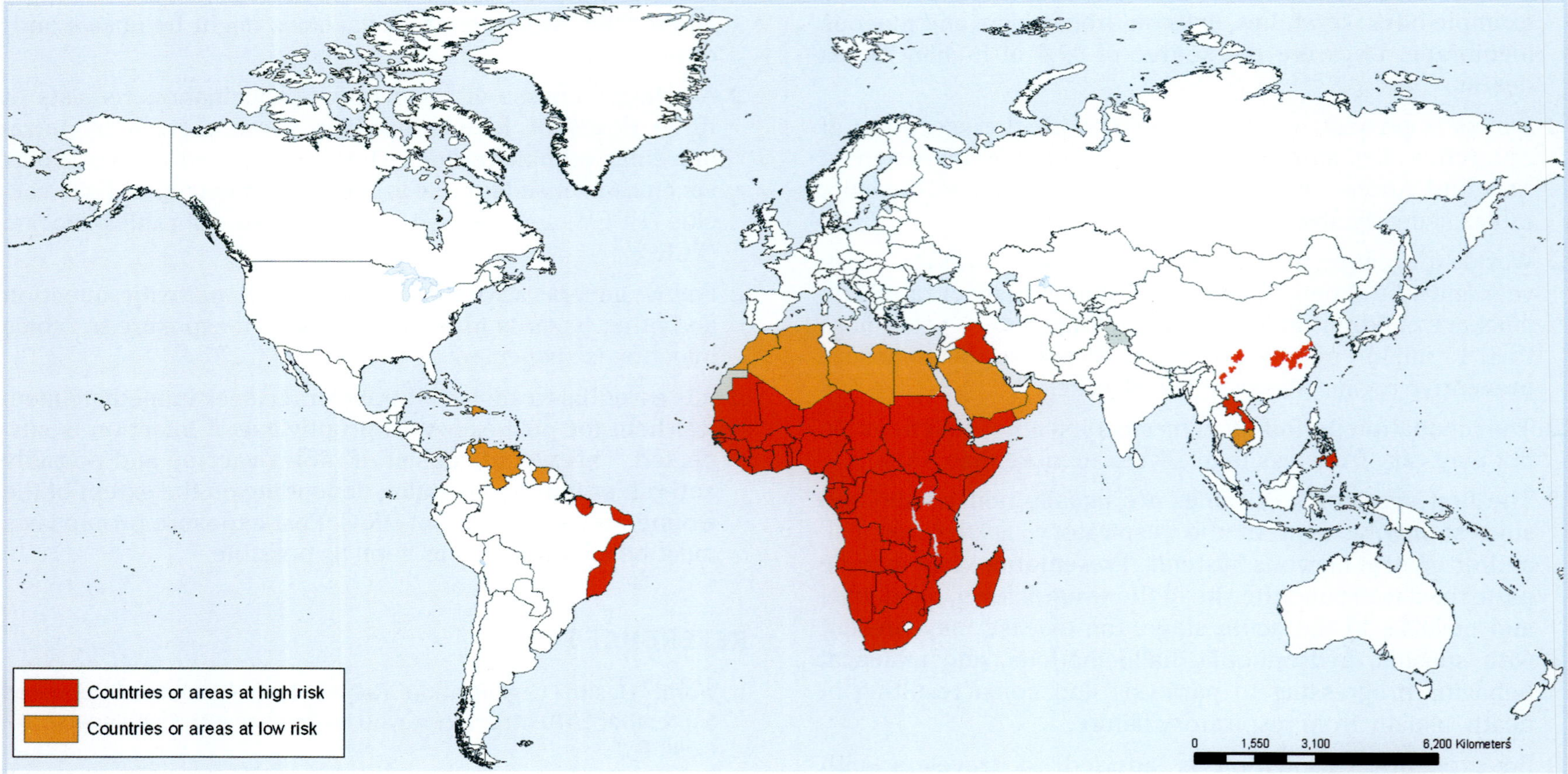

DATA SOURCE: World Health Organization; accessed May 2011. MAP PRODUCTION: Public Health Information and Geographic Information System (GIS) World Health Organization.

SCHISTOSOMIASIS (BILHARZIA)

- It is estimated that at least 207 million people around the world are afflicted with schistosomiasis with an estimated 700 million at risk in 74 endemic countries. It ranks second behind malaria in terms of socio-economic and public health importance in tropical and subtropical areas.[1]

- Schistosomiasis or Bilharzia is infection with a parasitic worm which spends part of its life cycle in fresh water snails and the other part in a human host.

- There are three major species of schistosomes:[1]
  1. *Schistosoma haemtobium* found mainly in Africa and also the Middle East
  2. *Schistosoma mansoni* found in Africa, the Middle East, the Caribbean, Brazil, Venezuela, and Suriname.
  3. *Schistosoma japonicum* which is found in China, Indonesia, and the Philippines.

- Schistosomiasis is a very serious problem in Africa where 85% of the 207 million cases live.

- Incubation period is typically 14–84 days for acute schistosomiasis, but chronic infection can remain asymptomatic for years.[2]

- The transmission cycle is by the excretion of eggs from the infected human host into a fresh water lake or stream, in which certain snails live. The eggs hatch to liberate larvae which infect specific snails. Multiplication of the larvae occurs and they are released back into the water as cercariae to penetrate human skin. A rash may occur when this happens, known as "swimmers itch". A minimum of 2 to 3 weeks later, a toxemic illness may occur, called Katamaya fever. Whether or not Katayama fever occurs, a chronic phase follows and once the infection becomes established, abdominal pain and blood in the urine or stool are common.

- Present day diagnosis and treatment can prevent progression of the disease, so that serious problems from chronic disease are rare in travelers.

- There is no available vaccine for this disease.

- Prevention is dependant upon avoidance of bathing and paddling in fresh water lakes and streams in an endemic country and travelers should never assume fresh water to be free from schistosomiasis in such areas.

REFERENCES

1. World Health Organization Factsheet No. 115 updated February 2010. Accessed at http://www.who.int/mediacentre/factsheets/fs115/en/index.html.
2. Centers for Disease Control and Prevention. CDC Health Information for International Travel 2010. Atlanta: U.S. Department of Health and Human Services, Public Health Service, 2009. Accessed at http://wwwnc.cdc.gov/travel/yellowbook/2010/chapter-5/schistosomiasis.aspx.

TUBERCULOSIS

ESTIMATED NEW CASES, 2009

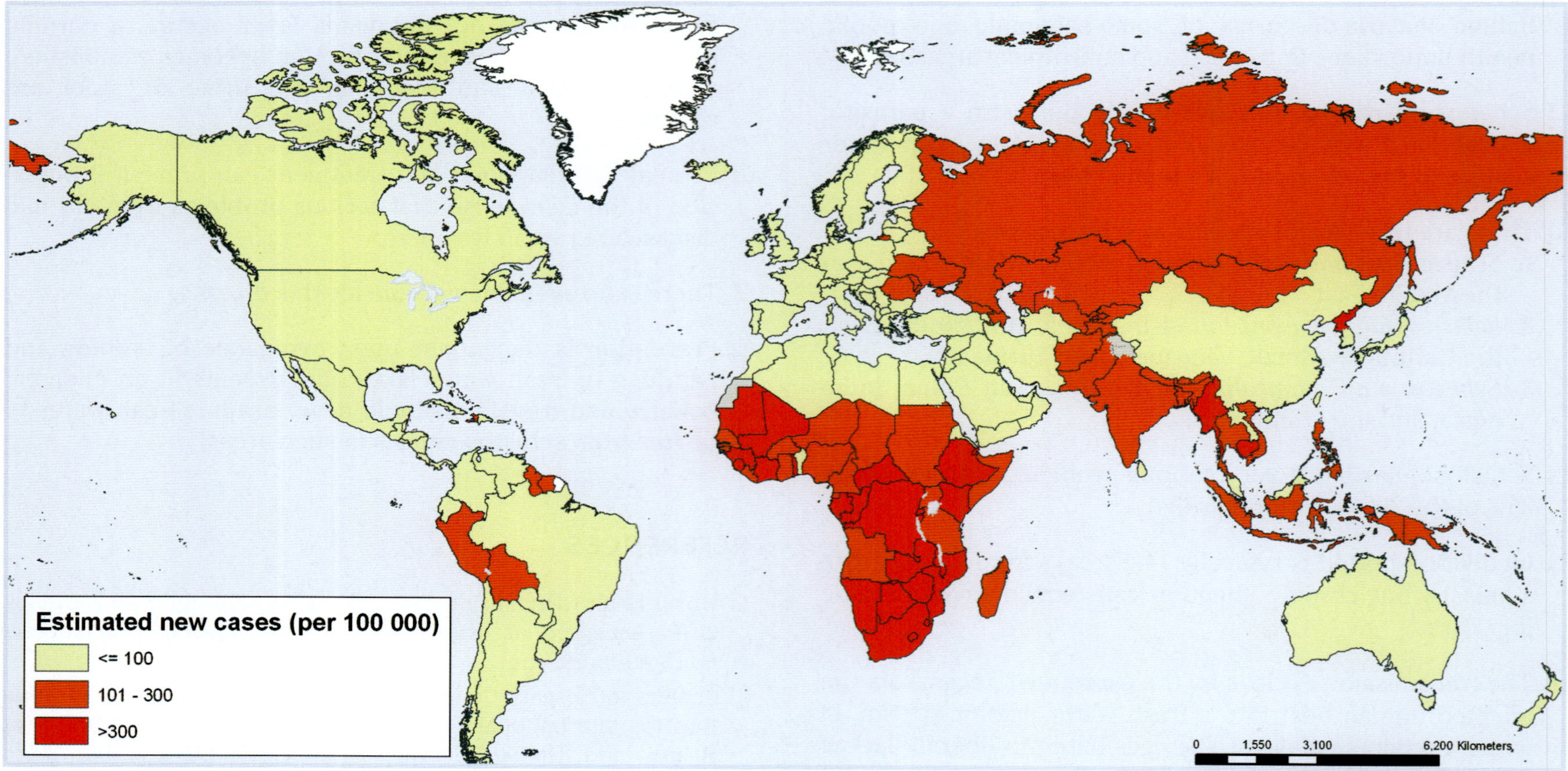

DATA SOURCE: World Health Organization; accessed May 2011. MAP PRODUCTION: Public Health Information and Geographic Information System (GIS) World Health Organization.

TUBERCULOSIS

- Tuberculosis (TB) is caused by *Mycobacterium tuberculosis* (MTB) in most cases. *M. africanum* and *M. canetti* occasionally cause disease in Africa, while *M. bovis* (the causative agent of bovine tuberculosis) still causes occasional human infections.[1]
- Tuberculosis is found worldwide. Approximately one-third of the world's population is infected with MTB; there are 9 million new cases and nearly 2 million deaths each year.[2]
- Infection is acquired by inhalation of mycobacteria in aerosols and dust or via ingestion of infected milk in the case of *M. bovis*. Approximately 30% of the global population is infected with tubercle bacilli, producing around two million deaths per year.
- The incubation period is 2 to 10 weeks for primary infection. Post-primary infection can present after years of asymptomatic latent infection.
- Primary tuberculosis begins in the lung. Many infections are asymptomatic, resulting in latent infection. Where primary tuberculosis results in clinical illness, fever and sweats, weight loss, and malaise occur. Disseminated infection (military tuberculosis) or spread to other organs may follow. Primary tuberculosis is more likely in those under 5 years of age and in the presence of HIV co-infection. The latent infection phase is asymptomatic and may remain so indefinitely. There is a 10% to 15% lifetime risk of reactivation.[2] Post-primary tuberculosis usually involves the lung with cough, malaise, night sweats, and weight loss, but may disseminate or spread as for primary tuberculosis.
- Diagnosis of TB may be on clinical suspicion supported by imaging, microbiology, and sometimes histopathology. Sputum or other clinical specimens are examined by Ziehl Neelsen stain and cultured for acid-fast bacilli. Molecular diagnosis (e.g., by PCR) is available in reference centers. Latent infection can be detected by tuberculin skin testing, though host anergy or previous BCG vaccination can make interpretation problematic. Interferon gamma release assays provide an alternative means of assessing cell-mediated immunity and are unaffected by previous immunization with BCG.[1]
- Treatment is with antituberculous medication for at least 6 months. Choice of agent and duration of treatment depend upon the type of disease present, drug sensitivity testing, and whether or not there is underlying immunodeficiency. UK treatment regimens are summarized in the British National Formulary.[3]
- Prevention advice includes avoidance of close contact with infectious pulmonary tuberculosis. Respiratory precautions should be undertaken by healthcare workers. Policy for the use of BCG vaccine varies between countries. For travelers, the UK recommends vaccination for:
  - Previously unvaccinated individuals under the age of 16 years planning to live for more than 3 months in a country with an annual incidence of tuberculosis of greater than or equal to 40 per 100,000.
  - Healthcare workers under 35 years old planning to travel to a country with an annual incidence of tuberculosis of greater than or equal to 40 per 100,000 irrespective of duration of stay.
- Vaccination can be considered for healthcare workers over 35 years old at particular risk of tuberculosis after a thorough risk assessment has been undertaken.[2]

REFERENCES

1. Ward KN, et al. Notes on Medical Microbiology. 2nd Edit. Edinburgh: Churchill Livingstone Elsevier; 2009 (597 pages).
2. Field VF, Ford L, Hill DR (Eds). Health Information for Overseas Travel. London: National Travel Health Network and Centre; 2010.
3. Joint Formulary Committee. British National Formulary. 60 ed. London: British Medical Association and Royal Pharmaceutical Society; 2010.

YELLOW FEVER

VACCINATION RECOMMENDATIONS, 2010:

IN THE AMERICAS

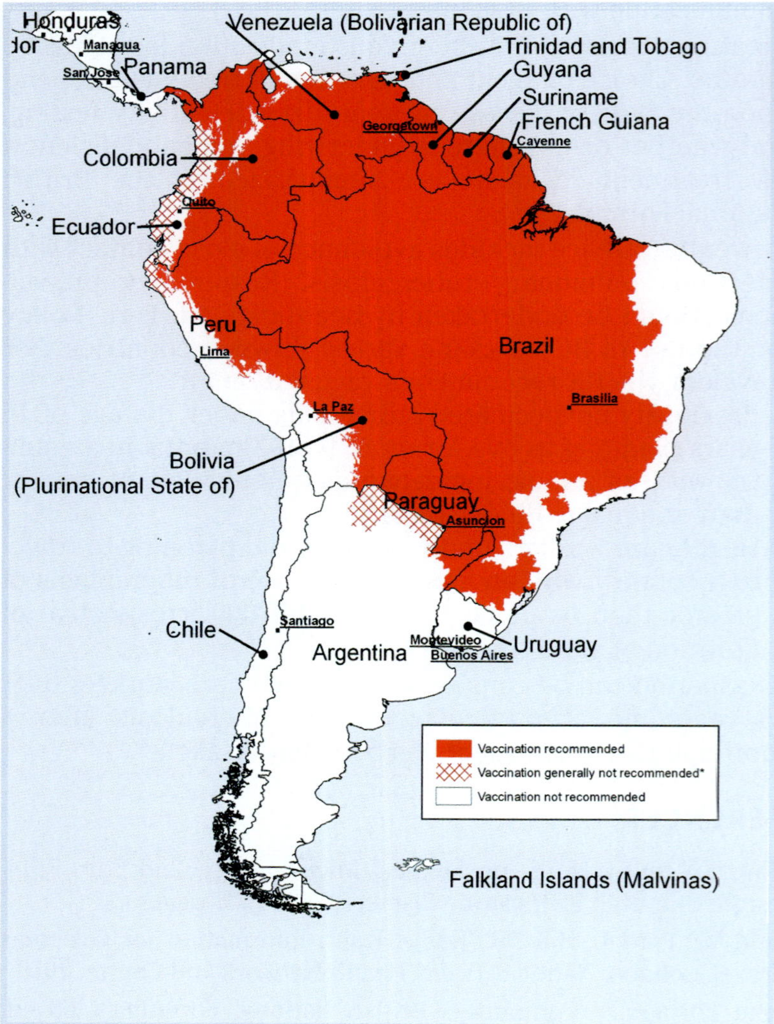

IN AFRICA

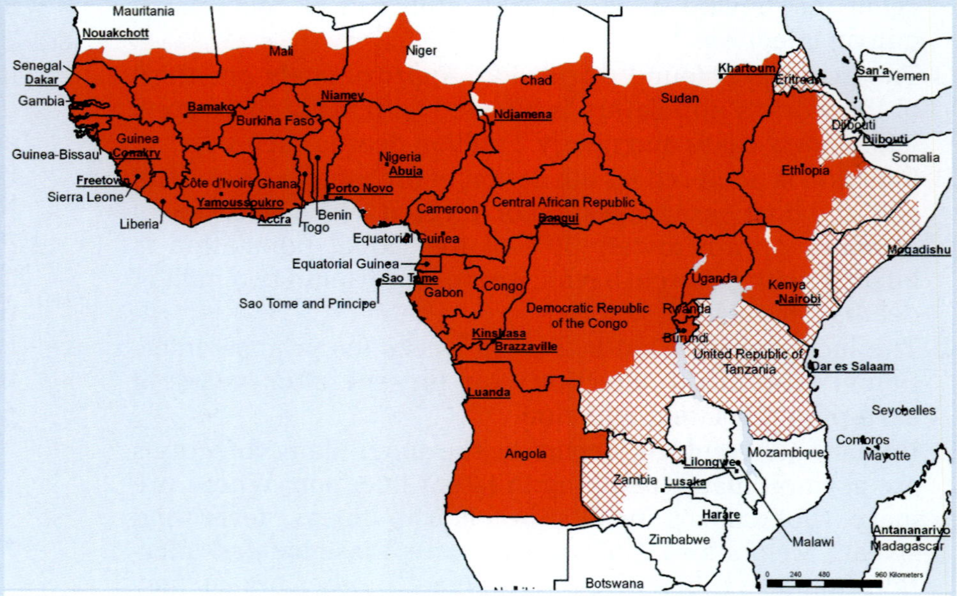

*Yellow Fever (YF) vaccination is generally not recommended in areas where there is low potential for YF virus exposure. However, vaccination might be considered for a small subset of travelers to these areas who are at increased risk for exposure to YFV because of prolonged travel, heavy exposure to mosquitoes, or inability to avoid mosquito bites. Consideration for vaccination of any traveler must take into account the traveler's risk of being infected with YF virus, country entry requirements, and individual risk factors for serious vaccine-associated adverse events (e.g., age, immune status).

DATA SOURCE: World Health Organization; accessed May 2011. MAP PRODUCTION: Public Health Information and Geographic Information System (GIS) World Health Organization.

LEGIONNAIRES' DISEASE

- Legionnaires' disease is a bacterial infection caused by *Legionella pneumophila*, usually serogroup 1, a gram negative rod.
- Legionella has a global distribution in the environment in both soil and water and may be present in domestic water and air conditioning units. It produces Legionnaires' disease, a type of atypical pneumonia which can be particularly severe in individuals with pre-existing medical conditions. It can also cause a non-specific febrile illness (Pontiac fever) or asymptomatic seroconversion.
- Infection is acquired by inhalation of contaminated aerosols, e.g., via air conditioning systems.[1] Sporadic cases or small outbreaks occur in travelers exposed in hotels or cruise ships. Therefore, legionellosis must be considered in the differential diagnosis of a pneumonic illness in recently returned travelers.
- Incubation period is 2 to 10 days.[2]
- Clinical features comprise cough, fever, shortness of breath, malaise, and myalgia. Confusion may also occur. Diarrhea is quite common and its presence should heighten suspicion of Legionella infection.
- Diagnosis involves clinical suspicion, imaging, culture from respiratory secretions. Detection of *L. pneumophila* serogroup 1 antigen in urine. (Serology requires paired samples and thus is unhelpful in the acute phase of illness.)
- Treatment is with antibiotics: macrolides (e.g., erythromycin, clarithromycin) or fluoroquinolones (e.g., ciprofloxacin). Supportive care is also required. The case fatality rate is 10% to 15% and can be higher in the elderly and in those with pre-existing lung disease or chronic medical conditions.[2]
- There is no vaccine available and travelers should be made aware of how Legionella is transmitted. Those at increased risk of severe or complicated infection should avoid using jacuzzis and whirlpool spas.

REFERENCES

1. Ward KN, et al. Notes on Medical Microbiology. 2nd Edit. Edinburgh: Churchill Livingstone Elsevier; 2009 (597 pages).
2. Field VF, Ford L, Hill DR (Eds). Health Information for Overseas Travel. London: National Travel Health Network and Centre; 2010.

MALARIA

- Malaria is a common and serious tropical disease. It is caused by a protozoan of the genus *Plasmodium*, transmitted to humans by the bite of an infected female Anopheles mosquito, usually between dusk and dawn. Five different species of *Plasmodium* can give rise to human malaria: *P. falciparum*, *P. vivax*, *P. ovale*, *P. malariae,* and *P. knowlesi*. *Plasmodium falciparum* is the most serious, responsible for most of the deaths which occur. Prevention and treatment of *P. falciparum* malaria has become increasingly difficult because its resistance to antimalarial drugs has increased and it has become more widespread. In recent years, human cases of malaria have also occurred with *Plasmodium knowlesi*, a monkey malaria that occurs in certain forested areas of Southeast Asia.[1]
- Globally in 2008 there were 247 million cases of malaria and nearly one million deaths, mostly among children living in Africa. One child dies from malaria every 45 seconds in Africa and the disease accounts for 20% of all childhood deaths.[1]
- Malaria is both preventable and curable.
- In 2010, 1761 cases of malaria were reported in the UK, including 7 deaths.[2]
- Every case of malaria in a traveler represents a failure: (1) of public health and the travel industry to promote awareness of the risk; (2) of the traveler to seek pre-travel health advice; (3) of the health care provider to provide appropriate advice; (4) of the traveler to adhere to appropriate recommendations for preventing infection.[3]
- There are four principles of malaria prevention that should receive attention from both travelers and their advisers, which are essential to prevent suffering due to malaria in travelers.[4]

1. ***Awareness—know about the risks***. This entails the traveler needing to know: whether or not malaria is transmitted in the country and area that they are visiting; whether or not chloroquine or other drug resistant malaria is present; the transmission season and the level of transmission.

2. ***Bites by mosquitoes—prevent or avoid.*** This will have a significant impact upon malaria transmission. This entails ensuring that the traveler is aware that bite prevention is as important as taking chemoprophylaxis. Refer to *Section 1, page 4* for advice on bite prevention.

3. ***Compliance with appropriate chemoprophylaxis.*** This entails choosing the appropriate drug suitable for the traveler's destination and their health assessment; ensuring compliance with medication—that the chosen chemoprophylaxis is taken at the appropriate time interval prior to entering the malarious area, all the time there, and for the correct time after leaving the malarious area; depending on the choice of chemoprophylaxis selected, ensuring that administration of the chosen chemoprophylaxis is correct. Educating the traveler to be aware that no chemoprophylaxis is 100% effective while pointing out the benefits of taking it.

4. ***Diagnose breakthrough malaria swiftly and obtain treatment promptly.*** It is impossible to distinguish early falciparum malaria from influenza on clinical grounds. Travelers visiting malarious areas need to be aware of the need to seek medical advice promptly for any febrile or flu-like illness occurring within a year and especially within three months of returning from an endemic area.

REFERENCES

1. World Health Organization Malaria Factsheet no. 94 April 2010. Accessed at http://www.who.int/mediacentre/factsheets/fs094/en/index.html.
2. Imported malaria cases and deaths, United Kingdom: 1991–2010 Data from the HPA Malaria Reference Laboratory. Accessed at http://www.hpa.org.uk/web/HPAweb&HPAwebStandard/HPAweb_C/1195733773780.
3. Keystone J, Kozarsky P. In: Schlagenhauf-Lawlor P. Travelers' Malaria, 2nd edit. 2008;26: 288–393.
4. Chiodini P, et al. Guidelines for malaria prevention in travelers from the United Kingdom. London, Health Protection Agency, January 2007. Accessed at http://www.hpa.org.uk/Topics/InfectiousDiseases/InfectionsAZ/Malaria/Guidelines/.

Delivering Appropriate Advice and Using the Malaria Risk Area Maps Within This Atlas

Specific information about appropriate malaria chemoprophylaxis has not been included within this atlas. This information should be obtained from other reference sources as described in the *Introduction*. Advisers may also find the *Guidelines for the Prevention of Malaria in Travelers from the United Kingdom* (see Ref. 4 above) extremely useful to read, which includes guidance on the advice that should be given to travelers including:

- ❑ Emphasizing the ABCD of malaria prevention.
- ❑ Emphasizing that while no drug regiment is 100% effective, the combination of preventive measures advised will give significant protection against malaria.
- ❑ Making use of visual aids, especially malaria distribution maps, examples of preventive measures for bite prevention.
- ❑ Discussing the choice of chemoprophylaxis regimens and their individual advantages and disadvantages, including cost.
- ❑ Providing the traveler with written information.

Maps of countries where malaria is endemic are shown in *Section 3* for the following countries:

- Afghanistan
- Algeria
- Angola
- Argentina
- Armenia
- Azerbaijan
- Bangladesh
- Belize
- Bolivia
- Botswana
- Brazil
- Cambodia
- Cameroon
- Central African Republic
- China
- Colombia
- Costa Rica
- Democratic Republic of Congo
- Dominican Republic
- East Timor
- Ecuador, including the Galapagos Islands
- Ethiopia
- Gabon
- Gambia
- Ghana
- Guatemala
- Guyana
- Haiti
- Honduras
- Hong Kong Sar
- India
- Indonesia (including Bali)
- Iran
- Iraq
- Jamaica
- Kenya
- Korea, Democratic Peoples Republic of North Korea
- Korea, Republic of South Korea
- Laos People's Democratic Republic
- Madagascar
- Malawi
- Malaysia
- Mali
- Mexico
- Mozambique
- Myanmar
- Namibia
- Nepal
- Nicaragua
- Niger
- Nigeria
- Pakistan
- Panama
- Papua New Guinea
- Paraguay
- Peru
- Philippines
- Rwanda
- Saudi Arabia
- Senegal
- Somalia
- South Africa
- Sri Lanka
- Sudan
- Tajikistan
- Tanzania
- Thailand
- Turkey
- Turkmenistan
- Uganda
- Venezuela, including Margarita Island
- Vietnam
- Yemen
- Zambia
- Zimbabwe

TETANUS

- Tetanus is an acute disease caused by the action of tetanus toxin, released following infection by the bacterium *Clostridium tetani*. a spore-forming Gram-positive anaerobic bacillus.
- *Clostridium tetani* is found worldwide and inhabits the intestine of animals, especially horses and is thus widely found in the soil. Tetanus can never be eradicated because of its presence in the environment. The spores may be introduced into the body through a puncture wound, burn or scratch—which may go unnoticed. Neonatal tetanus is due to infection of the baby's umbilical stump. As a result, devitalized tissue permits anaerobic bacterial growth. Intravenous drug users can acquire *C. tetani* via contaminated injection paraphernalia.
- The incubation period of tetanus is between 4 and 21 days (most commonly about 10 days).[1]
- Clinical features of tetanus are due to tetanospasmin, a powerful neurotoxin produced by *C. tetani* growing anaerobically in a contaminated wound.[2] Such clinical features include: trismus (lock jaw) due to spasm of the jaw muscles; risus sardonicus due to spasm of the facial muscles; generalized tetanus with uncontrolled muscle spasms (e.g., producing opisthotonus). Involvement of the autonomic nervous system can result in sweating, tachycardia, and labile blood pressure. Even with intensive care the mortality is around 10%, but is as high as 50% in the absence of good medical facilities.[3]
- Diagnosis is often on clinical signs. Bacterial culture of the wound often fails to isolate *C. tetani*.
- Human tetanus immunoglobulin is given as treatment, intravenously (IV) or intramuscularly at multiple sites if IV administration is not feasible, to neutralize toxin already produced. Radical wound debridement to remove devitalized tissue may be performed. Metronidazole can be given to kill *C. tetani* and thus prevent further toxin production. Intensive care support may be required.
- An episode of tetanus does not confer immunity to the disease, so vaccination with tetanus toxoid is required post-recovery.
- All travelers should ensure they are vaccinated to prevent tetanus. While 5 doses in the national immunization program provides protection for life within the UK, booster doses at 10 yearly intervals continue to be recommended to travelers at risk, as a routine measure.[1] The current presentation of tetanus vaccine is only available in the UK combined with antigens of diphtheria and polio.

REFERENCES

1. Department of Health. Immunization Against Infectious Disease—"the Green Book". London: The Stationery Office. London; 2006. Updated online August 2009. Accessed at http://www.dh.gov.uk/prod_consum_dh/groups/dh_digitalassets/@dh/@en/documents/digitalasset/dh_103982.pdf.
2. Ward KN, et al. Notes on Medical Microbiology. 2nd Edit. Edinburgh: Churchill Livingstone Elsevier: 2009 (597 pages).
3. Field VF, Ford L, Hill DR (Eds). Health Information for Overseas Travel. London: National Travel Health Network and Centre; 2010.

TICK-BORNE ENCEPHALITIS

- Tick-borne encephalitis (TBE) is caused by a flavivirus transmitted by the tick vector *Ixodes ricinus* or, less commonly, by ingestion of unpasteurized milk from infected animals, especially goats.
- There are three subtypes of TBE: the European subtype is present in large parts of central and eastern Europe, particularly Austria, southern Germany, and northern Switzerland, the Baltic states (Estonia, Latvia, Lithuania), the Czech Republic, Hungary, and Poland; the Far Eastern subtype is found from north-eastern Europe to China and Japan; the Siberian subtype is found from northern Europe to Siberia. The disease is seasonal, with most cases occurring during April through November. The risk is highest in forested areas up to an altitude of about 1400 m.[1]
- The incubation period of TBE is from 2 to 28 days.[2]
- The ratio of asymptomatic to symptomatic infection is about 250 to 1. Two-thirds of symptomatic patients develop a flu-like illness which is self-limiting. One third of these patients may proceed to a second phase of the illness with sudden fever, central nervous system involvement with headache and meningitis. Progression to encephalitis is more common in those over 40 years of age.[3]
- Risk is mainly to those working, walking, or camping in rural areas where ticks are prevalent. Transmission season is from April to November; the Eastern subtype is more common in the spring and the Western subtypes in autumn.
- Prevention is by taking precautions against tick bite (see *Section 1, page 4*), avoidance of consumption of unpasteurized dairy products, and by vaccination.
- Any ticks which are found should be removed as soon as possible with tweezers, as close to the skin attachment as possible, by pulling steadily, but not jerking or twisting. Medical advice should be sought as soon as possible to advise on treatment.
- Both adult and pediatric formulations of a licensed inactivated virus vaccine are available in the UK for those considered at risk.

REFERENCES

1. World Health Organization International Travel And Health Geneva: WHO, 2011. Accessed at www.who.int/ith.
2. Department of Health. Immunization Against Infectious Disease—“the Green Book”. London: The Stationery Office; 2006. Accessed at http://www.dh.gov.uk/prod_consum_dh/groups/dh_digitalassets/@dh/@en/documents/digitalasset/dh_063662.pdf.
3. Field VF, Ford L, Hill DR (Eds). Health Information for Overseas Travel. London: National Travel Health Network and Centre; 2010.

TRAVELERS' DIARRHEA

- ❑ Diarrhea is the most common illness reported in international travelers, particularly in those traveling from high-income countries to low income regions where hygiene and sanitary infrastructure may be less robust.
- ❑ Certain regions of the world such as Africa, South and Southeast Asia, South and Central America, and the Middle East are particularly high risk.[1]
- ❑ Travelers' diarrhea is caused by ingestion of the causative organisms which can be bacterial, viral, or parasitic. The most common sources of travelers' diarrhea are contaminated food and, to a lesser extent, water. Enteropathogens survive in ice and swimming pools. Sea water, heavily contaminated with sewage and fecal microorganisms, is another source.
- ❑ Classical travelers' diarrhea (TD) is defined as three or more unformed stools in a 24-hour period, often accompanied by at least one of the following: fever, nausea, vomiting, cramps, tenesmus, or bloody stools (dysentery), with symptoms usually starting during or shortly after a period of foreign travel. The illness is often described as mild and self-limiting, usually lasting 3–5 days; however, illness severity can vary depending on the individual and the etiological cause of the illness. In some cases, it can cause serious illness or be extremely unpleasant and disruptive to a holiday or business trip. It can also have an important economic impact on international tourism.[1]
- ❑ Prevention is behavioral (see *General Advice: Food, Water, and Personal Hygiene* in *Section 1, page 2*). There is no vaccine yet available to give protection against travelers' diarrhea, although development of vaccines against some of the causes is underway.
- ❑ The mainstay of treatment is rehydration. The use of rehydration solution is extremely useful, especially in severe cases and particularly for children and the elderly. Rehydration solution in sachets is available commercially (e.g., Dioralyte®, Electrolade®) .
- ❑ Anti-motility drugs can be useful (e.g., Imodium® or Lomotil®) but these should never be used in children under 4 years of age, and only on prescription for children aged 4 to 12 years. None of these tablets should ever be used if the person has a fever or has blood in the stool.
- ❑ Medical help should be sought if the affected person has a fever, blood in the diarrhea, diarrhea for more than 48 hours (or 24 hours in children), or becomes confused.
- ❑ In very special circumstances, antibiotics are sometimes used for chemoprophylaxis, but this must be reviewed by the patient's doctor.
- ❑ Remember to inform female travelers taking the oral contraceptive pill, that full contraceptive protection may be lost if they suffer diarrhea and vomiting and they will need to use extra protection.

REFERENCES

1. Health Protection Agency. Foreign travel-associated illness—a focus on travelers' diarrhea. 2010 report. London: Health Protection Agency; 2010 (*see also,* www.hpa.org.uk).

TYPHOID

- ❑ Typhoid fever is a systemic infection caused by the Gram negative bacillus *Salmonella typhi*. (Do not confuse this with *S. typhimurium* which is a non-typhoidal Salmonella causing a diarrheal illness).
- ❑ Typhoid fever is spread by the fecal-oral route, usually through food or drink that has been contaminated with the excreta of a human case or carrier. Flies may also transfer infection to foods resulting in contamination which may be sufficient to cause human infection.[1]
- ❑ Symptoms of this septicemic illness include fever, headache, abdominal discomfort, constipation, often a dry cough, and sometimes confusion. After 7–10 days, the fever reaches a peak, rose spots may appear, and diarrhea begins.
- ❑ Treatment is with antibiotics. If untreated, complications can develop, the most common being intestinal bleeding or perforation which can cause severe illness and death.
- ❑ Around 2% to 5% of those who contract typhoid fever become chronic carriers, as bacteria persist in the biliary tract after symptoms have resolved.[1]
- ❑ Typhoid is predominantly a disease of countries with poor sanitation and poor standards of personal and food hygiene, especially in Africa, Asia, Central and South America, and Southeast Europe.
- ❑ An estimated 22 million cases of typhoid fever and 200000 related deaths occur worldwide every year.[2]
- ❑ Vaccination is available against typhoid in injectable and oral forms, but it must be remembered that the vaccines are not 100% effective.
- ❑ Travelers should still adhere to food, water, and personal hygiene advice.

REFERENCE

1. World Health Organization. International Travel and Health Geneva: WHO, 2011. Accessed at www.who.int/ith.
2. Centers for Disease Control and Prevention. CDC Health Information for International Travel 2010. Atlanta: U.S. Department of Health and Human Services, Public Health Service, 2009.

SECTION 3 Countries

Country-specific general and immunization advice, malaria advice and precautions, maps, and weather charts:

AFGHANISTAN

General Advice

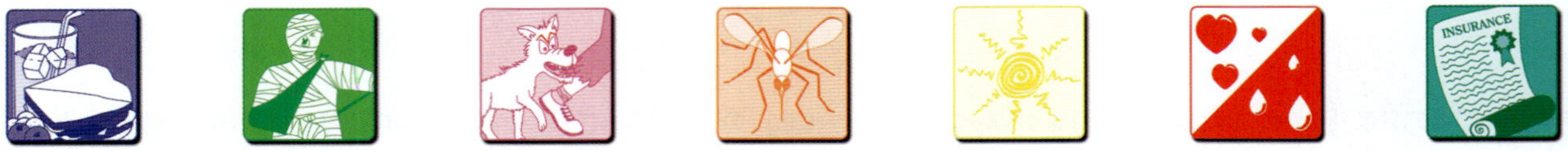

Immunization Advice

- ❑ Immunizations recommended for life should be up to date, especially those for children and boosters of tetanus for adults.
- ❑ Courses or boosters of diphtheria and hepatitis A, poliomyelitis and typhoid are usually advised.
- ❑ Vaccines sometimes advised are: BCG, cholera, hepatitis B, rabies.
- ❑ A yellow fever certificate is required if entering from an infected country.

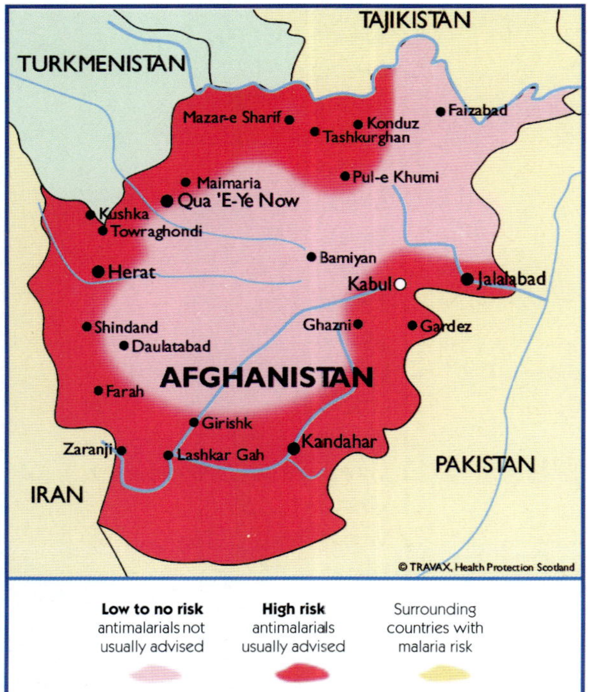

This map is only intended as a guide since mosquitoes do not respect boundaries and the risk areas shown may not be exact. **Reproduced with permission from Fitfortravel, Health Protection Scotland's Travel website www.fitfortravel.nhs.uk.**

Malaria Advice

- ❑ Malaria is a serious and sometimes fatal disease transmitted by mosquitoes. You cannot be vaccinated against malaria.

MALARIA PRECAUTIONS

- ❑ Malaria precautions are essential in areas below 2000 m from May to November. Avoid mosquito bites by covering up with clothing such as long sleeves and long trousers especially after sunset, using insect repellents on exposed skin and, when necessary, sleeping under a mosquito net.
- ❑ Check with your doctor or nurse about suitable antimalarial tablets.
- ❑ Prompt investigation of fever is essential.

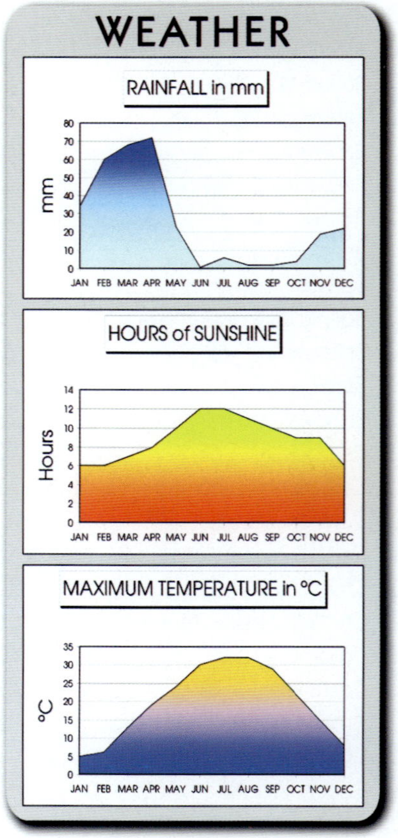

ALBANIA

General Advice

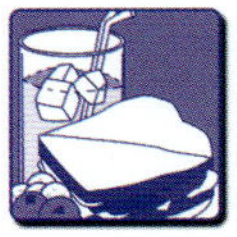
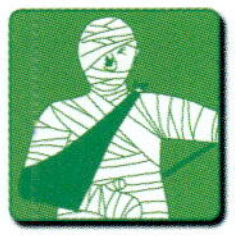
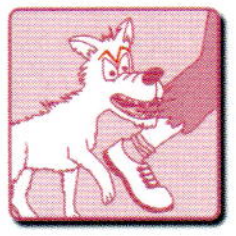
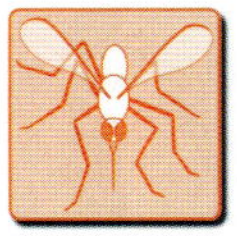
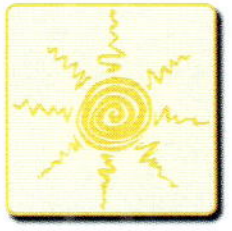

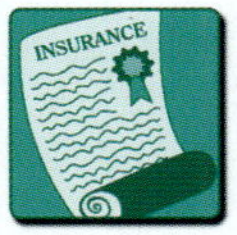

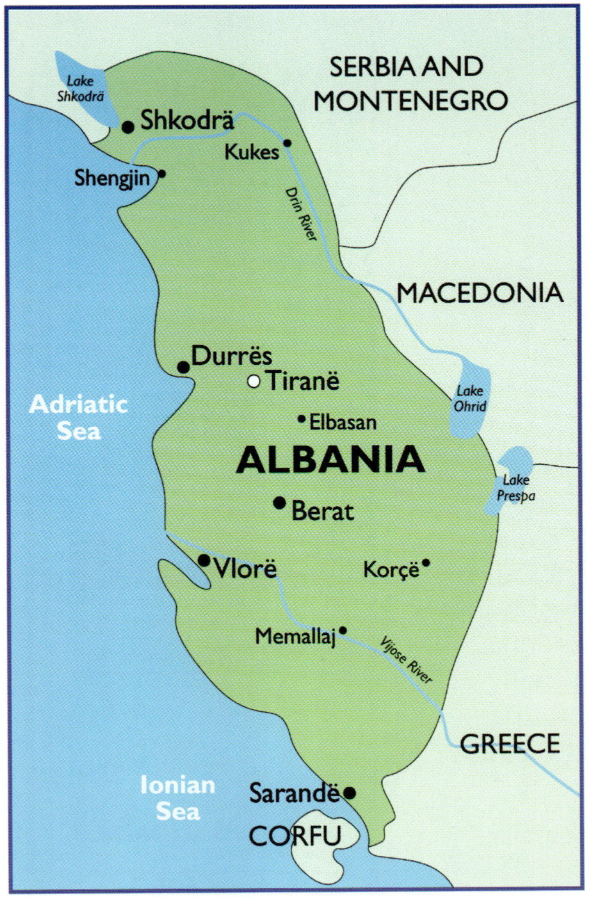

Immunization Advice

- ❑ Immunizations recommended for life should be up to date, especially those for children and boosters of tetanus for adults.
- ❑ Courses or boosters of hepatitis A are usually advised.
- ❑ Vaccines sometimes advised are: diphtheria, hepatitis B, rabies, tickborne encephalitis.
- ❑ A yellow fever certificate is required if aged over 1 year old and entering from an infected country.

Malaria Advice

- ❑ Malaria is not normally present.

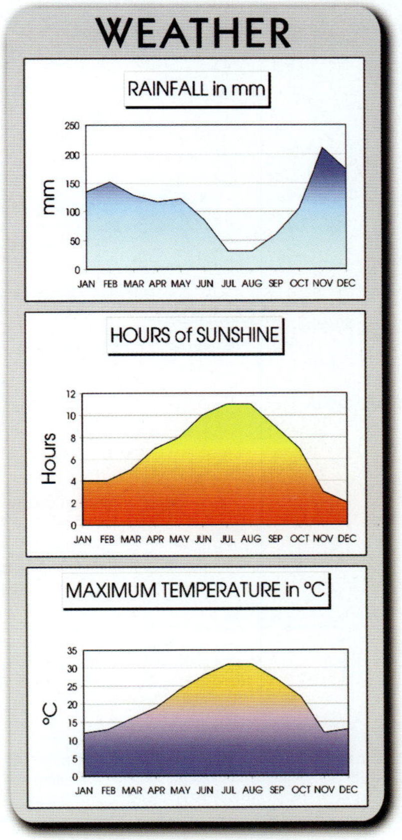

ALGERIA

General Advice

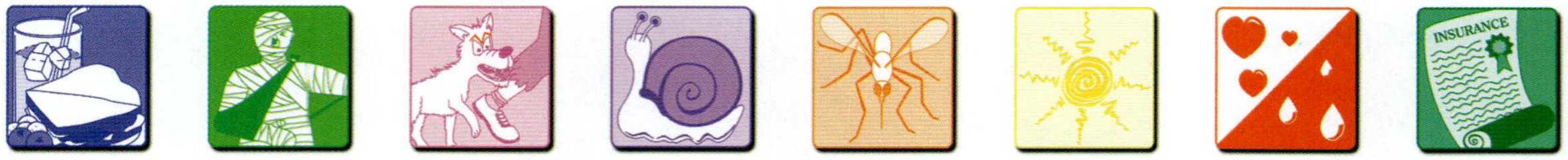

Immunization Advice

- ❑ Immunizations recommended for life should be up to date, especially those for children and boosters of tetanus for adults.

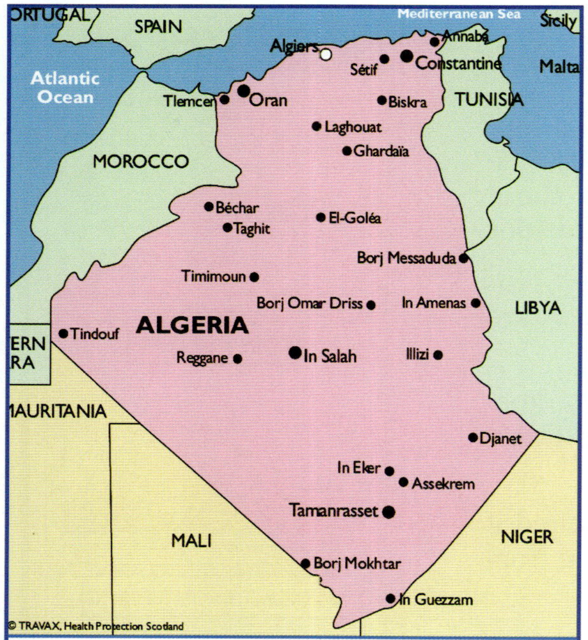

Low to no risk antimalarials not usually advised

Surrounding countries with malaria risk

This map is only intended as a guide since mosquitoes do not respect boundaries and the risk areas shown may not be exact. **Reproduced with permission from Fitfortravel, Health Protection Scotland's Travel website www.fitfortravel.nhs.uk.**

- ❑ Courses or boosters of diphtheria, hepatitis A, and typhoid are usually advised.
- ❑ Vaccines sometimes advised are: BCG, hepatitis B, rabies.
- ❑ A yellow fever certificate is required if aged over 1 year old and entering from an infected country.

Malaria Advice

- ❑ Malaria is a serious and sometimes fatal disease transmitted by mosquitoes. You cannot be vaccinated against malaria.

MALARIA PRECAUTIONS

- ❑ Malaria precautions are essential in one small focus in the southeast (Ihrir) all year round. Avoid mosquito bites by covering up with clothing such as long sleeves and long trousers especially after sunset, using insect repellents on exposed skin and, when necessary, sleeping under a mosquito net.
- ❑ Antimalarial tablets are not normally recommended.
- ❑ Prompt investigation of fever is essential.

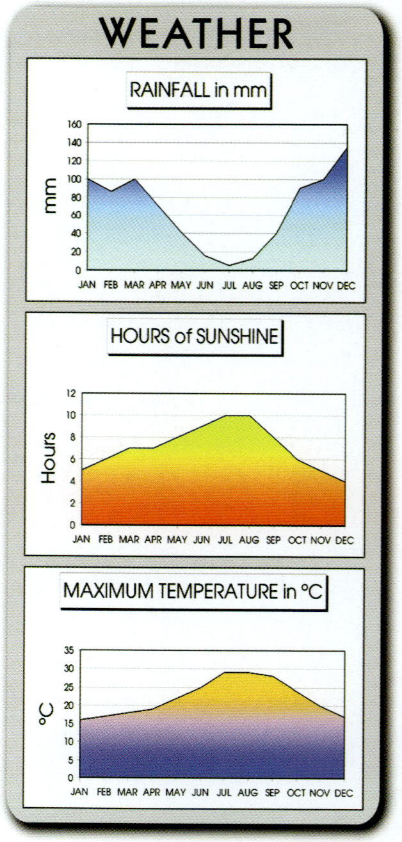

ANGOLA

General Advice

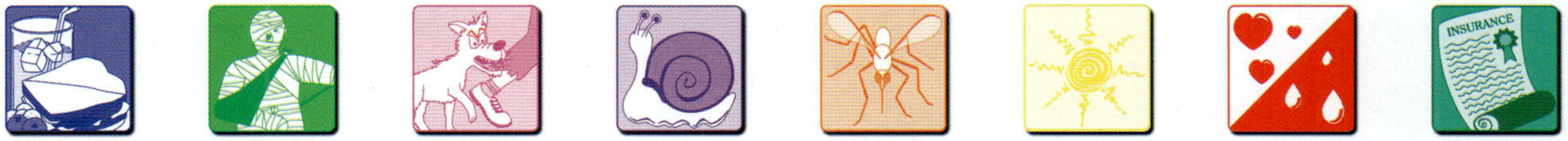

Immunization Advice

- ❑ Immunizations recommended for life should be up to date, especially those for children and boosters of tetanus for adults.

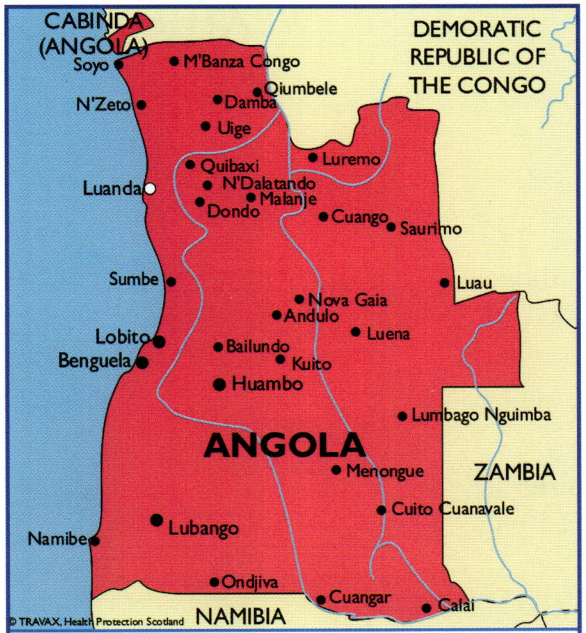

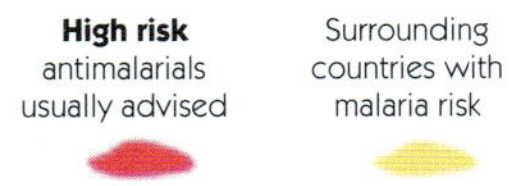

This map is only intended as a guide since mosquitoes do not respect boundaries and the risk areas shown may not be exact. **Reproduced with permission from Fitfortravel, Health Protection Scotland's Travel website www.fitfortravel.nhs.uk.**

- ❑ Courses or boosters of diphtheria, hepatitis A, poliomyelitis, typhoid, and yellow fever are usually advised.
- ❑ Vaccines sometimes advised are: BCG, cholera, hepatitis B, rabies.
- ❑ A yellow fever certificate is required for all travelers aged over 1 year.

Malaria Advice

- ❑ Malaria is a serious and sometimes fatal disease transmitted by mosquitoes. You cannot be vaccinated against malaria.

MALARIA PRECAUTIONS

- ❑ Malaria precautions are essential in all areas all year round. Avoid mosquito bites by covering up with clothing such as long sleeves and long trousers especially after sunset, using insect repellents on exposed skin and, when necessary, sleeping under a mosquito net.
- ❑ Check with your doctor or nurse about suitable antimalarial tablets.
- ❑ Prompt investigation of fever is essential.

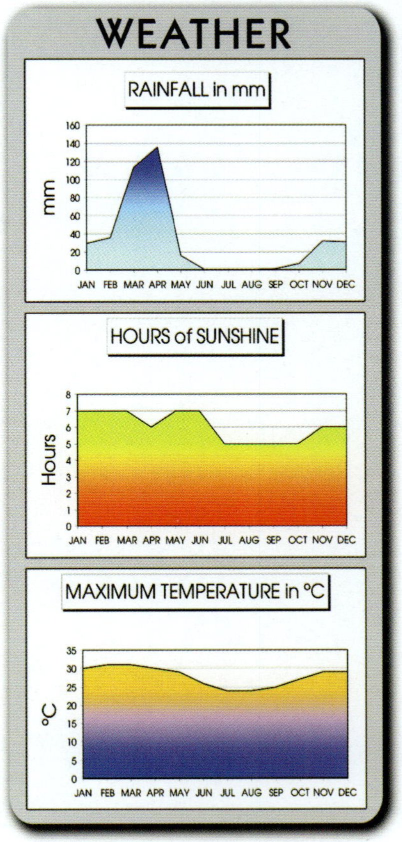

ANTIGUA and BARBUDA

General Advice

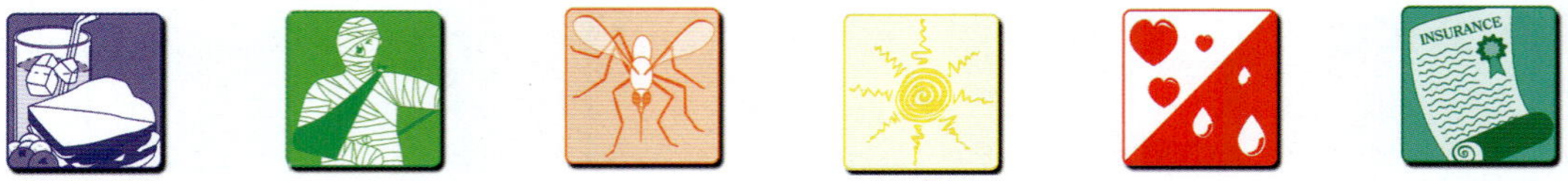

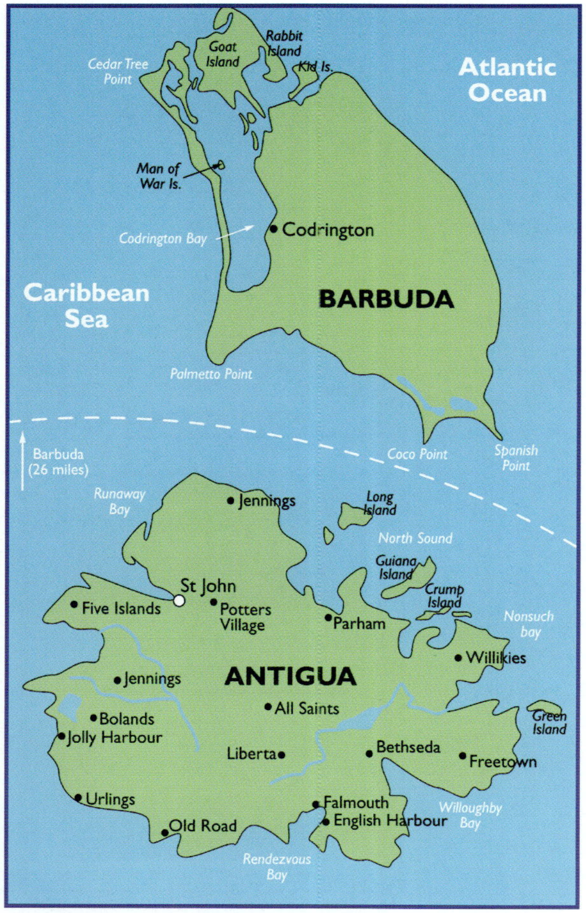

Immunization Advice

- ❑ Immunizations recommended for life should be up to date, especially those for children and adults boosters of tetanus.
- ❑ Vaccines sometimes advised are: diphtheria, hepatitis A, hepatitis B.
- ❑ A yellow fever certificate is required if aged over 1 year old and entering from an infected country.

Malaria Advice

- ❑ Malaria is not normally present.

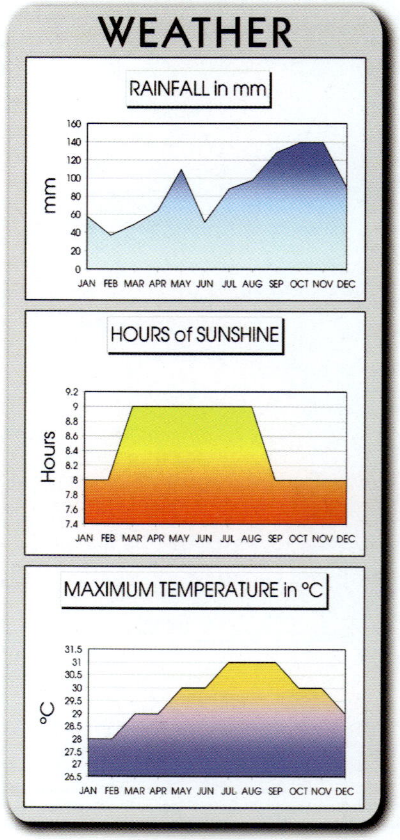

ARGENTINA

General Advice

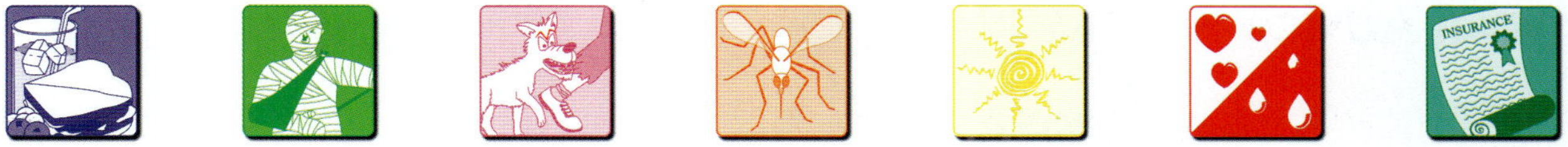

Immunization Advice

- ❑ Immunizations recommended for life should be up to date, especially those for children and boosters of tetanus for adults.
- ❑ Courses or boosters of hepatitis A are usually advised.
- ❑ Vaccines sometimes advised are: hepatitis B, rabies, typhoid, yellow fever (for north and northeastern forested areas including Iguacu Falls and border areas of Brazil and Paraguay; see yellow fever map).
- ❑ No certificate of vaccination for yellow fever is required.

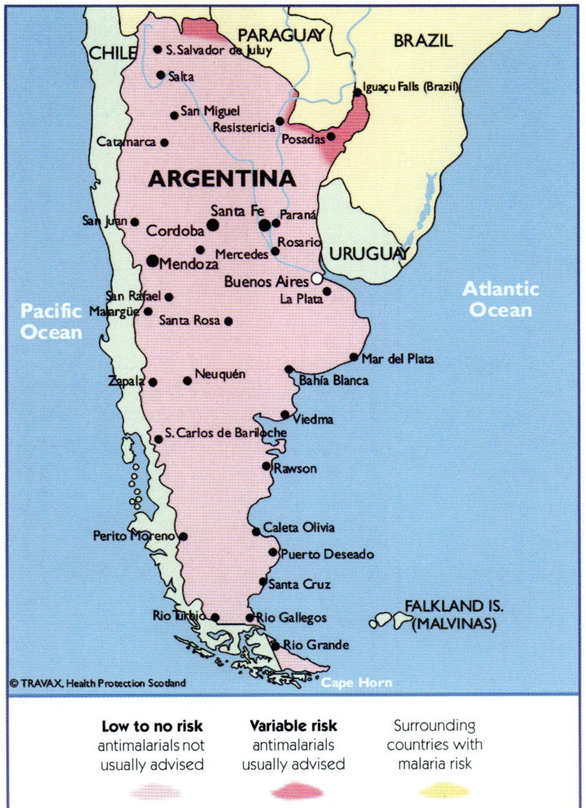

This map is only intended as a guide since mosquitoes do not respect boundaries and the risk areas shown may not be exact. **Reproduced with permission from Fitfortravel, Health Protection Scotland's Travel website www.fitfortravel.nhs.uk.**

Malaria Advice

- ❑ Malaria is a serious and sometimes fatal disease transmitted by mosquitoes. You cannot be vaccinated against malaria.

MALARIA PRECAUTIONS

- ❑ Malaria precautions are essential in rural areas along the borders of Bolivia and the isthmus between Argentina/Paraguay/Brazil, all year round. There is minimal risk in the resort at Iguacu Falls with higher risk in nearby rural areas. Avoid mosquito bites by covering up with clothing such as long sleeves and long trousers especially after sunset, using insect repellents on exposed skin and, when necessary, sleeping under a mosquito net.
- ❑ Check with your doctor or nurse about suitable antimalarial tablets.
- ❑ Prompt investigation of fever is essential.

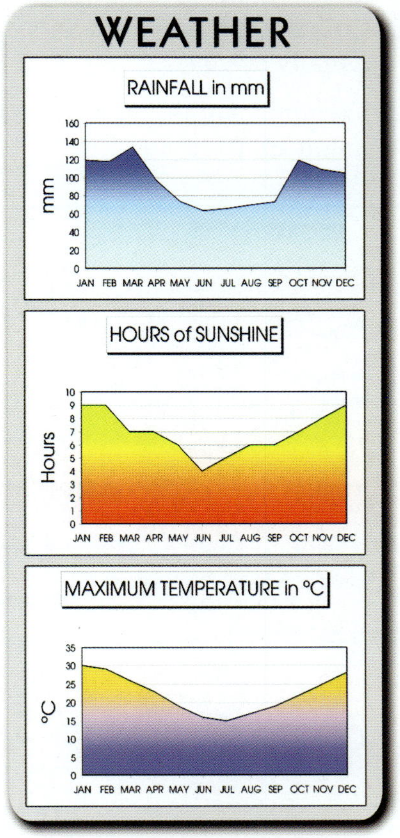

ARMENIA

General Advice

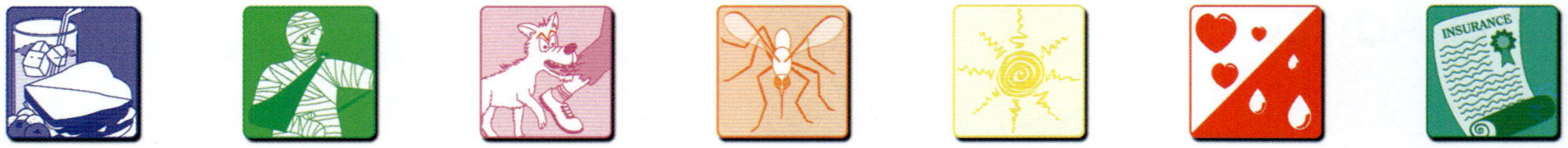

Immunization Advice

- ❑ Immunizations recommended for life should be up to date, especially those for children and boosters of tetanus for adults.
- ❑ Courses or boosters of hepatitis A are usually advised.
- ❑ Vaccines sometimes advised are: BCG, hepatitis B, rabies.

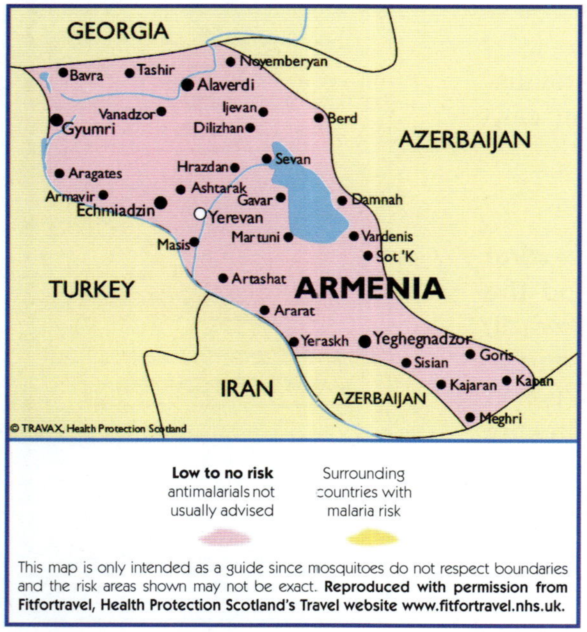

- ❑ No certificate of vaccination for yellow fever is required.

Malaria Advice

- ❑ Malaria is a serious and sometimes fatal disease transmitted by mosquitoes. You cannot be vaccinated against malaria.

MALARIA PRECAUTIONS

- ❑ Malaria precautions are essential in some villages in the Ararat Valley from June to October. There is no risk in the tourist areas. Avoid mosquito bites by covering up with clothing such as long sleeves and long trousers especially after sunset, using insect repellents on exposed skin and, when necessary, sleeping under a mosquito net.
- ❑ Check with your doctor or nurse about suitable antimalarial tablets.
- ❑ Prompt investigation of fever is essential.

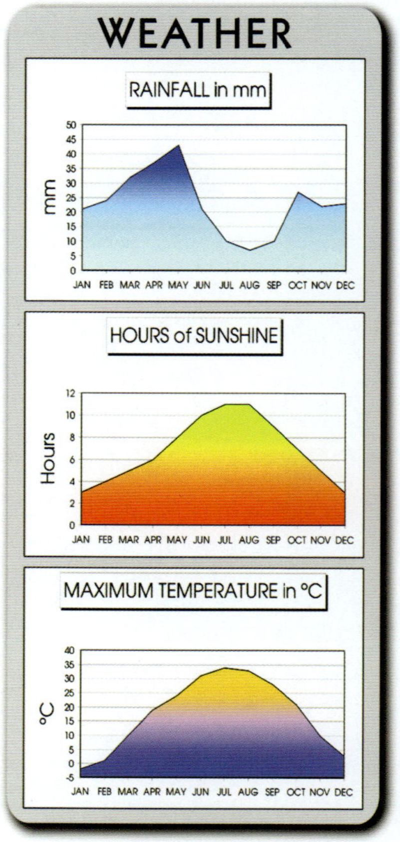

AUSTRALIA

General Advice

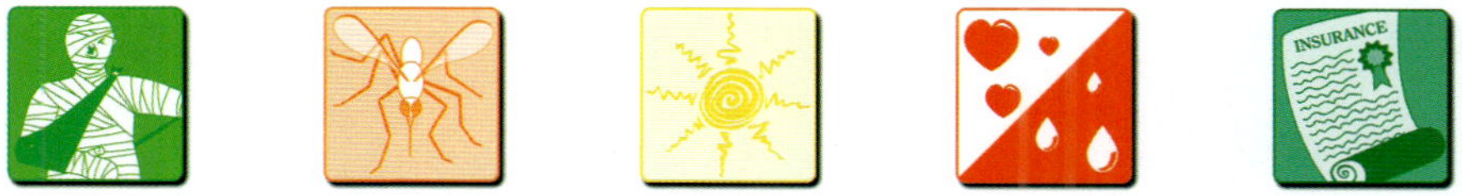

Immunization Advice

- ❑ Immunizations recommended for life should be up to date, especially those for children.
- ❑ Vaccines sometimes advised are: Japanese encephalitis (for long stays or frequent visits to rural areas of Badu Island in the Torres Strait).
- ❑ A yellow fever certificate is required if aged over 1 year old and entering Australia within 6 days of an overnight stay or longer in an infected country.

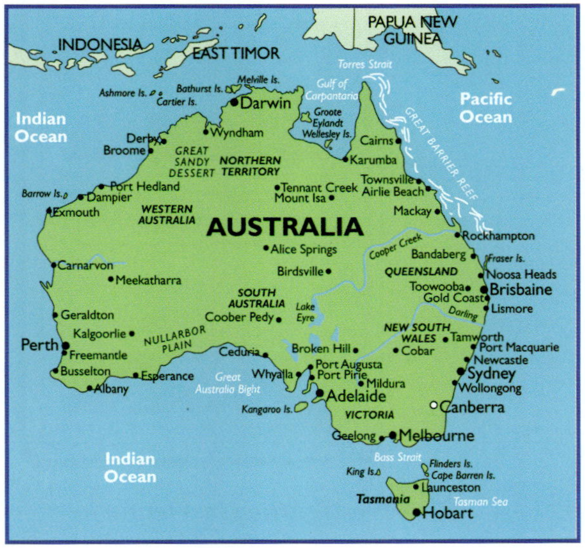

Malaria Advice

- ❑ Malaria is not normally present.

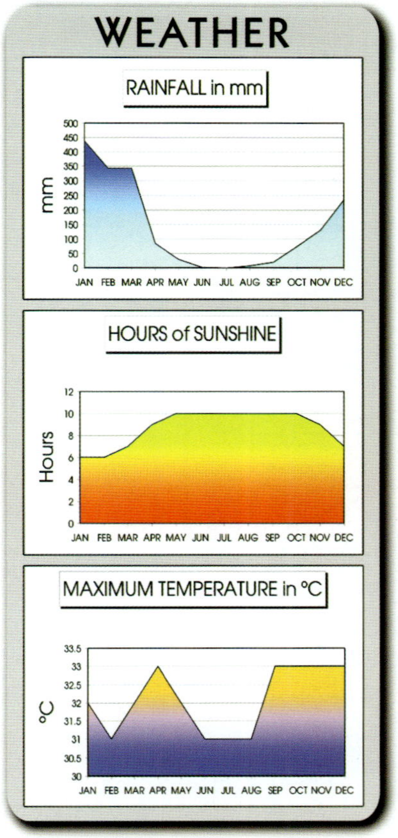

—Weather in Darwin—

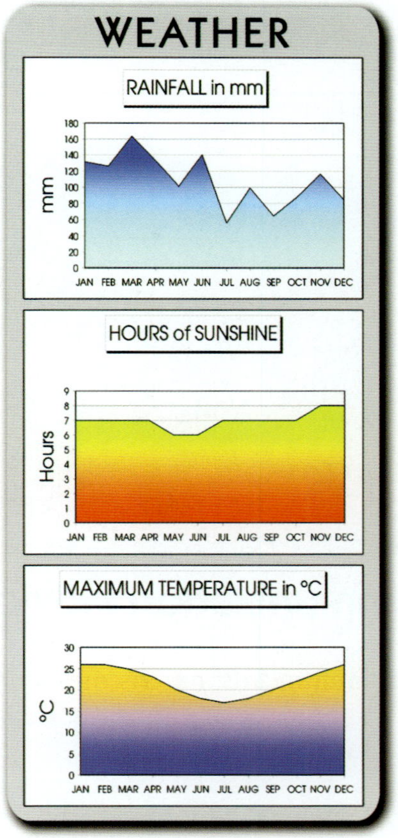

—Weather in Sidney—

AUSTRIA

General Advice

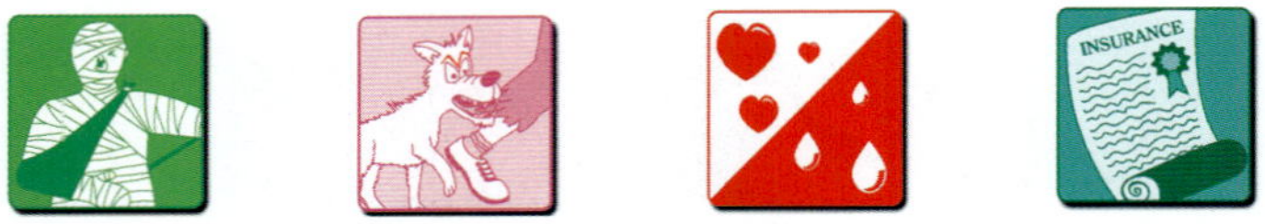

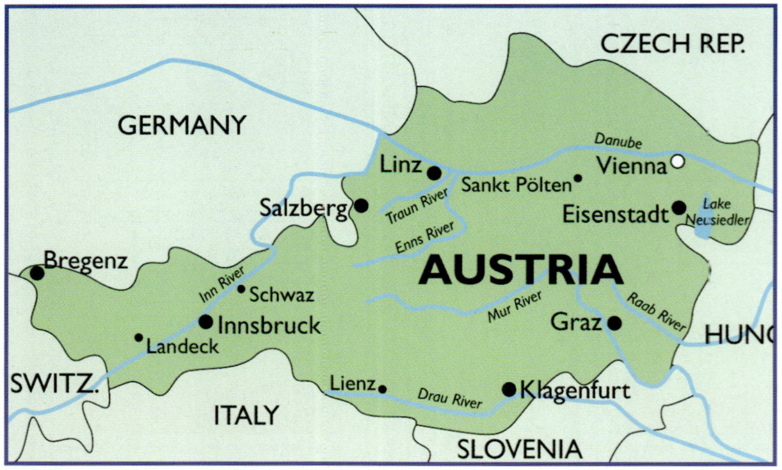

Immunization Advice

❑ Immunizations recommended for life should be up to date, especially those for children.

❑ Vaccines sometimes advised are: rabies, tick-borne encephalitis.

❑ No certificate of vaccination for yellow fever is required.

Malaria Advice

❑ Malaria is not normally present.

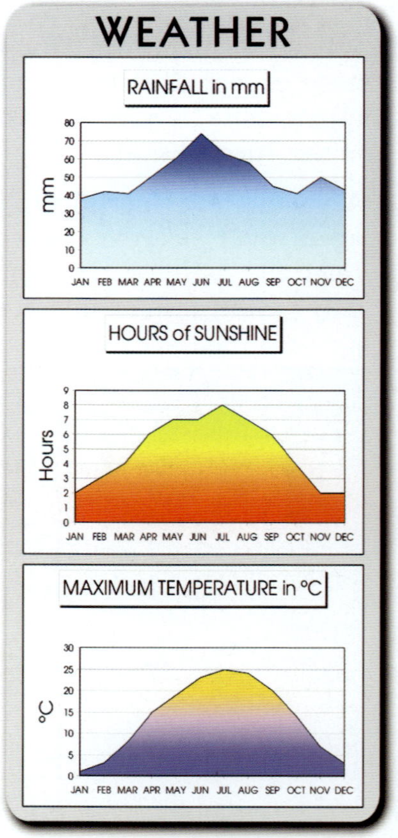

—Weather in Vienna—

AZERBAIJAN

General Advice

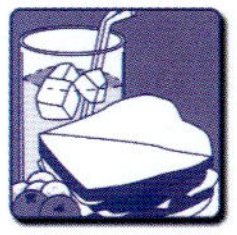 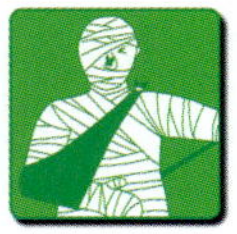 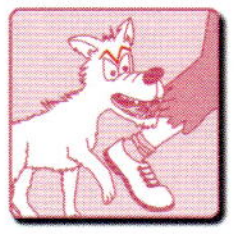 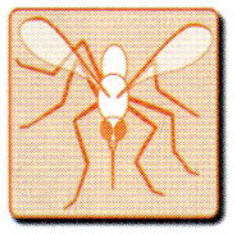 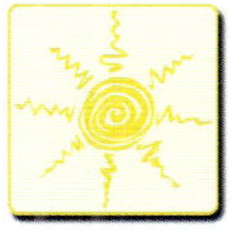  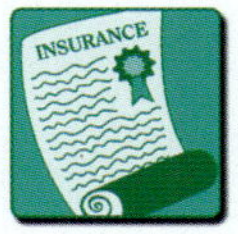

Immunization Advice

- ❑ Immunizations recommended for life should be up to date, especially those for children and boosters of tetanus for adults.

- ❑ Courses or boosters of hepatitis A are usually advised.

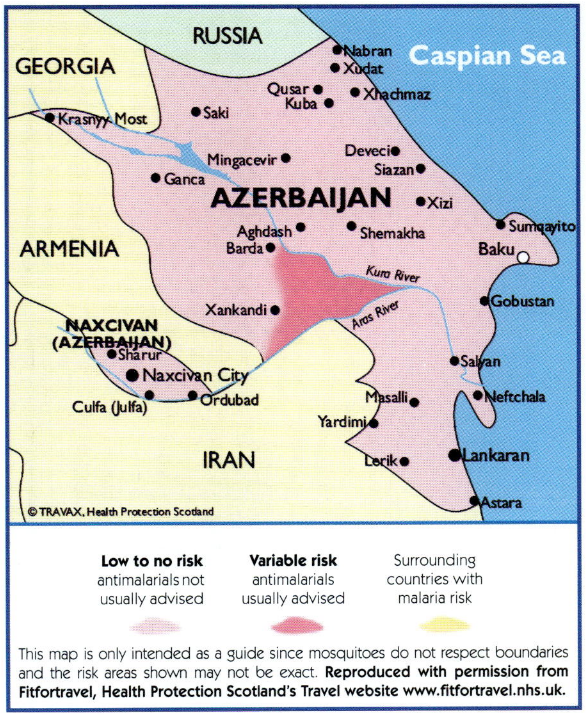

- ❑ Vaccines sometimes advised are: BCG, hepatitis B, rabies, typhoid.

- ❑ No certificate of vaccination for yellow fever is required.

Malaria Advice

- ❑ Malaria is a serious and sometimes fatal disease transmitted by mosquitoes. You cannot be vaccinated against malaria.

MALARIA PRECAUTIONS

- ❑ Malaria precautions are essential in some lowland areas between the Kura and Arax rivers from June to October. Avoid mosquito bites by covering up with clothing such as long sleeves and long trousers especially after sunset, using insect repellents on exposed skin and, when necessary, sleeping under a mosquito net.

- ❑ Check with your doctor or nurse about suitable antimalarial tablets.

- ❑ Prompt investigation of fever is essential.

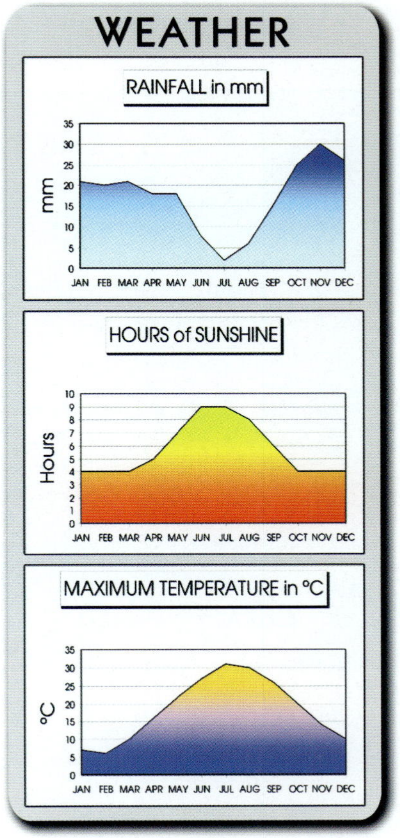

BAHAMAS

General Advice

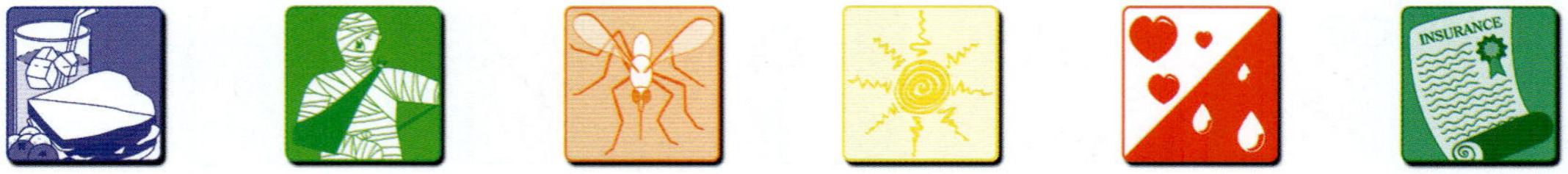

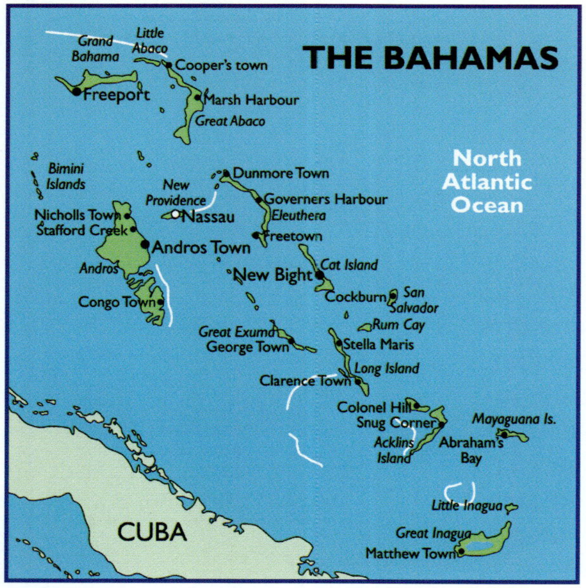

Immunization Advice

- ❑ Immunizations recommended for life should be up to date, especially those for children and boosters of tetanus for adults.
- ❑ Courses or boosters of hepatitis A are usually advised.
- ❑ Vaccines sometimes advised are: BCG, hepatitis B.
- ❑ A yellow fever certificate is required if aged over 1 year old and entering from an infected country.

Malaria Advice

- ❑ Malaria is not normally present.

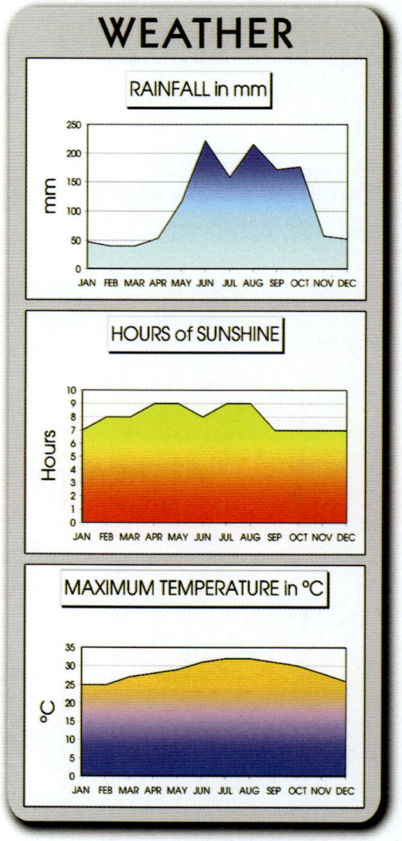

BAHRAIN

General Advice

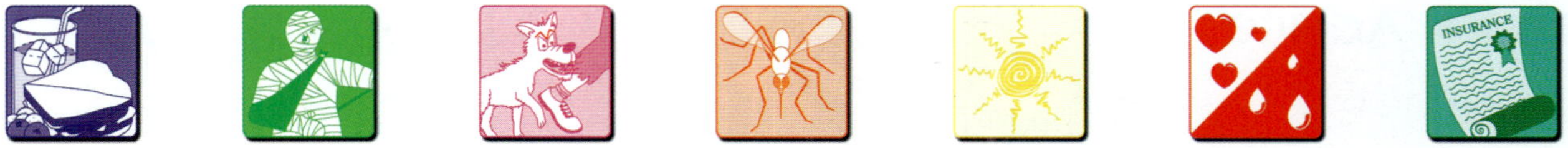

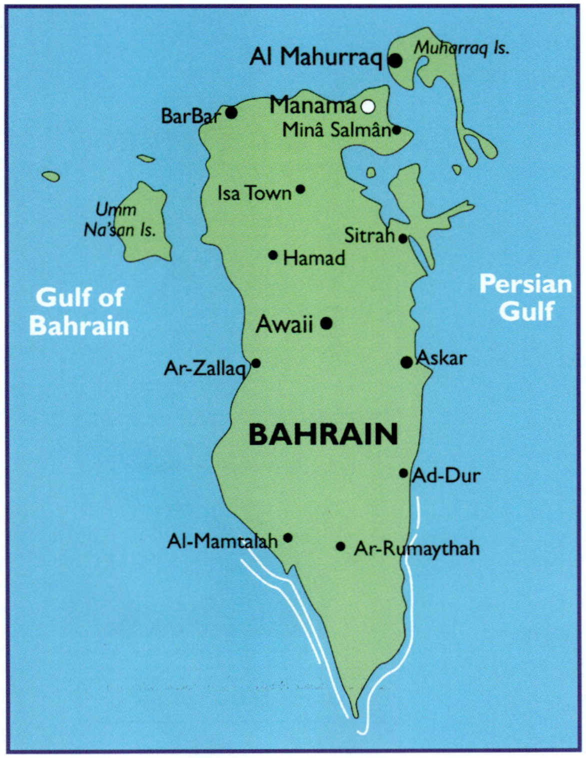

Immunization Advice

- ❑ Immunizations recommended for life should be up to date, especially those for children and boosters of tetanus for adults.
- ❑ Courses or boosters of hepatitis A are usually advised.
- ❑ Vaccines sometimes advised are: BCG, hepatitis B, rabies, typhoid.
- ❑ A yellow fever certificate is required if aged over 1 year old and entering from an infected country.

Malaria Advice

- ❑ Malaria is not normally present.

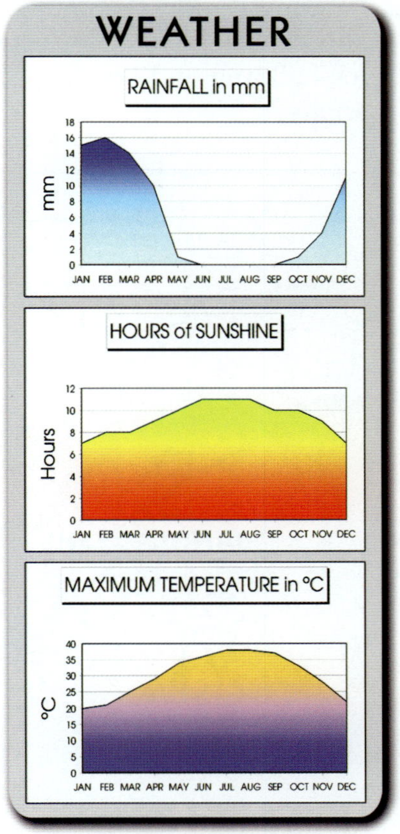

BANGLADESH

General Advice

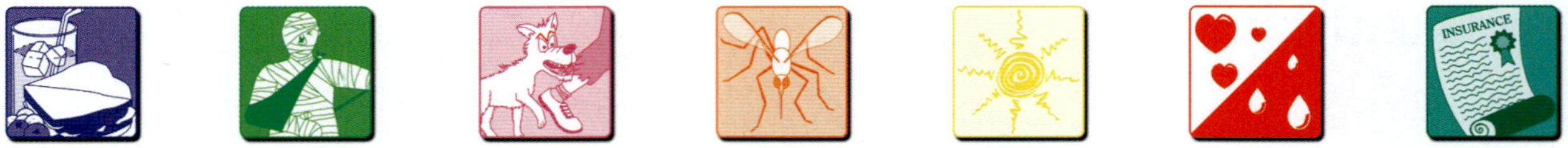

Immunization Advice

- ❑ Immunizations recommended for life should be up to date, especially those for children and boosters of tetanus for adults.
- ❑ Courses or boosters of diphtheria, hepatitis A and typhoid are usually advised.
- ❑ Vaccines sometimes advised are: BCG, cholera, hepatitis B, Japanese encephalitis, rabies.
- ❑ A yellow fever certificate is required if aged over 1 year old and entering from an infected country.

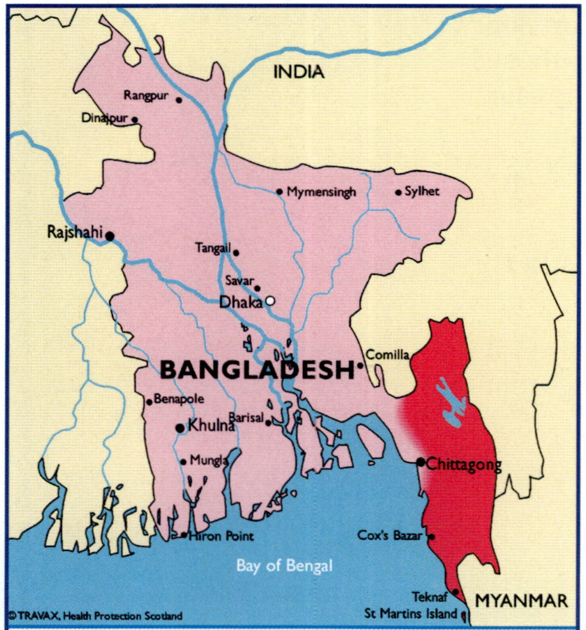

Low to no risk antimalarials not usually advised | **High risk** antimalarials usually advised | Surrounding countries with malaria risk

This map is only intended as a guide since mosquitoes do not respect boundaries and the risk areas shown may not be exact. **Reproduced with permission from Fitfortravel, Health Protection Scotland's Travel website www.fitfortravel.nhs.uk.**

Malaria Advice

- ❑ Malaria is a serious and sometimes fatal disease transmitted by mosquitoes. You cannot be vaccinated against malaria.

MALARIA PRECAUTIONS

- ❑ Malaria precautions are essential in most areas all year round. The highest risk is in the southeast. Avoid mosquito bites by covering up with clothing such as long sleeves and long trousers especially after sunset, using insect repellents on exposed skin and, when necessary, sleeping under a mosquito net.
- ❑ Check with your doctor or nurse about suitable antimalarial tablets.
- ❑ Prompt investigation of fever is essential.

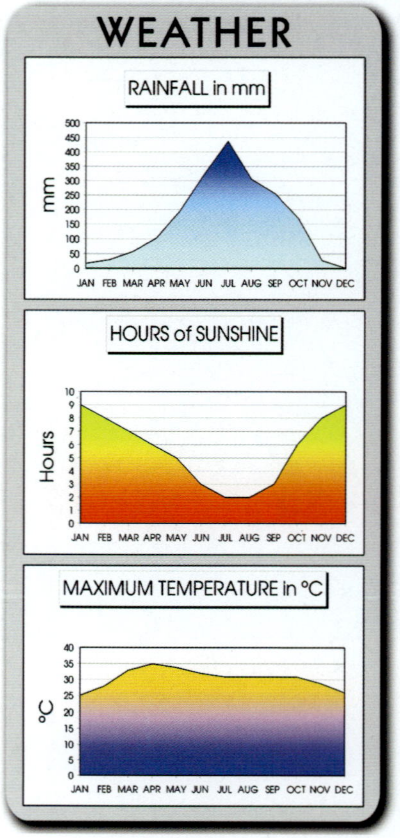

BARBADOS

General Advice

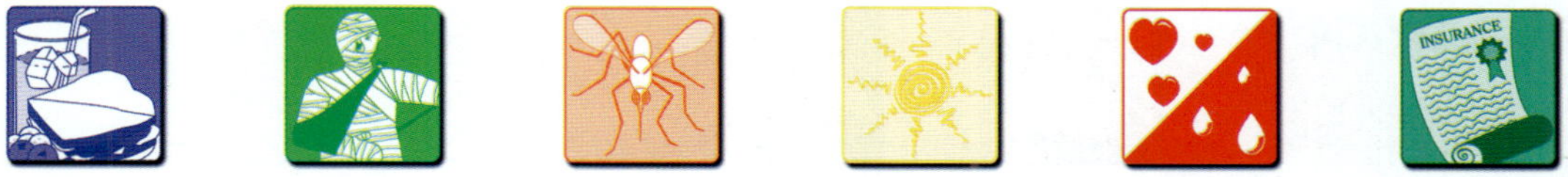

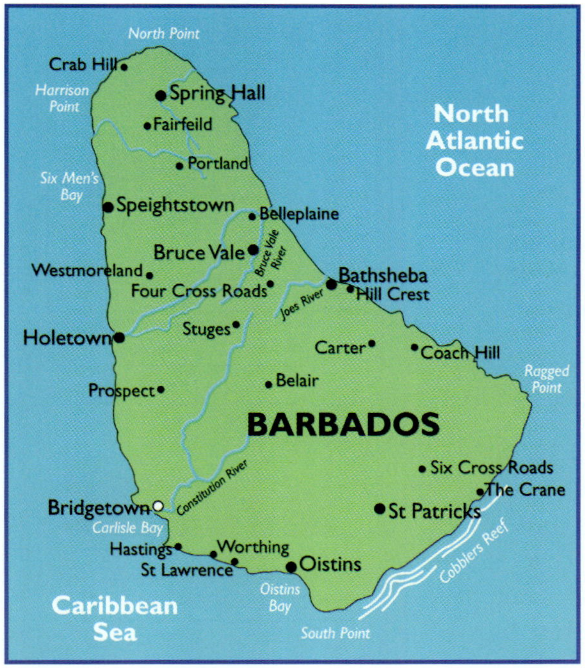

Immunization Advice

- ❑ Immunizations recommended for life should be up to date, especially those for children and boosters of tetanus for adults.
- ❑ Vaccines sometimes advised are: hepatitis A, hepatitis B.
- ❑ A yellow fever certificate is required if aged over 1 year old and entering from an infected country except Guyana and Trinidad and Tobago.

Malaria Advice

- ❑ Malaria is not normally present.

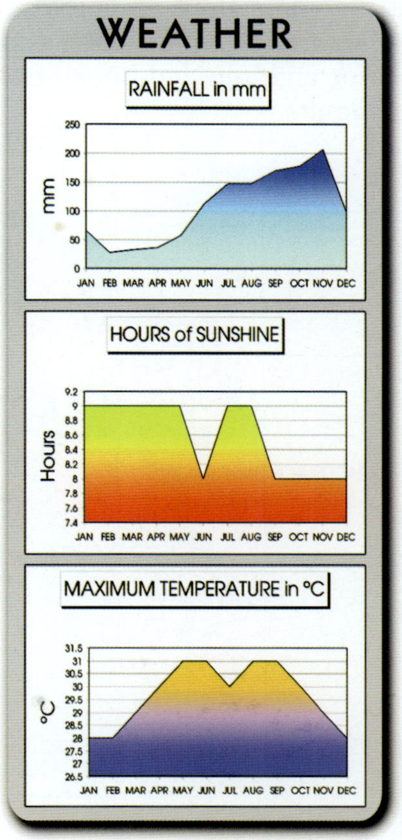

BELIZE

General Advice

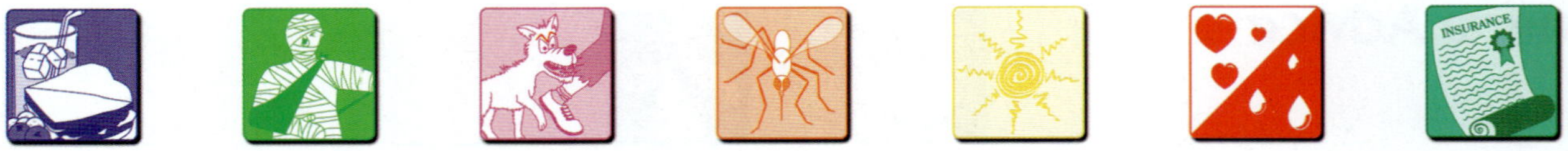

Immunization Advice

- ❑ Immunizations recommended for life should be up to date, especially those for children and boosters of tetanus for adults.
- ❑ Courses or boosters of hepatitis A are usually advised.
- ❑ Vaccines sometimes advised are: BCG, hepatitis B, rabies, typhoid.
- ❑ A yellow fever certificate is required if aged over 1 year old and entering from an infected country.

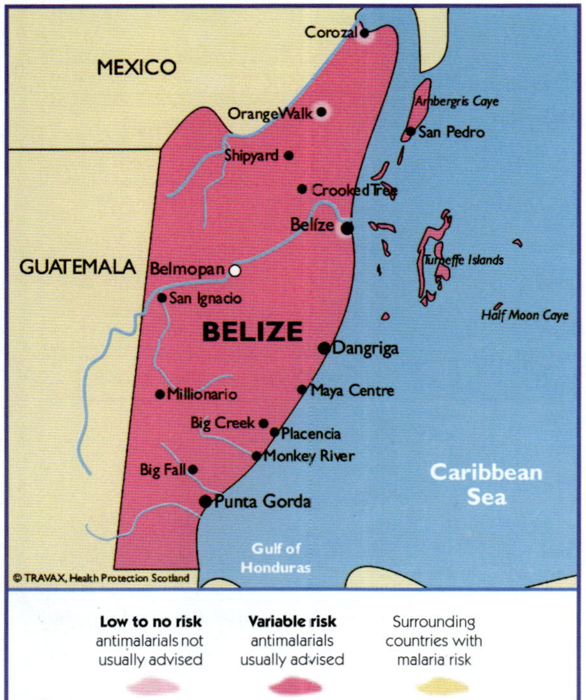

This map is only intended as a guide since mosquitoes do not respect boundaries and the risk areas shown may not be exact. **Reproduced with permission from Fitfortravel, Health Protection Scotland's Travel website www.fitfortravel.nhs.uk.**

Malaria Advice

- ❑ Malaria is a serious and sometimes fatal disease transmitted by mosquitoes. You cannot be vaccinated against malaria.

MALARIA PRECAUTIONS

- ❑ Malaria precautions are essential in all areas all year round. The highest risk is in Toledo and Stan Creek districts and is moderate in Cayo district. The risk is low in Belize district, Corozal, and Orange Walk. Avoid mosquito bites by covering up with clothing such as long sleeves and long trousers especially after sunset, using insect repellents on exposed skin and, when necessary, sleeping under a mosquito net.
- ❑ Check with your doctor or nurse about suitable antimalarial tablets.
- ❑ Prompt investigation of fever is essential.

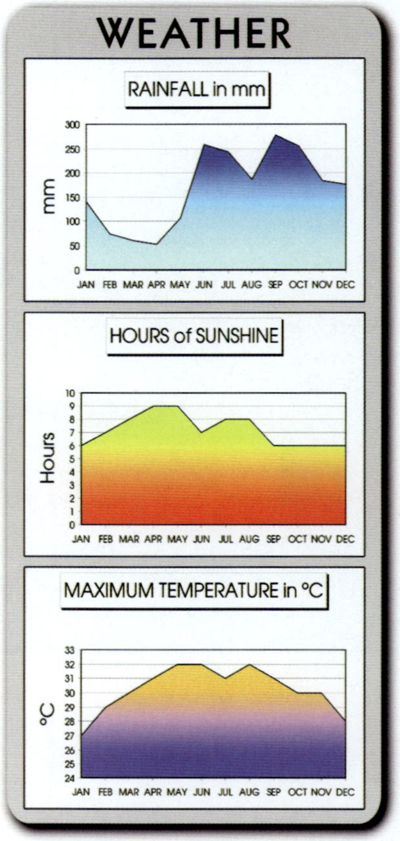

BERMUDA

General Advice

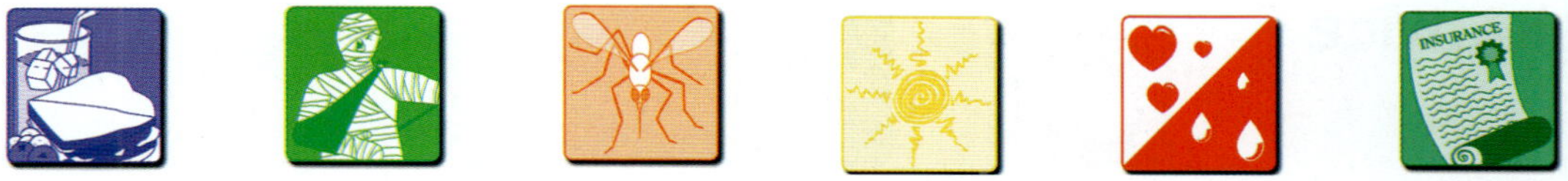

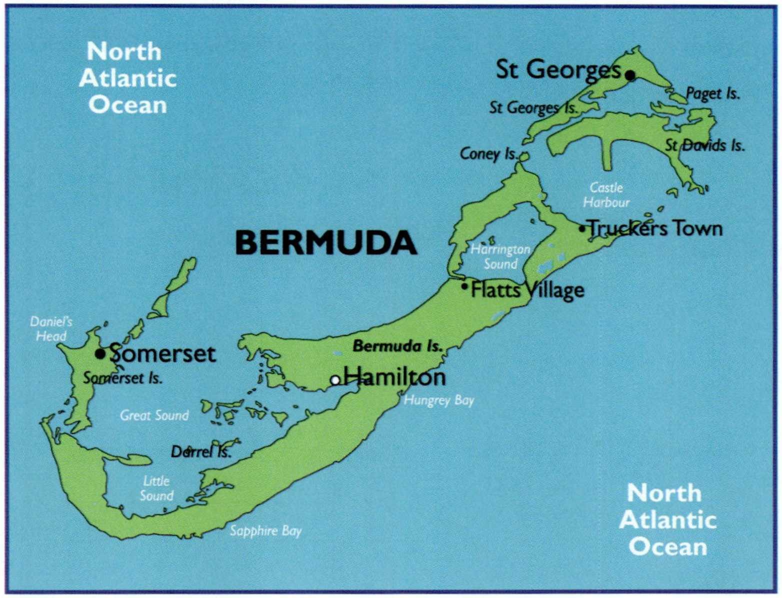

Immunization Advice

- ❑ Immunizations recommended for life should be up to date, especially those for children and boosters of tetanus for adults.
- ❑ Vaccines sometimes advised are: hepatitis A, hepatitis B.
- ❑ No certificate of vaccination for yellow fever is required.

Malaria Advice

- ❑ Malaria is not normally present.

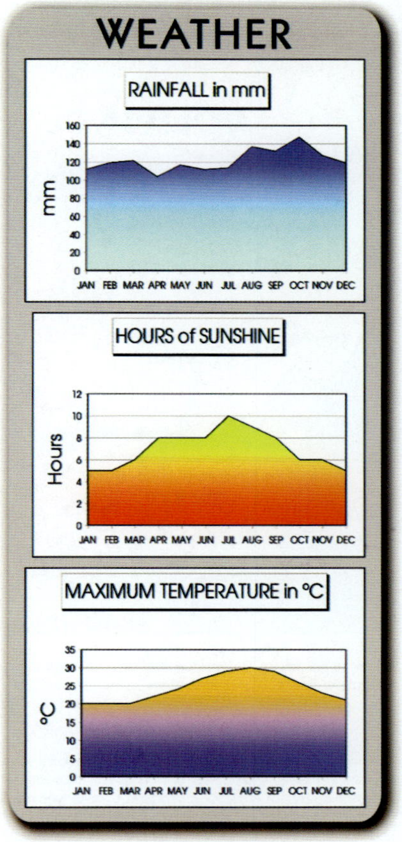

BOLIVIA

General Advice

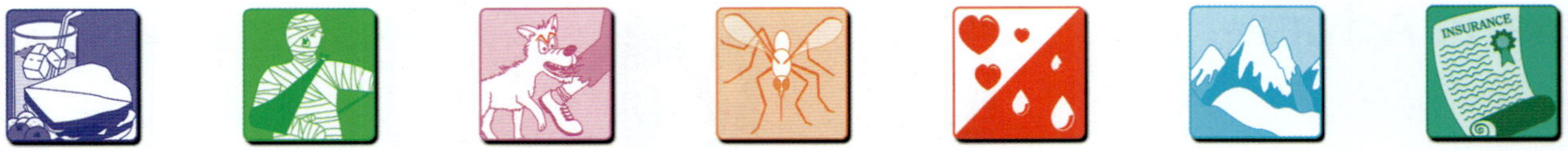

Immunization Advice

- ❑ Immunizations recommended for life should be up to date, especially those for children and boosters of tetanus for adults.
- ❑ Courses or boosters of hepatitis A and typhoid are usually advised.
- ❑ Vaccines sometimes advised are: BCG, hepatitis B, rabies, yellow fever (see yellow fever map).
- ❑ A yellow fever certificate is required if aged over 1 year old and entering from an infected country.

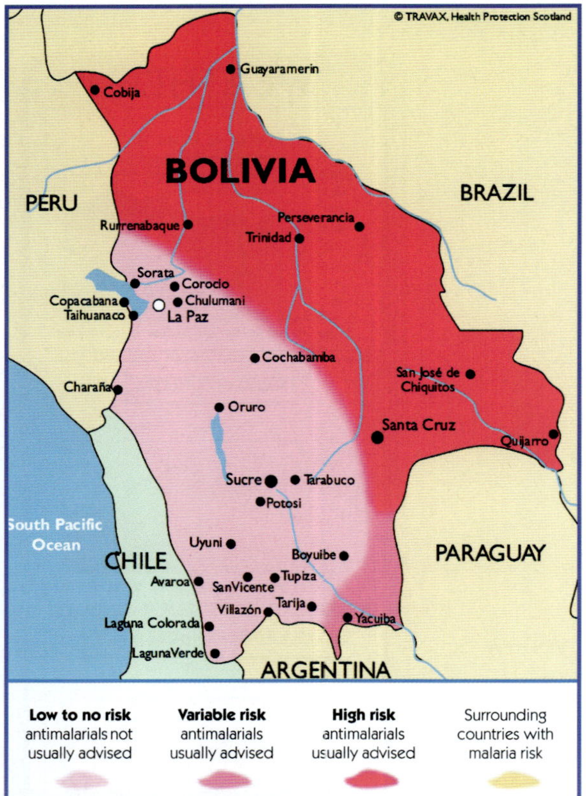

This map is only intended as a guide since mosquitoes do not respect boundaries and the risk areas shown may not be exact. **Reproduced with permission from Fitfortravel, Health Protection Scotland's Travel website www.fitfortravel.nhs.uk.**

Malaria Advice

- ❑ Malaria is a serious and sometimes fatal disease transmitted by mosquitoes. You cannot be vaccinated against malaria.

MALARIA PRECAUTIONS

- ❑ Malaria precautions are essential in all areas below 2500 m all year round. The risk is highest in the departments of Santa Cruz, northern Beni, and Pando. Avoid mosquito bites by covering up with clothing such as long sleeves and long trousers especially after sunset, using insect repellents on exposed skin and, when necessary, sleeping under a mosquito net.
- ❑ Check with your doctor or nurse about suitable antimalarial tablets.
- ❑ Prompt investigation of fever is essential.

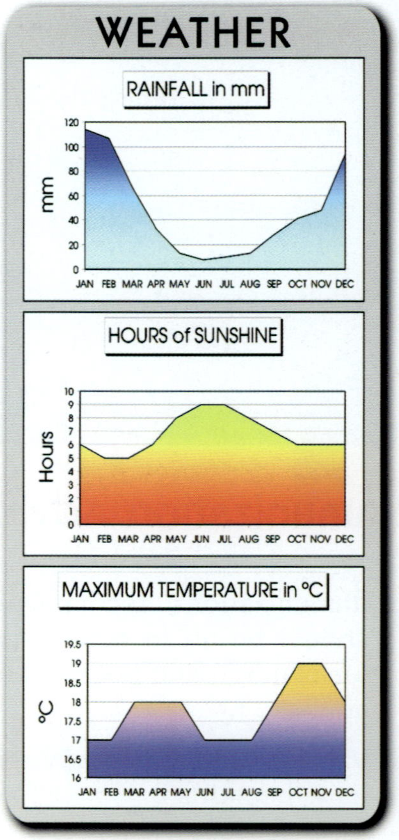

BOSNIA and HERZEGOVINA

General Advice

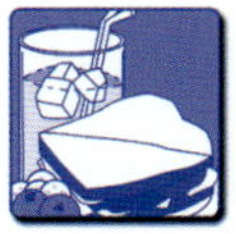
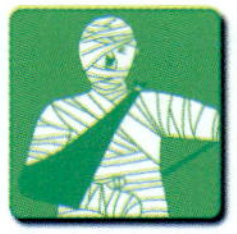
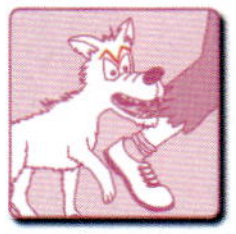
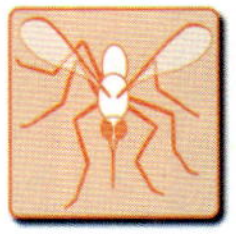
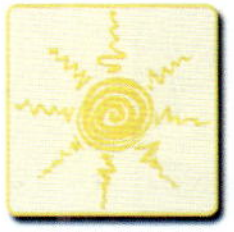

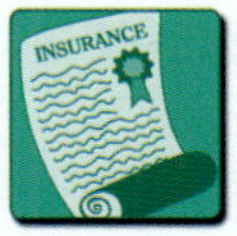

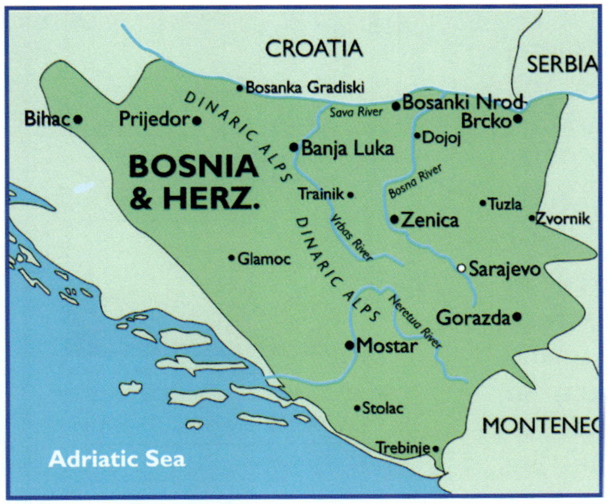

Immunization Advice

- ❑ Immunizations recommended for life should be up to date, especially those for children and boosters of tetanus for adults.
- ❑ Courses or boosters of hepatitis A are usually advised.
- ❑ Vaccines sometimes advised are: BCG, hepatitis B, rabies, tick-borne encephalitis.
- ❑ No certificate of vaccination for yellow fever is required.

Malaria Advice

- ❑ Malaria is not normally present.

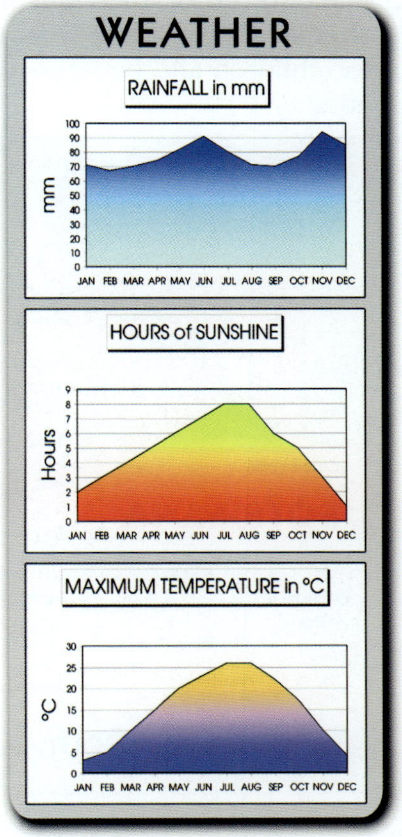

BOTSWANA

General Advice

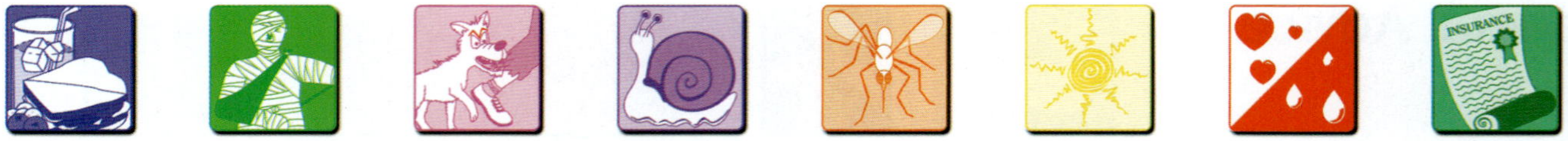

Immunization Advice

❑ Immunizations recommended for life should be up to date, especially those for children and boosters of tetanus for adults.

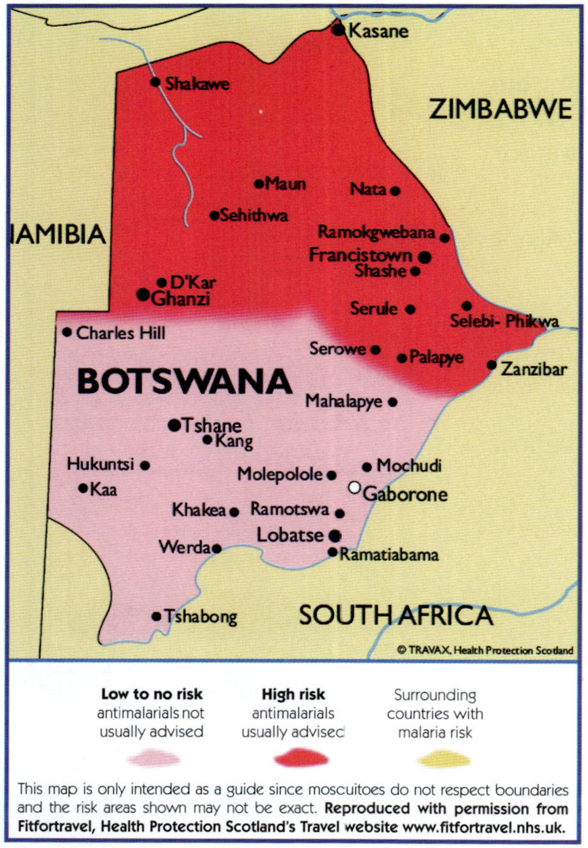

❑ Courses or boosters of hepatitis A and typhoid are usually advised.

❑ Vaccines sometimes advised are: BCG, cholera, hepatitis B, rabies.

❑ A yellow fever certificate is required if aged over 1 year old and entering from an infected country.

Malaria Advice

❑ Malaria is a serious and sometimes fatal disease transmitted by mosquitoes. You cannot be vaccinated against malaria.

MALARIA PRECAUTIONS

❑ Malaria precautions are essential in northern areas, along the Zimbabwean border, the Zambezi river, and game parks north of the Kalihari desert, all year round, but especially from November to June. Avoid mosquito bites by covering up with clothing such as long sleeves and long trousers especially after sunset, using insect repellents on exposed skin and, when necessary, sleeping under a mosquito net.

❑ Check with your doctor or nurse about suitable antimalarial tablets.

❑ Prompt investigation of fever is essential.

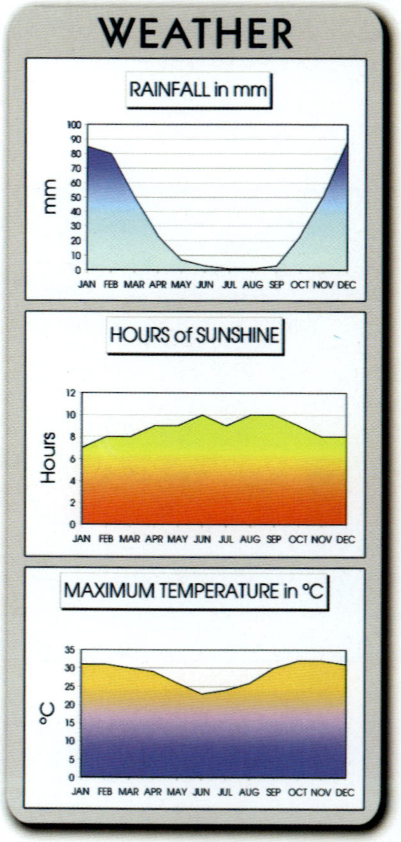

BRAZIL

General Advice

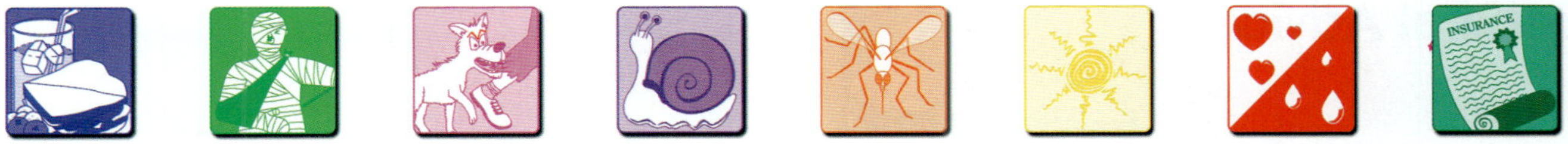

Immunization Advice

- ❑ Immunizations recommended for life should be up to date, especially those for children and boosters of tetanus for adults.

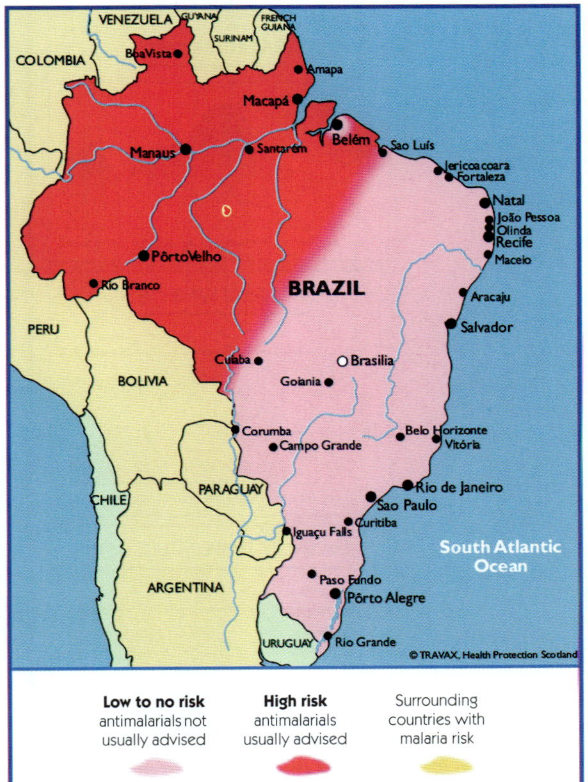

This map is only intended as a guide since mosquitoes do not respect boundaries and the risk areas shown may not be exact. **Reproduced with permission from Fitfortravel, Health Protection Scotland's Travel website www.fitfortravel.nhs.uk.**

- ❑ Courses or boosters of diphtheria and hepatitis A are usually advised.
- ❑ Vaccines sometimes advised are: BCG, hepatitis B, rabies, typhoid, yellow fever (see yellow fever map).
- ❑ No certificate of vaccination for yellow fever is required.

Malaria Advice

- ❑ Malaria is a serious and sometimes fatal disease transmitted by mosquitoes. You cannot be vaccinated against malaria.

MALARIA PRECAUTIONS

- ❑ Malaria precautions are essential in forested areas below 900 m and within "legal Amazonia" all year round. There is minimal risk in the resort at Iguacu Falls with higher risk in nearby rural areas. Risk is minimal outside Amazonia states including coastal areas south of Belem. There can be a risk for those on Amazon cruises (see map). Avoid mosquito bites by covering up with clothing such as long sleeves and long trousers especially after sunset, using insect repellents on exposed skin and, when necessary, sleeping under a mosquito net.
- ❑ Check with your doctor or nurse about suitable anti-malarial tablets.
- ❑ Prompt investigation of fever is essential.

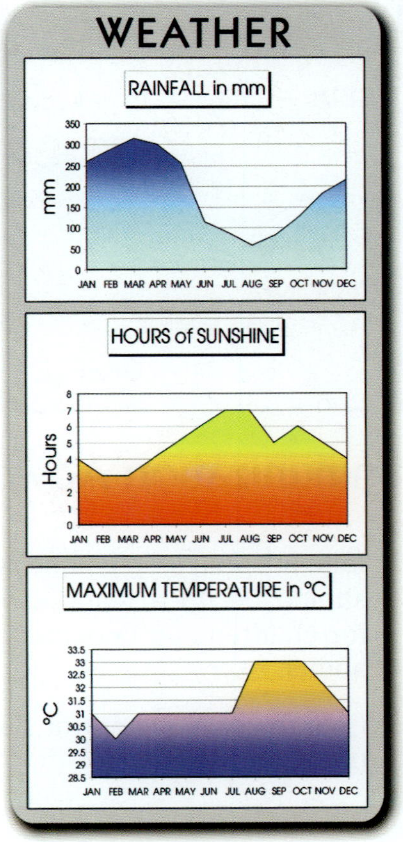

BULGARIA

General Advice

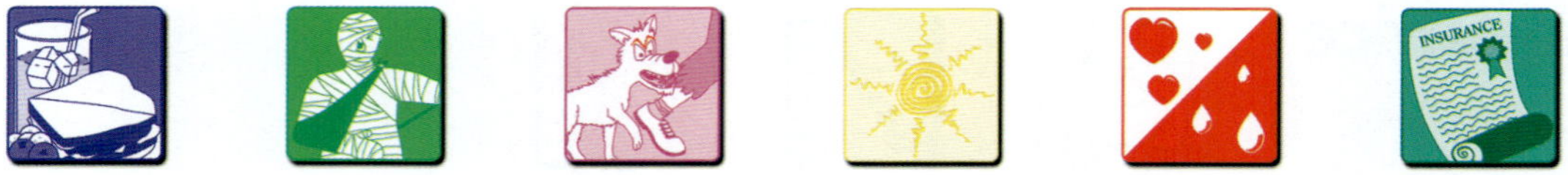

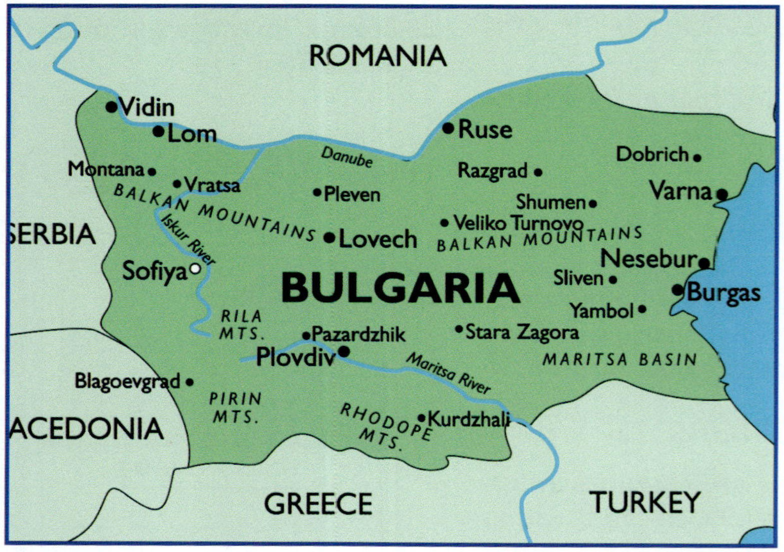

Immunization Advice

- ❑ Immunizations recommended for life should be up to date, especially those for children and boosters of tetanus for adults.
- ❑ Courses or boosters of hepatitis A are usually advised.
- ❑ Vaccines sometimes advised are: BCG, hepatitis B, rabies.
- ❑ No certificate of vaccination for yellow fever is required.

Malaria Advice

- ❑ Malaria is not normally present.

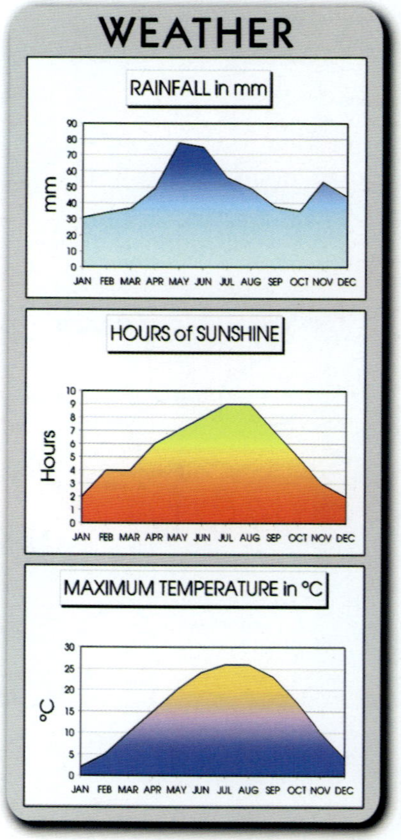

CAMBODIA

General Advice

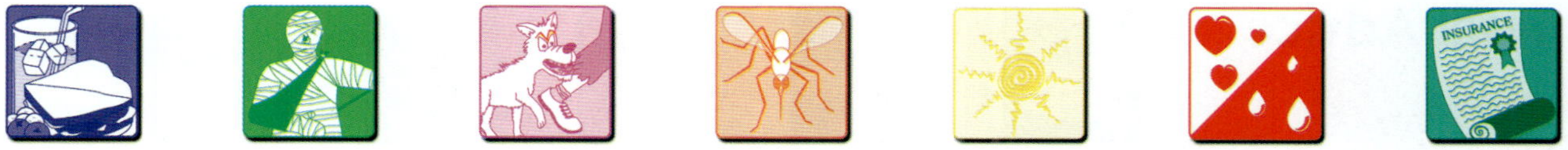

Immunization Advice

- ❑ Immunizations recommended for life should be up to date, especially those for children and boosters of tetanus for adults.
- ❑ Courses or boosters of diphtheria, hepatitis A and typhoid are usually advised.

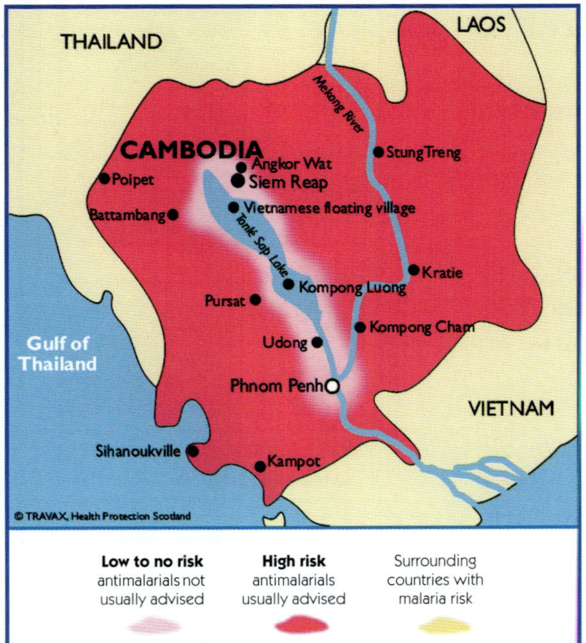

This map is only intended as a guide since mosquitoes do not respect boundaries and the risk areas shown may not be exact. **Reproduced with permission from Fitfortravel, Health Protection Scotland's Travel website www.fitfortravel.nhs.uk.**

- ❑ Vaccines sometimes advised are: BCG, cholera, hepatitis B, Japanese encephalitis, rabies.
- ❑ A yellow fever certificate is required if aged over 1 year old and entering from an infected country.

Malaria Advice

- ❑ Malaria is a serious and sometimes fatal disease transmitted by mosquitoes. You cannot be vaccinated against malaria.

MALARIA PRECAUTIONS

- ❑ Malaria precautions are essential in all areas, all year round. The risk is minimal in Phnom Penh, close to Tonle Sap and around Angkor Wat. Avoid mosquito bites by covering up with clothing such as long sleeves and long trousers especially after sunset, using insect repellents on exposed skin and, when necessary, sleeping under a mosquito net.
- ❑ Check with your doctor or nurse about suitable antimalarial tablets.
- ❑ Prompt investigation of fever is essential.

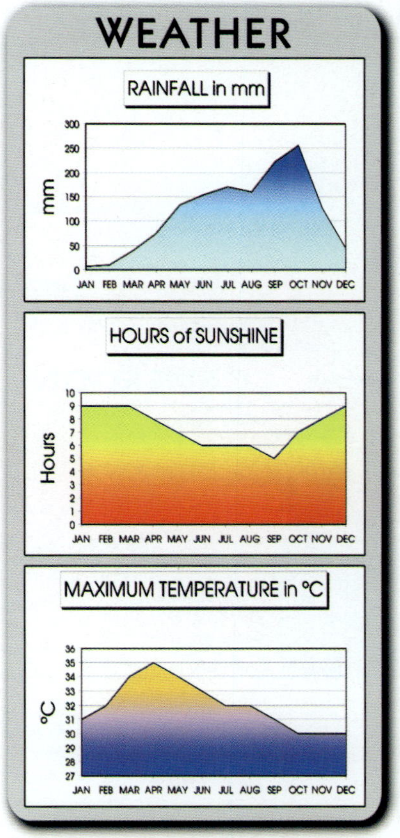

CAMEROON

General Advice

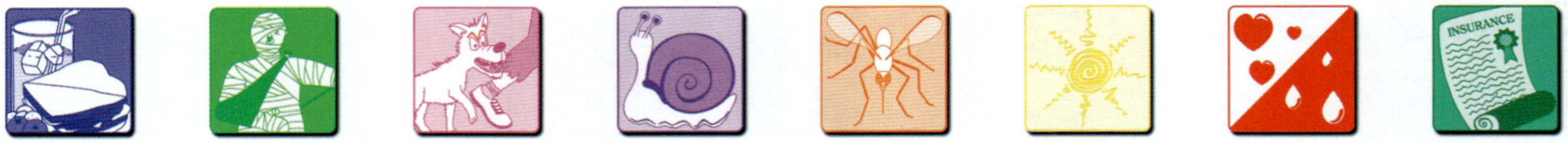

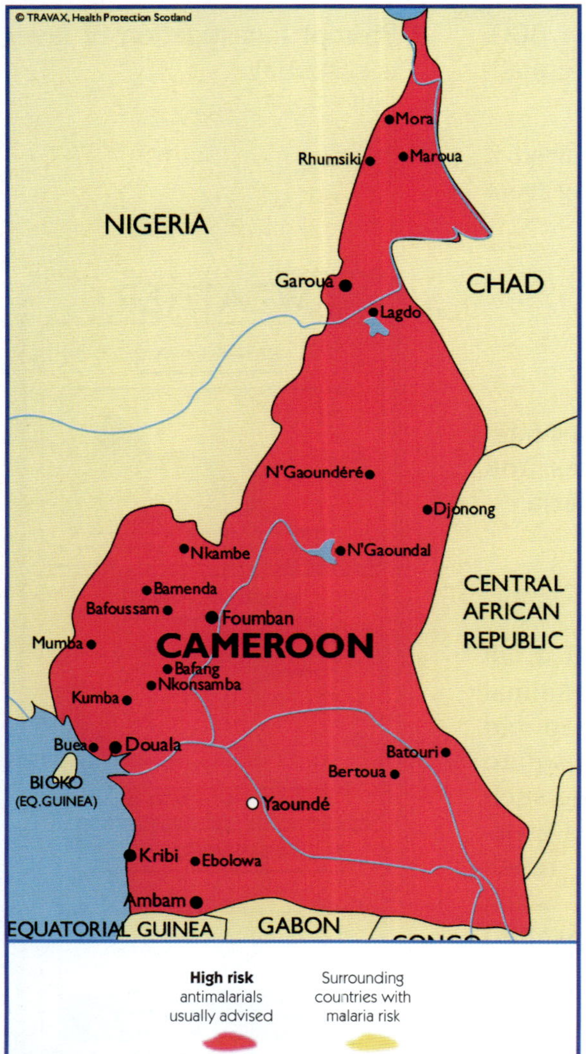

This map is only intended as a guide since mosquitoes do not respect boundaries and the risk areas shown may not be exact. **Reproduced with permission from Fitfortravel, Health Protection Scotland's Travel website www.fitfortravel.nhs.uk.**

Immunization Advice

- ❑ Immunizations recommended for life should be up to date, especially those for children and boosters of tetanus for adults.
- ❑ Courses or boosters of hepatitis A, poliomyelitis, typhoid, and yellow fever are usually advised.
- ❑ Vaccines sometimes advised are: BCG, cholera, hepatitis B, meningococcal A and C, and rabies.
- ❑ A yellow fever certificate is required for all travelers aged over 1 year.

Malaria Advice

- ❑ Malaria is a serious and sometimes fatal disease transmitted by mosquitoes. You cannot be vaccinated against malaria.

MALARIA PRECAUTIONS

- ❑ Malaria precautions are essential in all areas all year round. Avoid mosquito bites by covering up with clothing such as long sleeves and long trousers especially after sunset, using insect repellents on exposed skin and, when necessary, sleeping under a mosquito net.
- ❑ Check with your doctor or nurse about suitable antimalarial tablets.
- ❑ Prompt investigation of fever is essential.

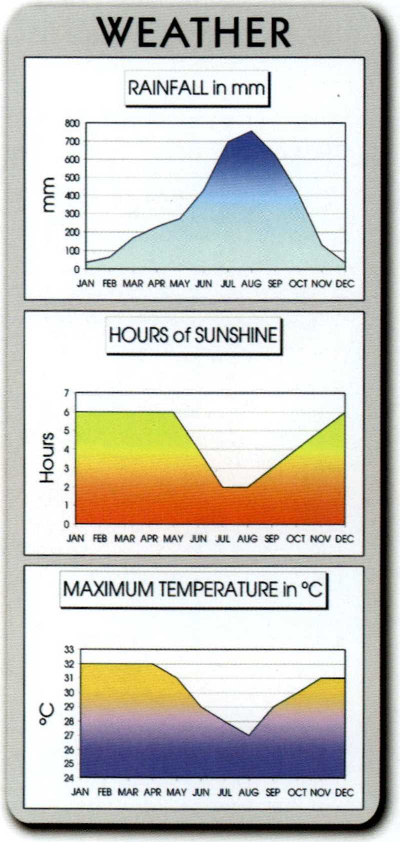

CAYMAN ISLANDS

General Advice

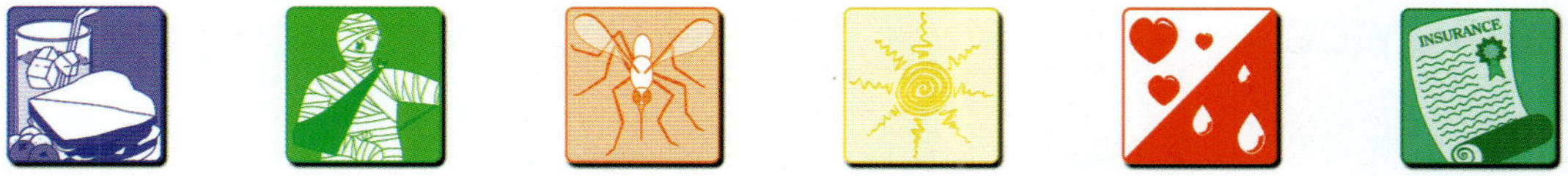

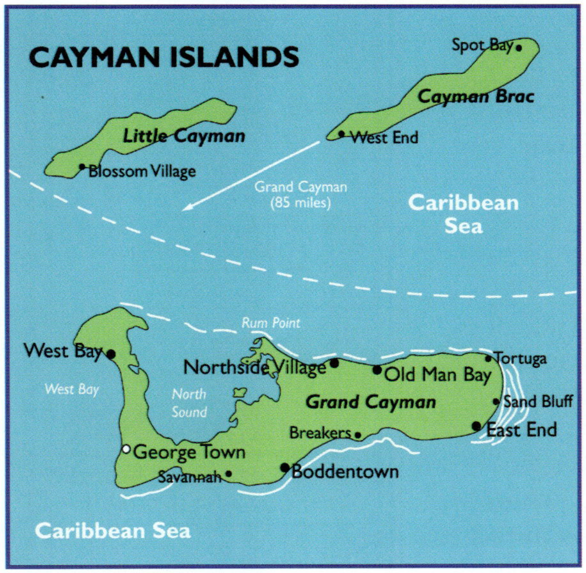

Immunization Advice

- ❑ Immunizations recommended for life should be up to date, especially those for children and boosters of tetanus for adults.
- ❑ Vaccines sometimes advised are: hepatitis A, hepatitis B.
- ❑ No certificate of vaccination for yellow fever is required.

Malaria Advice

- ❑ Malaria is not normally present.

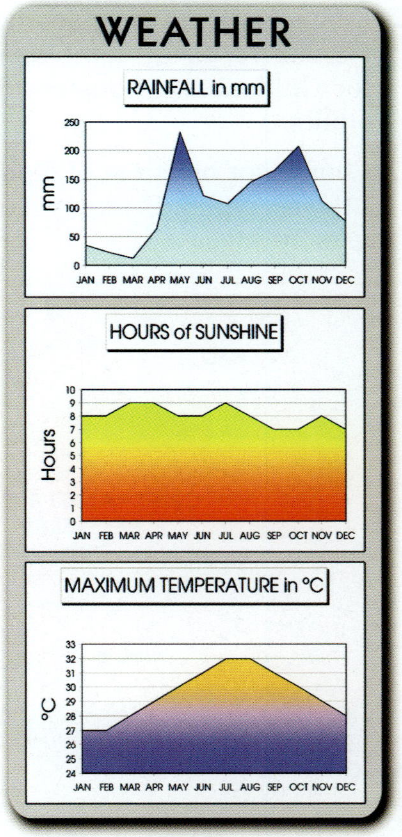

CENTRAL AFRICAN REPUBLIC

General Advice

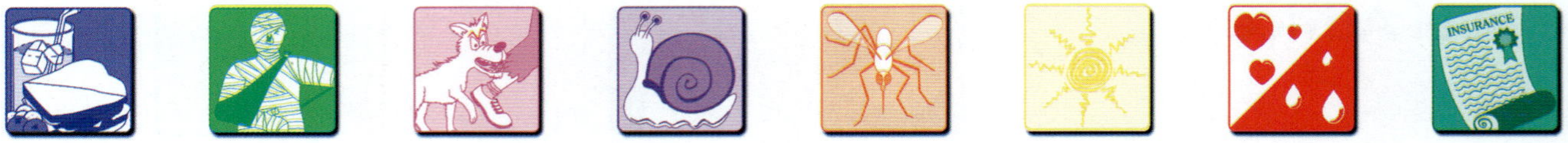

Immunization Advice

❑ Immunizations recommended for life should be up to date, especially those for children and boosters of tetanus for adults.

❑ Courses or boosters of diphtheria, hepatitis A, typhoid, and yellow fever are usually advised.

❑ Vaccines sometimes advised are: BCG, cholera, hepatitis B, meningococcal A and C, and rabies.

❑ A yellow fever certificate is required for all travelers aged over 1 year.

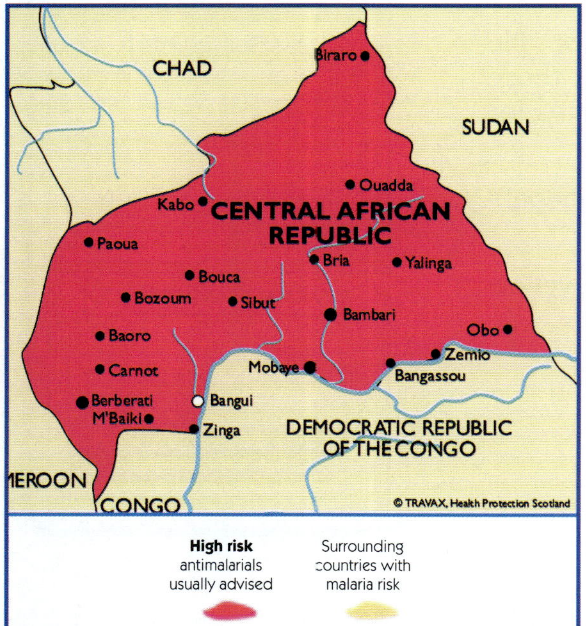

This map is only intended as a guide since mosquitoes do not respect boundaries and the risk areas shown may not be exact. **Reproduced with permission from Fitfortravel, Health Protection Scotland's Travel website www.fitfortravel.nhs.uk.**

Malaria Advice

❑ Malaria is a serious and sometimes fatal disease transmitted by mosquitoes. You cannot be vaccinated against malaria.

MALARIA PRECAUTIONS

❑ Malaria precautions are essential in all areas all year round. Avoid mosquito bites by covering up with clothing such as long sleeves and long trousers especially after sunset, using insect repellents on exposed skin and, when necessary, sleeping under a mosquito net.

❑ Check with your doctor or nurse about suitable antimalarial tablets.

❑ Prompt investigation of fever is essential.

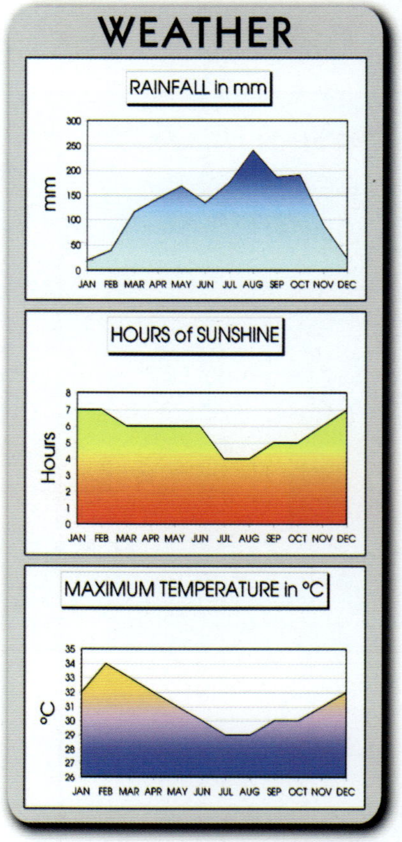

CHILE

General Advice

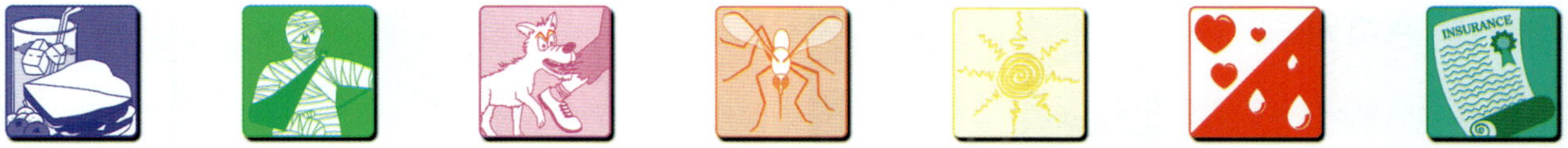

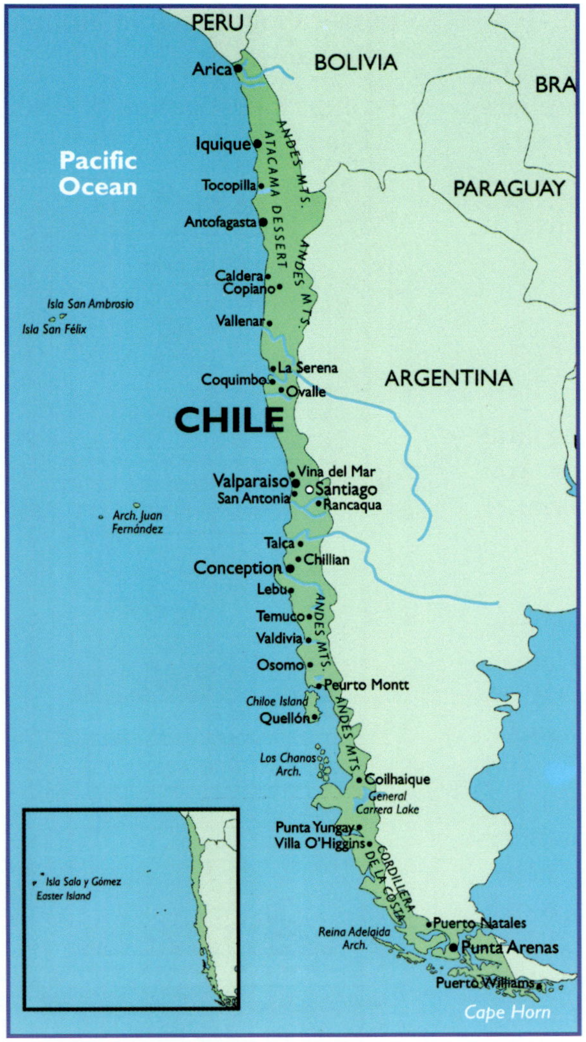

Immunization Advice

- ❑ Immunizations recommended for life should be up to date, especially those for children and boosters of tetanus for adults.
- ❑ Courses or boosters of hepatitis A are usually advised.
- ❑ Vaccines sometimes advised are: hepatitis B, rabies, typhoid.
- ❑ No certificate of vaccination for yellow fever is required.

Malaria Advice

- ❑ Malaria is not normally present.

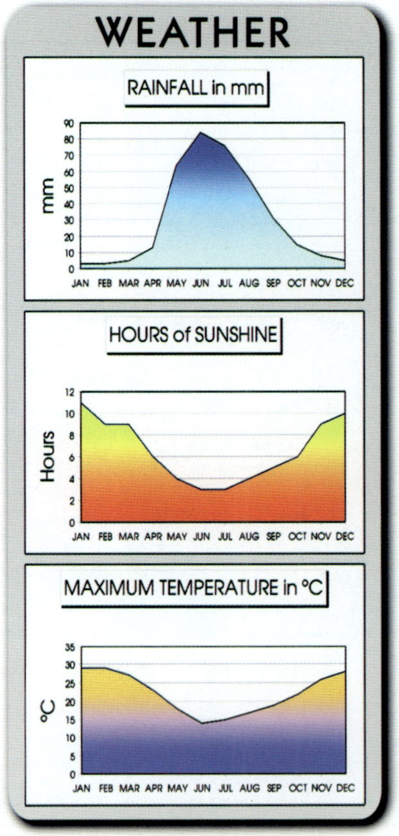

CHINA and TAIWAN

General Advice

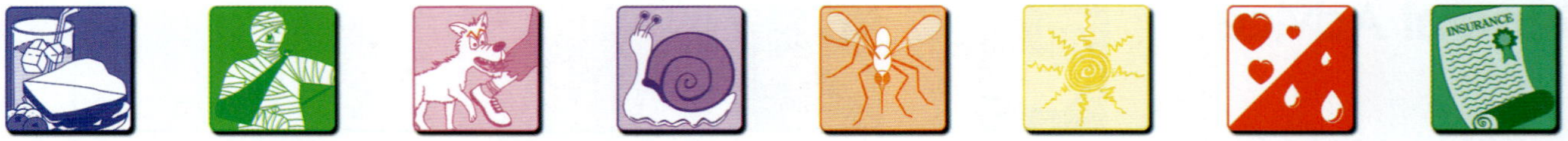

Immunization Advice

- ❑ Immunizations recommended for life should be up to date, especially those for children and boosters of tetanus for adults.
- ❑ Courses or boosters of diphtheria and hepatitis A are usually advised.
- ❑ Vaccines sometimes advised are: BCG, cholera, hepatitis B, Japanese encephalitis, rabies, tick-borne encephalitis, typhoid.
- ❑ A yellow fever certificate is required if entering from an infected country.

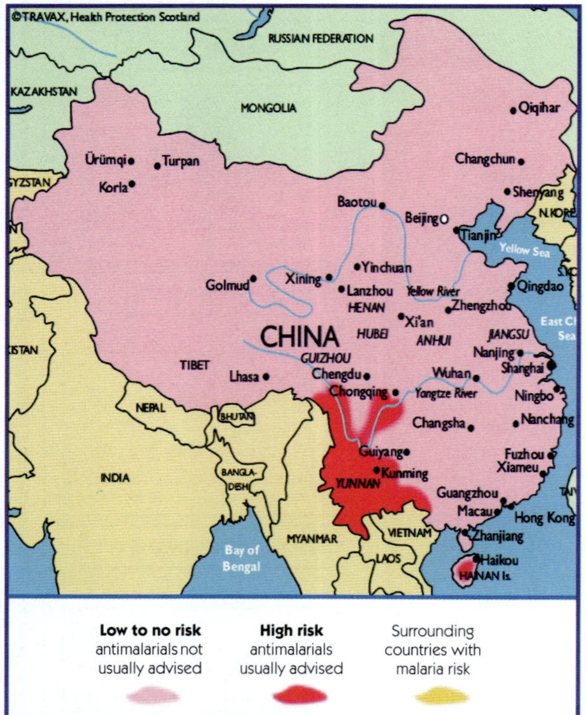

This map is only intended as a guide since mosquitoes do not respect boundaries and the risk areas shown may not be exact. **Reproduced with permission from Fitfortravel, Health Protection Scotland's Travel website www.fitfortravel.nhs.uk.**

Malaria Advice

- ❑ Malaria is a serious and sometimes fatal disease transmitted by mosquitoes. You cannot be vaccinated against malaria.

MALARIA PRECAUTIONS

- ❑ Malaria precautions are essential in Yunnan province and the interior of Hainan all year round. There is a very low risk in Anhui, Ghuizhou, Hubei, and Jiangsu. There is low to no risk on Yellow and Yangtse cruises. Avoid mosquito bites by covering up with clothing such as long sleeves and long trousers especially after sunset, using insect repellents on exposed skin and, when necessary, sleeping under a mosquito net.
- ❑ Check with your doctor or nurse about suitable antimalarial tablets.
- ❑ Prompt investigation of fever is essential.

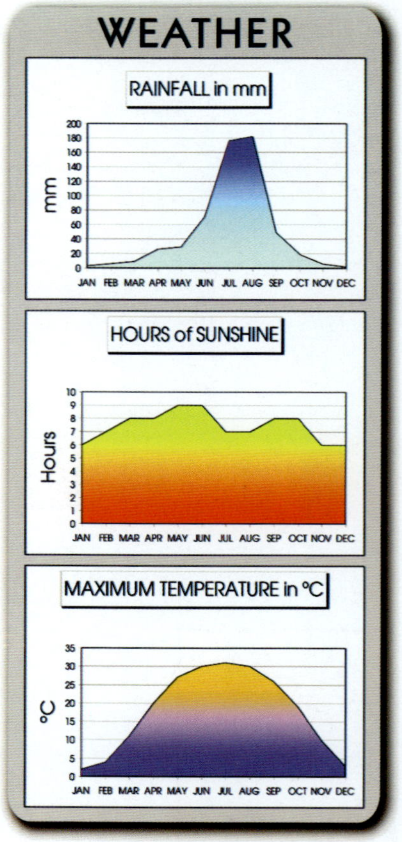

—Weather in Beijing—

COLOMBIA

General Advice

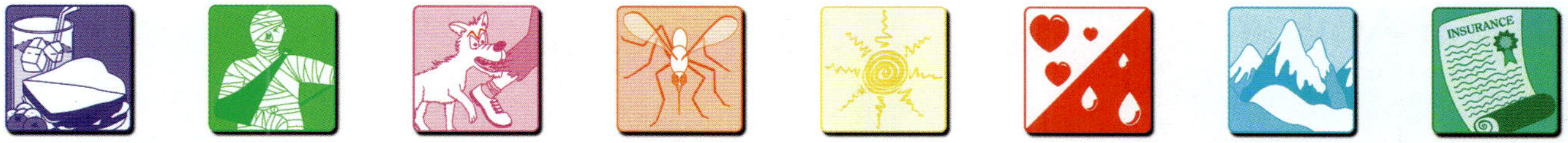

Immunization Advice

- ❑ Immunizations recommended for life should be up to date, especially those for children and boosters of tetanus for adults.

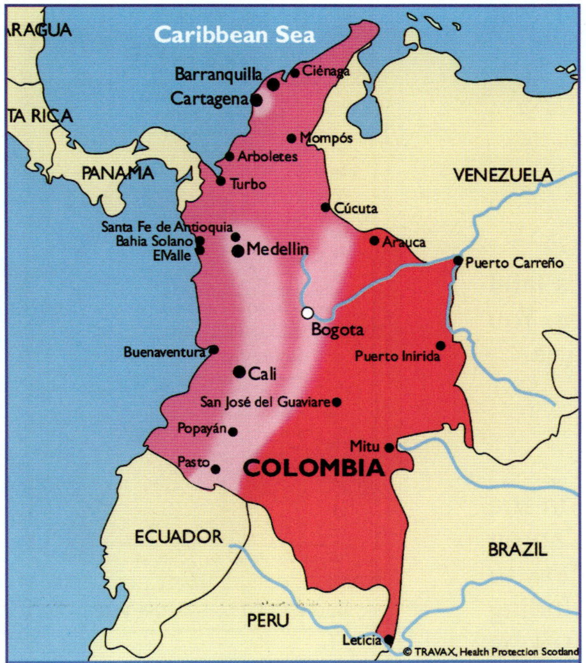

Low to no risk antimalarials not usually advised	**Variable risk** antimalarials usually advised	**High risk** antimalarials usually advised	Surrounding countries with malaria risk

This map is only intended as a guide since mosquitoes do not respect boundaries and the risk areas shown may not be exact. **Reproduced with permission from Fitfortravel, Health Protection Scotland's Travel website www.fitfortravel.nhs.uk.**

- ❑ Courses or boosters of hepatitis A are usually advised.
- ❑ Vaccines sometimes advised are: hepatitis B, rabies, typhoid, yellow fever (see yellow fever map).
- ❑ No certificate of vaccination for yellow fever is required.

Malaria Advice

- ❑ Malaria is a serious and sometimes fatal disease transmitted by mosquitoes. You cannot be vaccinated against malaria.

MALARIA PRECAUTIONS

- ❑ Malaria precautions are essential in rural and jungle areas below 1600 m in regions of Amazonia, Orinoquia, Pacifico and Uraba-Bajo Cauca, all year round. The risk is minimal in and around Bogota, Cartagena, and in areas above 1600 m. Avoid mosquito bites by covering up with clothing such as long sleeves and long trousers especially after sunset, using insect repellents on exposed skin and, when necessary, sleeping under a mosquito net.
- ❑ Check with your doctor or nurse about suitable anti-malarial tablets.
- ❑ Prompt investigation of fever is essential.

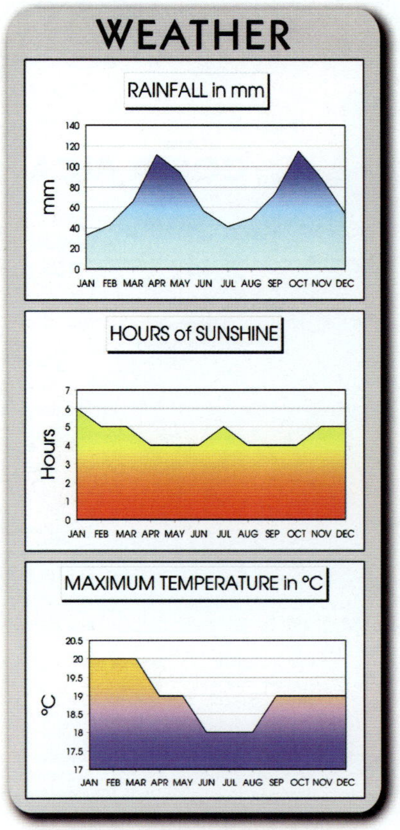

COSTA RICA

General Advice

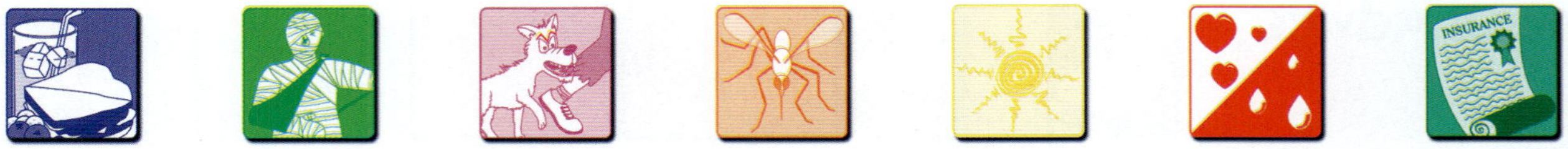

Immunization Advice

- ❑ Immunizations recommended for life should be up to date, especially those for children and boosters of tetanus for adults.

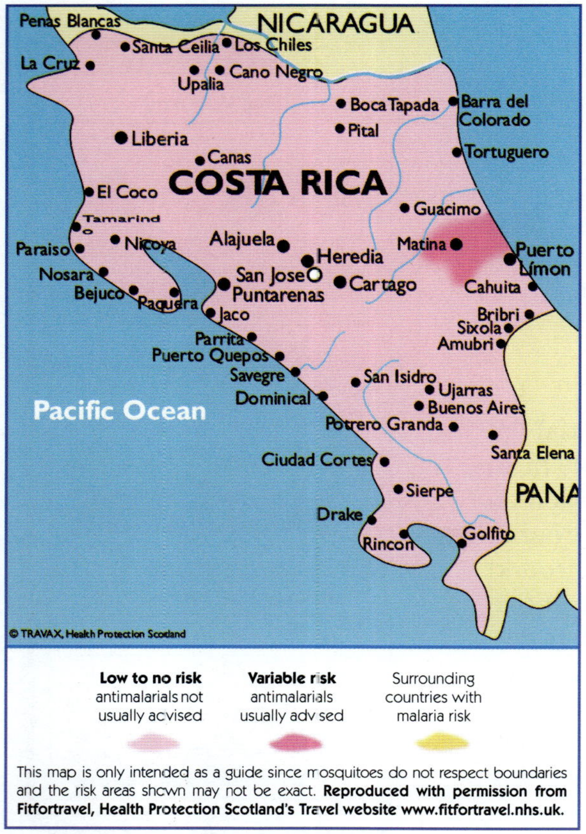

- ❑ Courses or boosters of hepatitis A are usually advised.
- ❑ Vaccines sometimes advised are: hepatitis B, rabies.
- ❑ A yellow fever certificate is required for all travelers aged over 9 months and entering from an infected country (except Argentina, Panama, and Trinidad and Tobago).

Malaria Advice

- ❑ Malaria is a serious and sometimes fatal disease transmitted by mosquitoes. You cannot be vaccinated against malaria.

MALARIA PRECAUTIONS

- ❑ Malaria precautions are essential in the Province of Limon, mainly in the Canton of Matina, all year round. There is low to no risk in all other areas including Puerto Limon. Avoid mosquito bites by covering up with clothing such as long sleeves and long trousers especially after sunset, using insect repellents on exposed skin and, when necessary, sleeping under a mosquito net.
- ❑ Check with your doctor or nurse about suitable anti-malarial tablets.
- ❑ Prompt investigation of fever is essential.

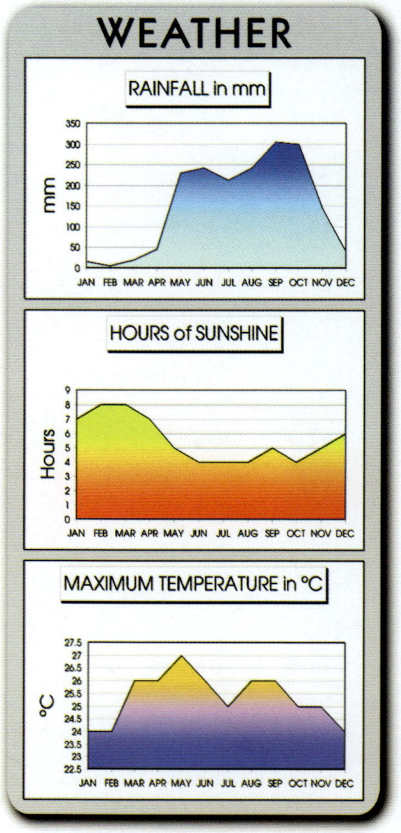

CROATIA

General Advice

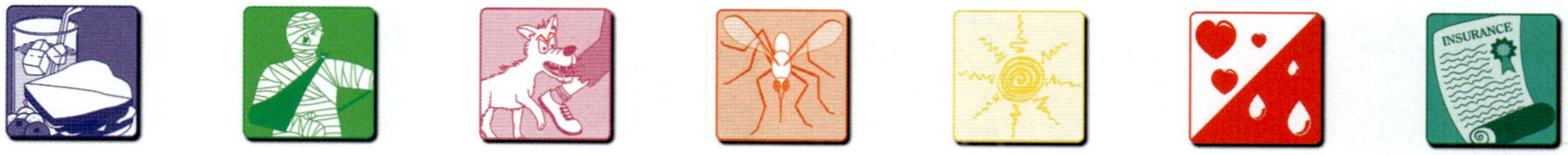

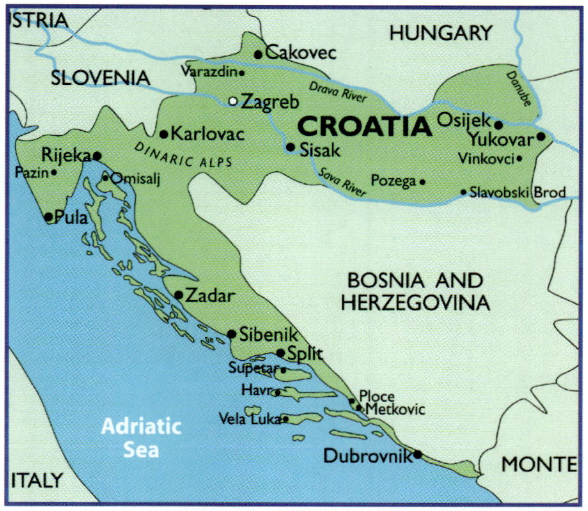

Immunization Advice

- ❑ Immunizations recommended for life should be up to date, especially those for children and boosters of tetanus for adults.
- ❑ Vaccines sometimes advised are: hepatitis A, hepatitis B, rabies, tick-borne encephalitis.
- ❑ No certificate of vaccination for yellow fever is required.

Malaria Advice

- ❑ Malaria is not normally present.

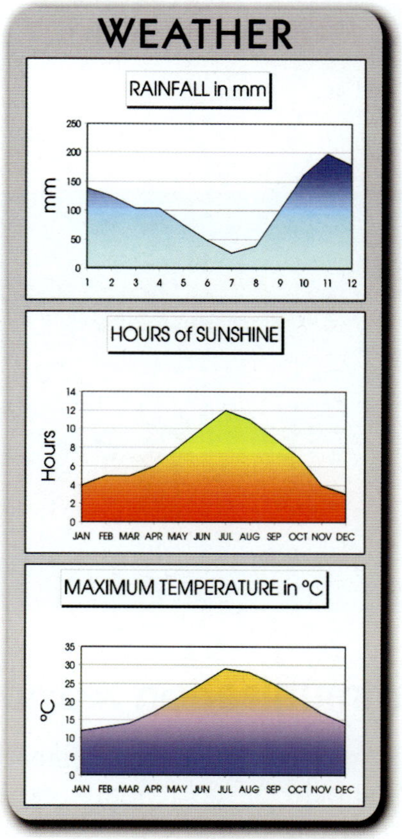

CUBA

General Advice

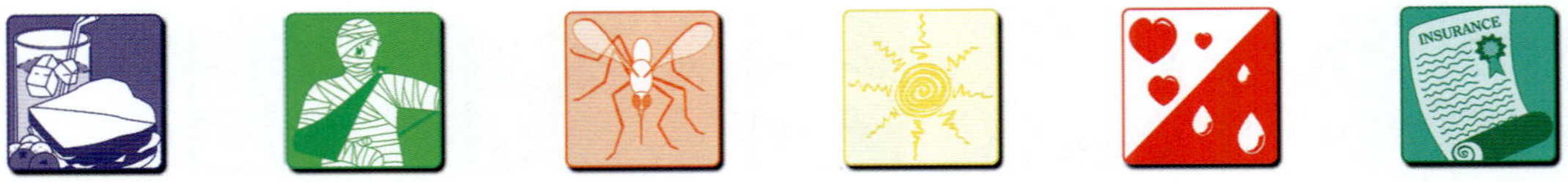

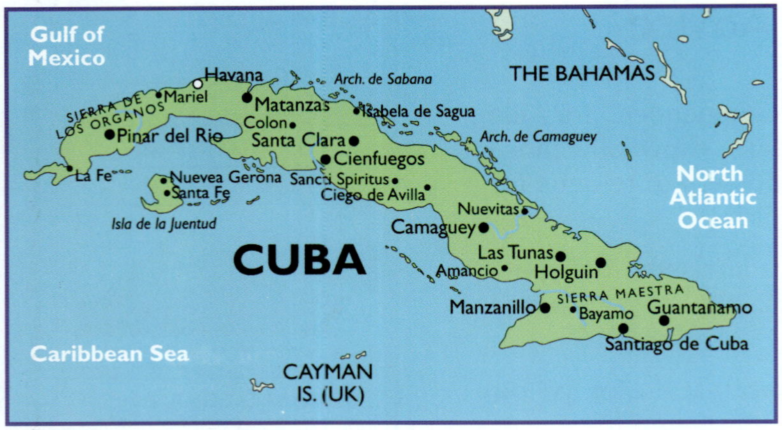

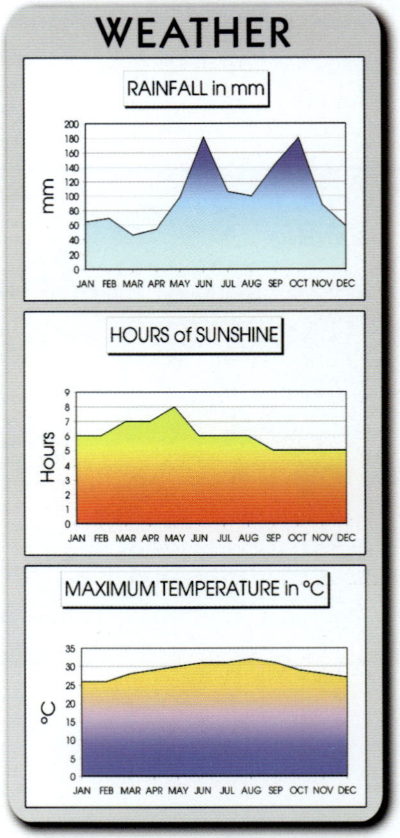

Immunization Advice

- ❑ Immunizations recommended for life should be up to date, especially those for children and boosters of tetanus for adults.
- ❑ Courses or boosters of hepatitis A are usually advised.
- ❑ Vaccines sometimes advised are: hepatitis B, rabies.
- ❑ No certificate of vaccination for yellow fever is required.

Malaria Advice

- ❑ Malaria is not normally present.

CZECH REPUBLIC

General Advice

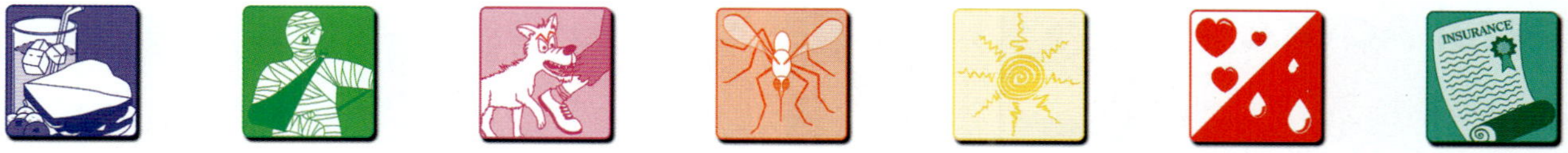

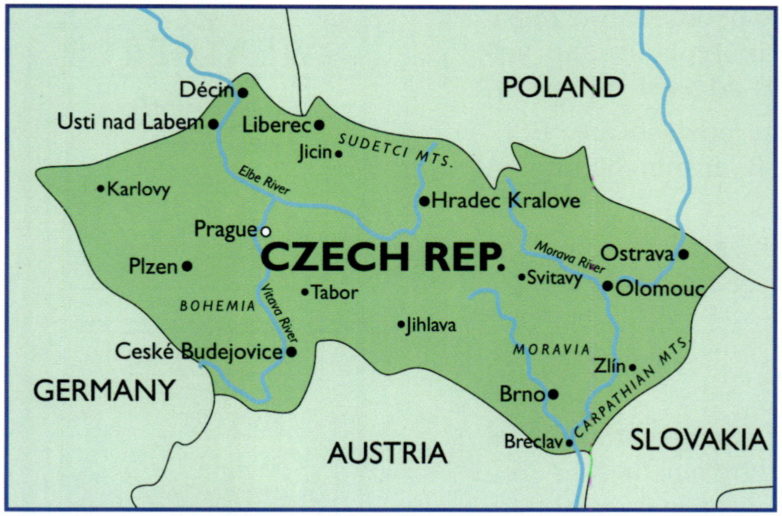

Immunization Advice

- ❑ Immunizations recommended for life should be up to date, especially those for children.
- ❑ Vaccines sometimes advised are: hepatitis A, rabies, tick-borne encephalitis.
- ❑ No certificate of vaccination for yellow fever is required.

Malaria Advice

- ❑ Malaria is not normally present.

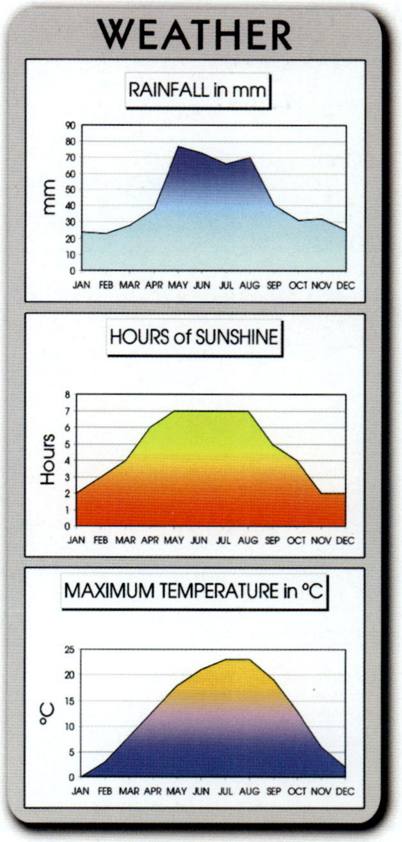

DEMOCRATIC REPUBLIC of the CONGO

General Advice

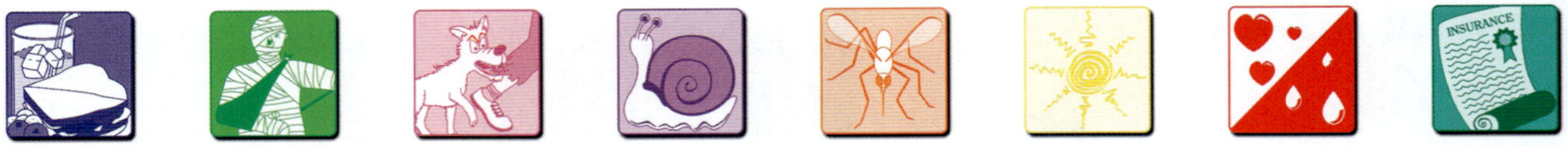

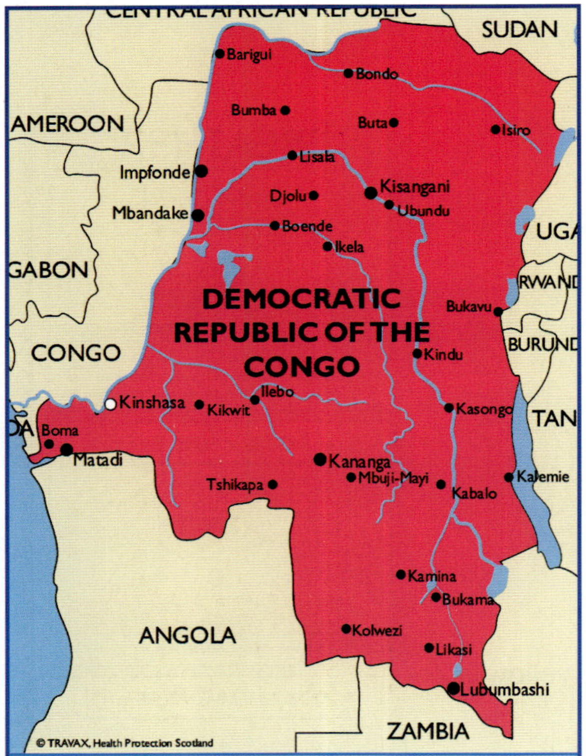

Low to no risk antimalarials not usually advised	**Variable risk** antimalarials usually advised	**High risk** antimalarials usually advised	Surrounding countries with malaria risk

This map is only intended as a guide since mosquitoes do not respect boundaries and the risk areas shown may not be exact. **Reproduced with permission from Fitfortravel, Health Protection Scotland's Travel website www.fitfortravel.nhs.uk.**

Immunization Advice

- ❑ Immunizations recommended for life should be up to date, especially those for children and boosters of tetanus for adults.
- ❑ Courses or boosters of diphtheria, hepatitis A, poliomyelitis, typhoid, and yellow fever are usually advised.
- ❑ Vaccines sometimes advised are: BCG, cholera, hepatitis B, meningococcal A and C, and rabies.
- ❑ A yellow fever certificate is required for all travelers aged over 1 year.

Malaria Advice

- ❑ Malaria is a serious and sometimes fatal disease transmitted by mosquitoes. You cannot be vaccinated against malaria.

MALARIA PRECAUTIONS

- ❑ Malaria precautions are essential in all areas all year round. Avoid mosquito bites by covering up with clothing such as long sleeves and long trousers especially after sunset, using insect repellents on exposed skin and, when necessary, sleeping under a mosquito net.
- ❑ Check with your doctor or nurse about suitable antimalarial tablets.
- ❑ Prompt investigation of fever is essential.

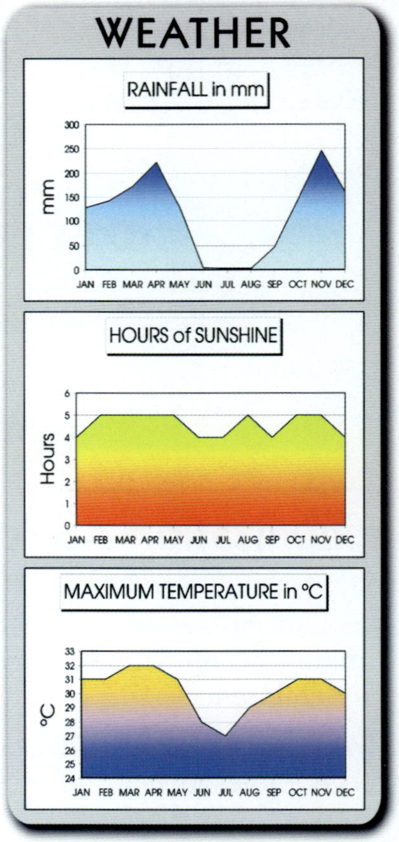

DOMINICA

General Advice

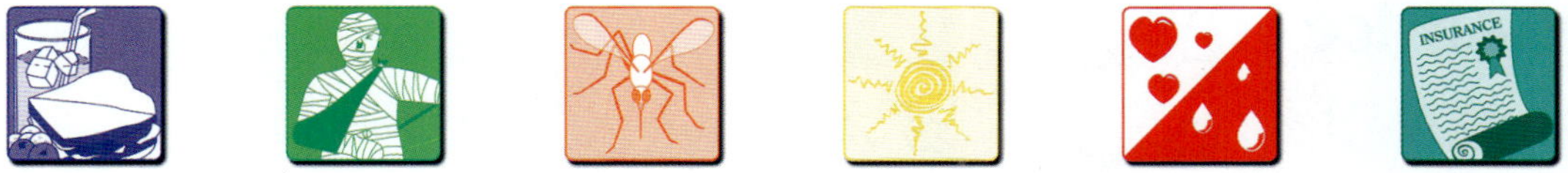

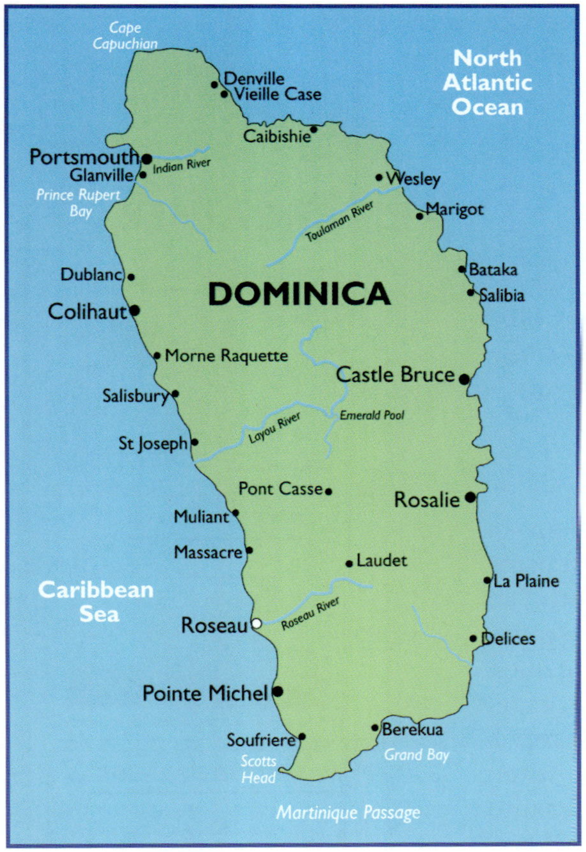

Immunization Advice

❑ Immunizations recommended for life should be up to date, especially those for children and boosters of tetanus for adults.

❑ Vaccines sometimes advised are: hepatitis A, hepatitis B.

❑ A yellow fever certificate is required for all travelers aged over 1 year.

Malaria Advice

❑ Malaria is not normally present.

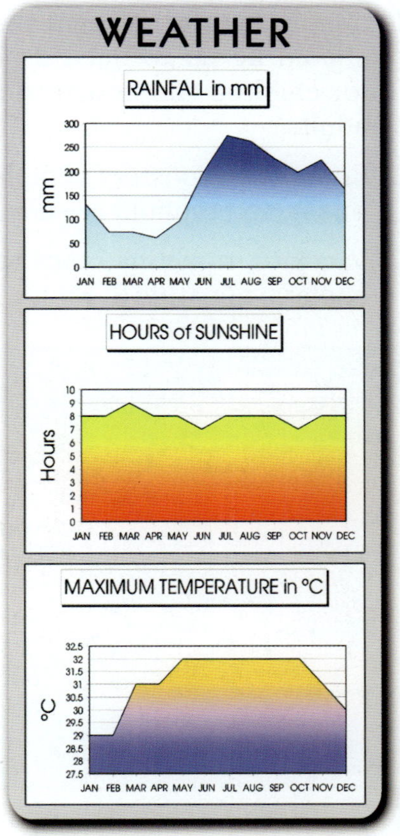

DOMINICAN REPUBLIC

General Advice

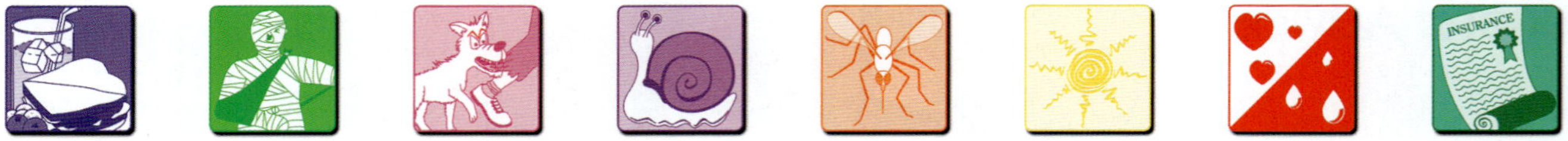

Immunization Advice

- ❑ Immunizations recommended for life should be up to date, especially those for children and boosters of tetanus for adults.
- ❑ Courses or boosters of diphtheria, hepatitis A, and typhoid are usually advised.
- ❑ Vaccines sometimes advised are: BCG, cholera, hepatitis B, rabies.
- ❑ No certificate of vaccination for yellow fever is required.

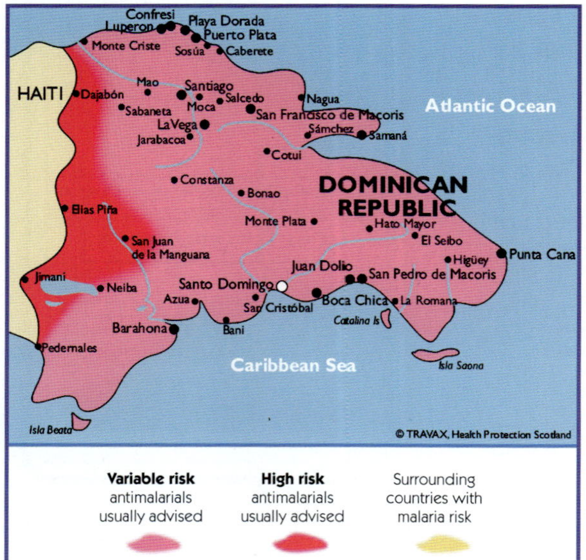

This map is only intended as a guide since mosquitoes do not respect boundaries and the risk areas shown may not be exact. **Reproduced with permission from Fitfortravel, Health Protection Scotland's Travel website www.fitfortravel.nhs.uk.**

Malaria Advice

- ❑ Malaria is a serious and sometimes fatal disease transmitted by mosquitoes. You cannot be vaccinated against malaria.

MALARIA PRECAUTIONS

- ❑ Malaria precautions are essential in all areas but risk is highest in western provinces of Dajabon, Elias Pina and San Juan, all year round. Avoid mosquito bites by covering up with clothing such as long sleeves and long trousers especially after sunset, using insect repellents on exposed skin and, when necessary, sleeping under a mosquito net.
- ❑ Check with your doctor or nurse about suitable antimalarial tablets.
- ❑ Prompt investigation of fever is essential.

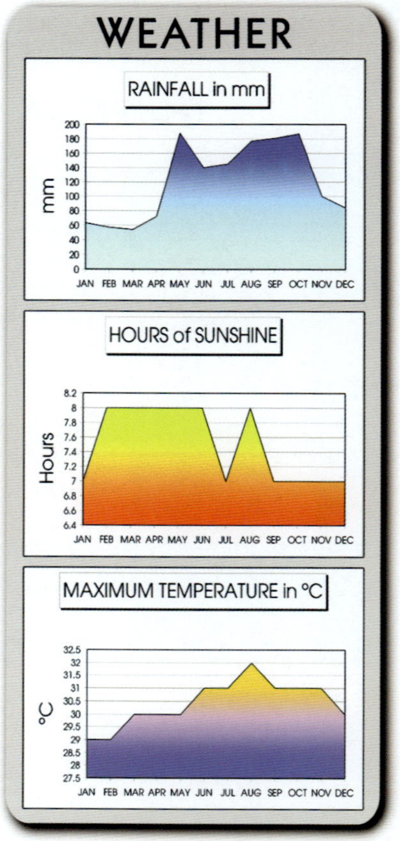

ECUADOR

General Advice

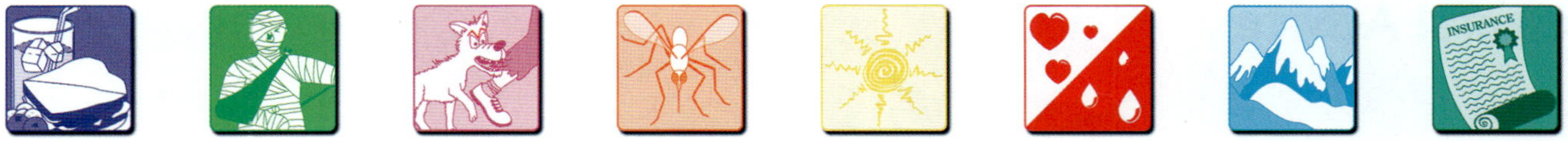

Immunization Advice

- ❑ Immunizations recommended for life should be up to date, especially those for children and boosters of tetanus for adults.
- ❑ Courses or boosters of hepatitis A and typhoid are usually advised.
- ❑ Vaccines sometimes advised are: BCG, hepatitis B, rabies, yellow fever (see yellow fever map).
- ❑ A yellow fever certificate is required if aged over 1 year old and entering from an infected country.
- ❑ Check with your doctor or nurse about suitable anti-malarial tablets.
- ❑ Prompt investigation of fever is essential.

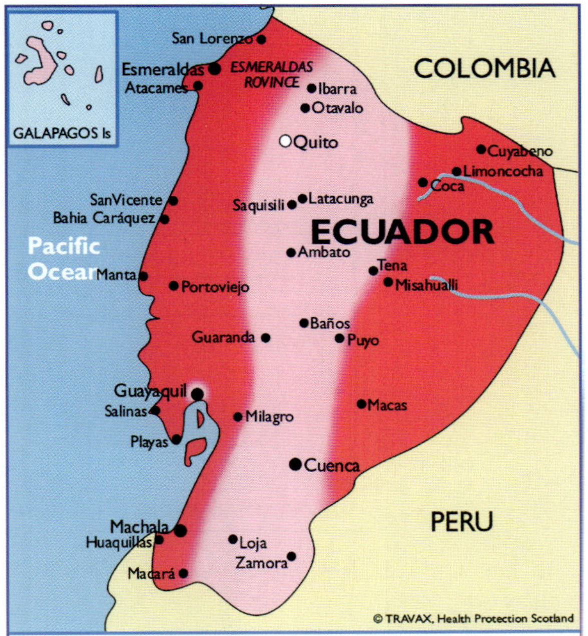

Low to no risk antimalarials not usually advised	**High risk** antimalarials usually advised	Surrounding countries with malaria risk

This map is only intended as a guide since mosquitoes do not respect boundaries and the risk areas shown may not be exact. **Reproduced with permission from Fitfortravel, Health Protection Scotland's Travel website www.fitfortravel.nhs.uk.**

Malaria Advice

- ❑ Malaria is a serious and sometimes fatal disease transmitted by mosquitoes. You cannot be vaccinated against malaria.

MALARIA PRECAUTIONS

- ❑ Malaria precautions are essential in most areas below 1500 m (see map), all year round. There is moderate risk in coastal provinces. There is no risk in Guayanquil, Quito, other cities in the inter-Andean region and the Galapagos islands. Avoid mosquito bites by covering up with clothing such as long sleeves and long trousers especially after sunset, using insect repellents on exposed skin and, when necessary, sleeping under a mosquito net.

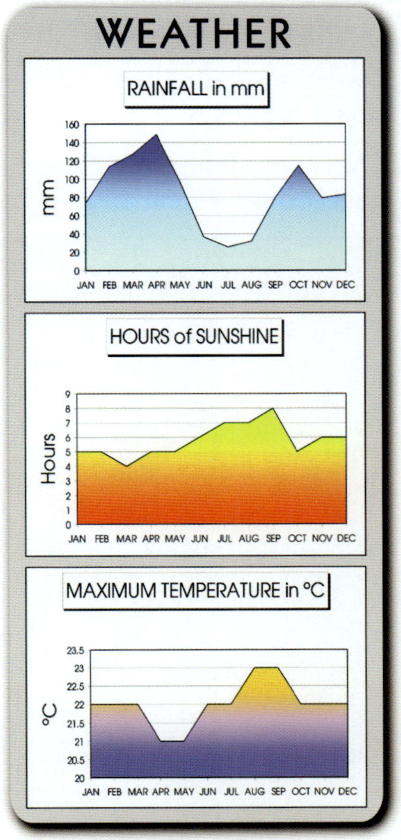

EGYPT

General Advice

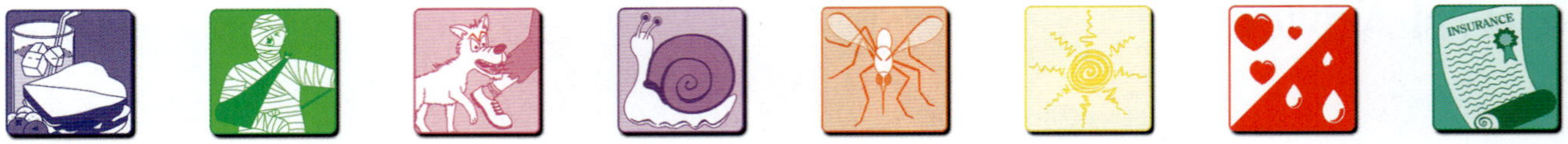

Immunization Advice

- ❑ Immunizations recommended for life should be up to date, especially those for children and boosters of tetanus for adults.
- ❑ Courses or boosters of hepatitis A and typhoid are usually advised.
- ❑ Vaccines sometimes advised are: hepatitis B, rabies.
- ❑ A yellow fever certificate is required if aged over 1 year old and entering from an infected country (Egypt may consider some additional countries to be yellow fever infected; check with an online resource).

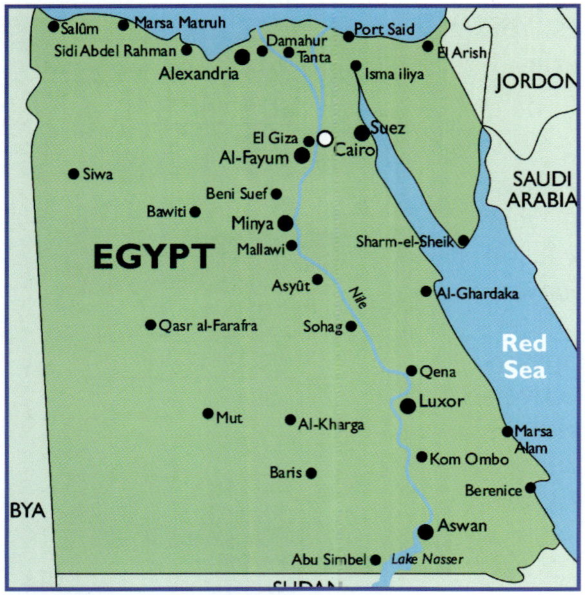

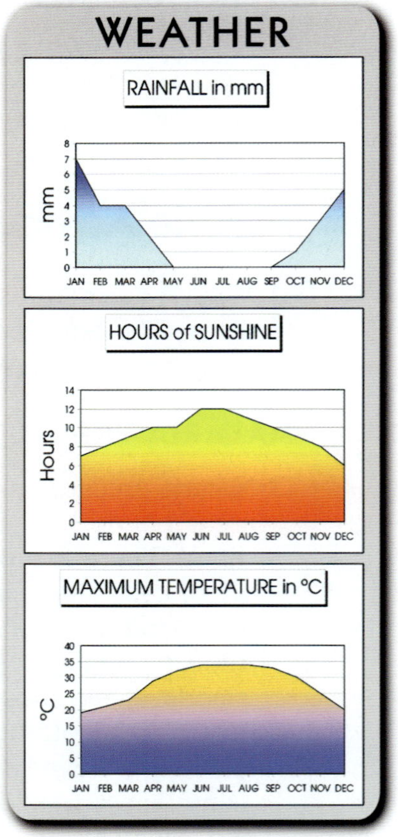

—Weather in Cairo—

Malaria Advice

- ❑ Malaria is not normally present.

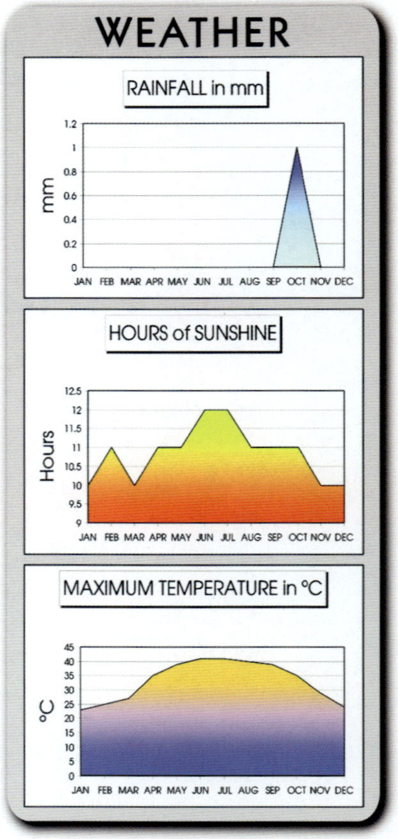

—Weather in Luxor—

ETHIOPIA

General Advice

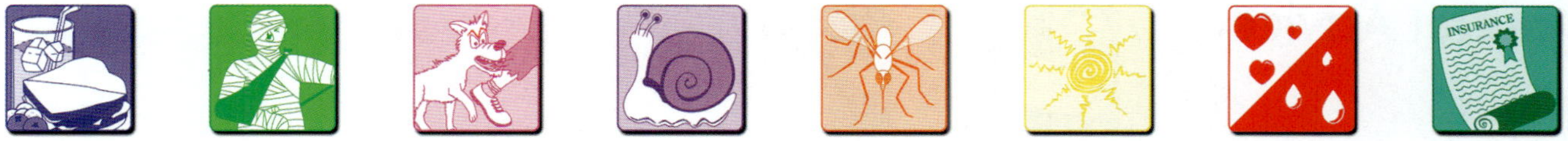

Immunization Advice

- ❑ Immunizations recommended for life should be up to date, especially those for children and boosters of tetanus for adults.
- ❑ Courses or boosters of diphtheria, hepatitis A, and typhoid are usually advised.
- ❑ Vaccines sometimes advised are: BCG, cholera, hepatitis B, meningococcal A and C, rabies, yellow fever (see yellow fever map).
- ❑ A yellow fever certificate is required if aged over 1 year old and entering from an infected country.

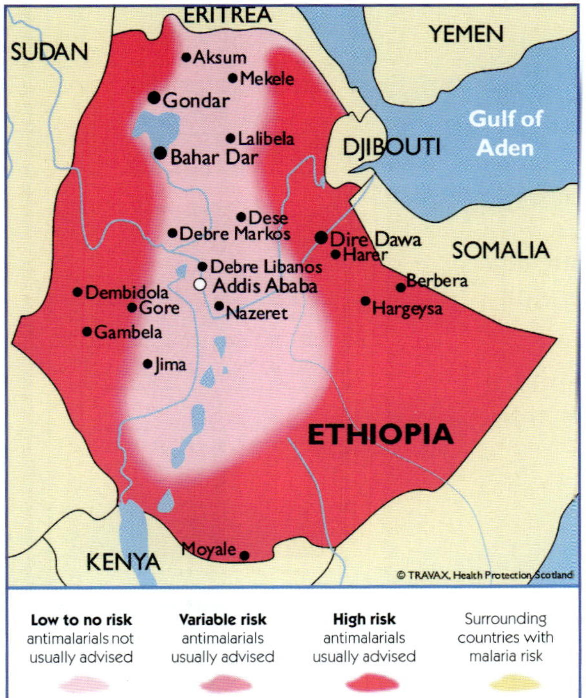

This map is only intended as a guide since mosquitoes do not respect boundaries and the risk areas shown may not be exact. **Reproduced with permission from Fitfortravel, Health Protection Scotland's Travel website www.fitfortravel.nhs.uk.**

Malaria Advice

- ❑ Malaria is a serious and sometimes fatal disease transmitted by mosquitoes. You cannot be vaccinated against malaria.

MALARIA PRECAUTIONS

- ❑ Malaria precautions are essential in all areas below 2000 m all year round. There is normally no risk in Addis Ababa. Avoid mosquito bites by covering up with clothing such as long sleeves and long trousers especially after sunset, using insect repellents on exposed skin and, when necessary, sleeping under a mosquito net.
- ❑ Check with your doctor or nurse about suitable anti-malarial tablets.
- ❑ Prompt investigation of fever is essential.

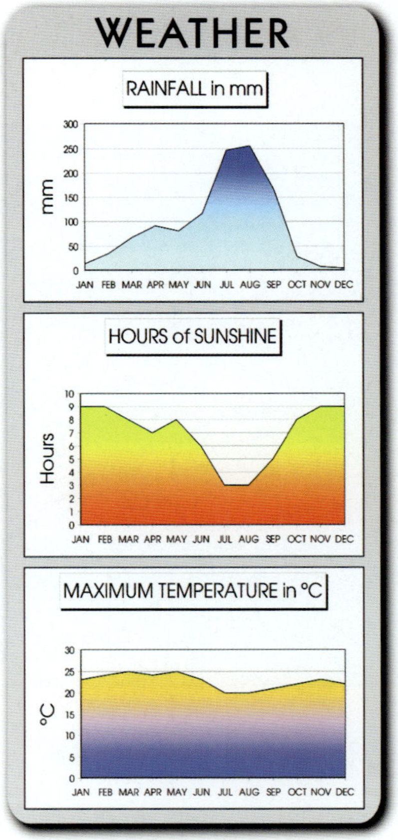

FIJI

General Advice

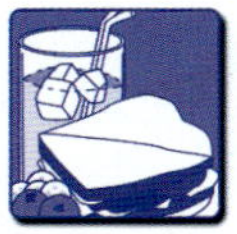
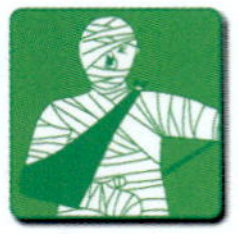
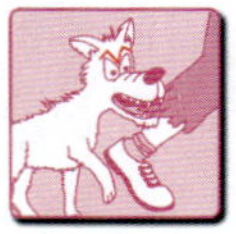
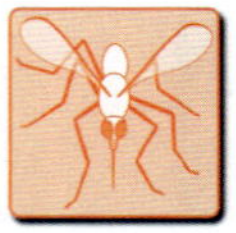
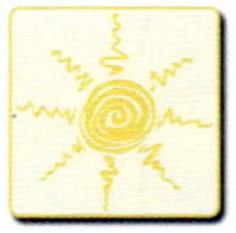

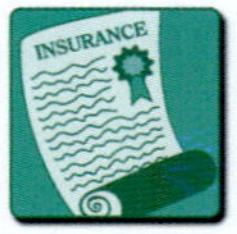

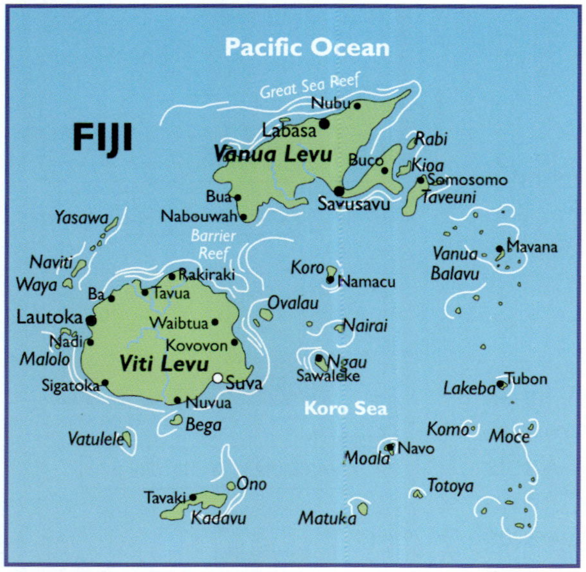

Immunization Advice

- ❑ Immunizations recommended for life should be up to date, especially those for children and boosters of tetanus for adults.
- ❑ Courses or boosters of hepatitis A are usually advised.
- ❑ Vaccines sometimes advised are: hepatitis B, typhoid.
- ❑ Rabies is not normally present but any animal or bat bite must be carefully assessed.
- ❑ A yellow fever certificate is required if aged over 1 year old and entering from an infected country.

Malaria Advice

- ❑ Malaria is not normally present.

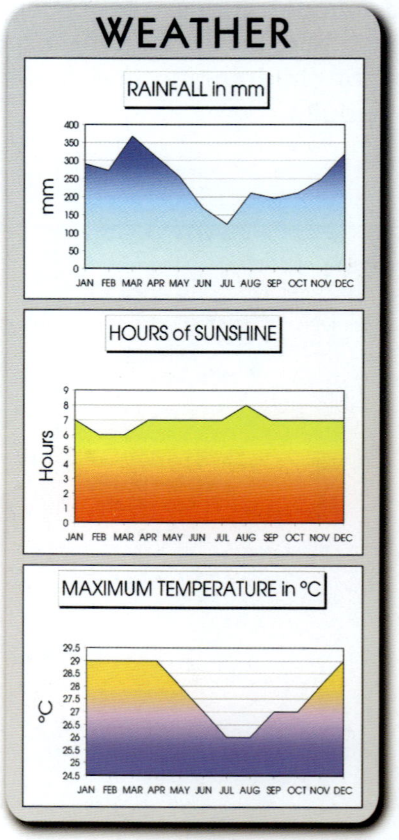

FINLAND

General Advice

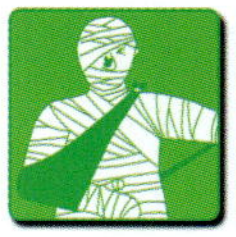
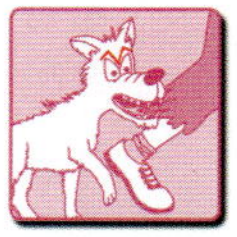

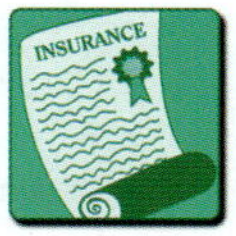

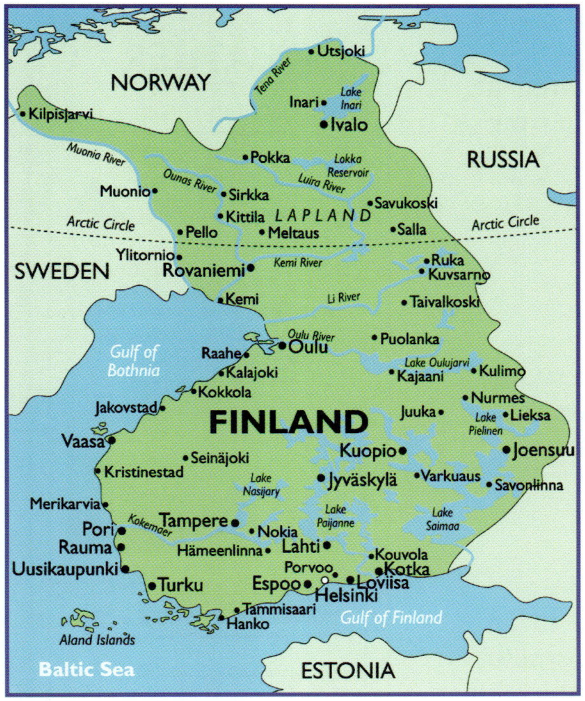

Immunization Advice

- ❑ Immunizations recommended for life should be up to date, especially those for children.
- ❑ Vaccines sometimes advised are: hepatitis B, rabies, tick-borne encephalitis.
- ❑ No certificate of vaccination for yellow fever is required.

Malaria Advice

- ❑ Malaria is not normally present.

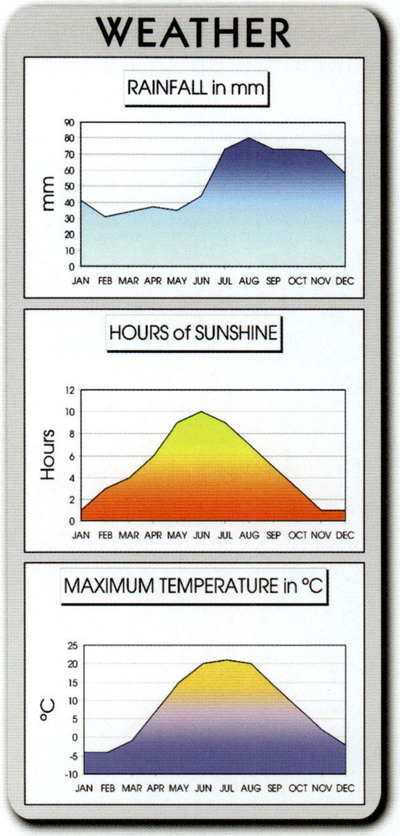

GABON

General Advice

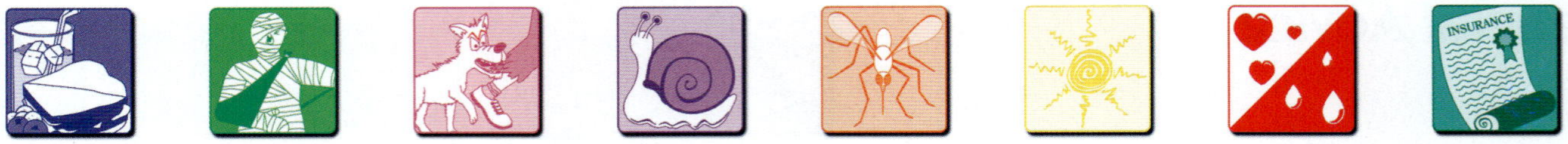

Immunization Advice

- ❑ Immunizations recommended for life should be up to date, especially those for children and boosters of tetanus for adults.
- ❑ Courses or boosters of diphtheria, hepatitis A, typhoid, and yellow fever are usually advised.
- ❑ Vaccines sometimes advised are: BCG, cholera, hepatitis B, rabies.
- ❑ A yellow fever certificate is required if aged over 1 year old and entering from an infected country.

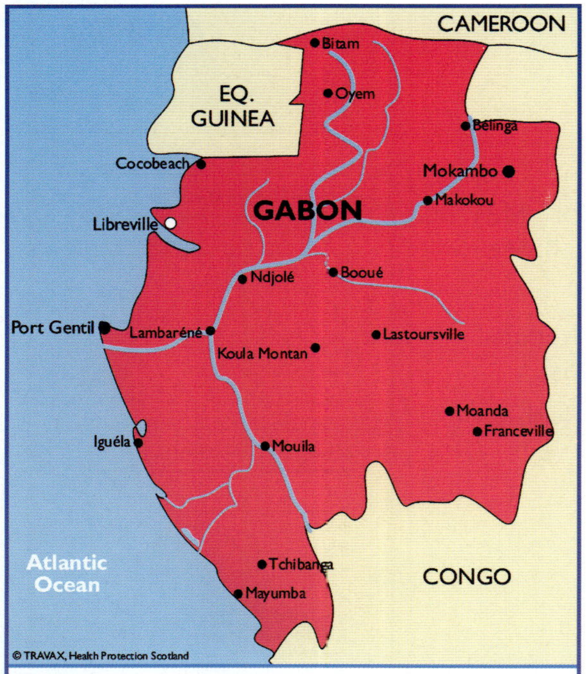

This map is only intended as a guide since mosquitoes do not respect boundaries and the risk areas shown may not be exact. **Reproduced with permission from Fitfortravel, Health Protection Scotland's Travel website www.fitfortravel.nhs.uk.**

Malaria Advice

- ❑ Malaria is a serious and sometimes fatal disease transmitted by mosquitoes. You cannot be vaccinated against malaria.

MALARIA PRECAUTIONS

- ❑ Malaria precautions are essential in all areas all year round. Avoid mosquito bites by covering up with clothing such as long sleeves and long trousers especially after sunset, using insect repellents on exposed skin and, when necessary, sleeping under a mosquito net.
- ❑ Check with your doctor or nurse about suitable antimalarial tablets.
- ❑ Prompt investigation of fever is essential.

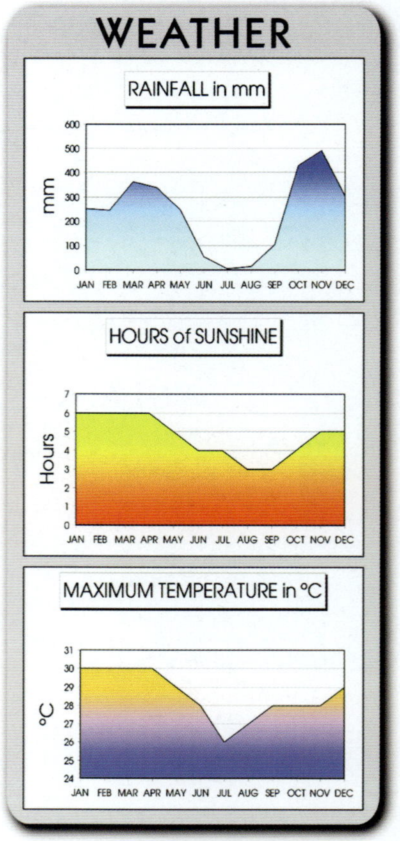

GAMBIA

General Advice

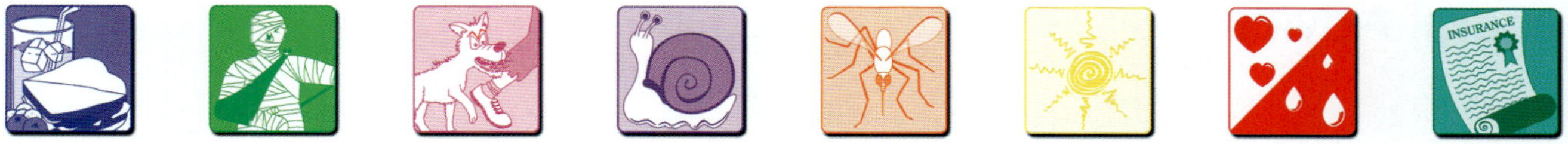

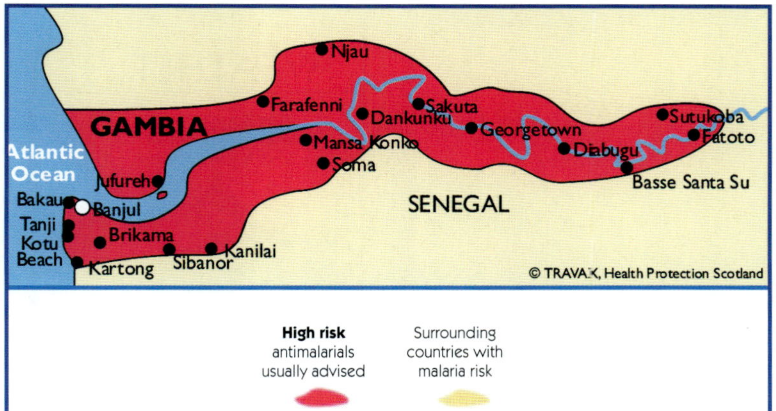

This map is only intended as a guide since mosquitoes do not respect boundaries and the risk areas shown may not be exact. **Reproduced with permission from Fitfortravel, Health Protection Scotland's Travel website www.fitfortravel.nhs.uk.**

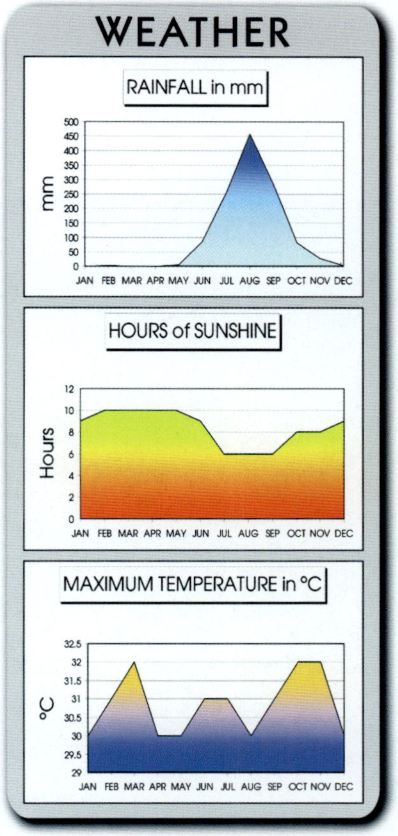

Immunization Advice

- ❑ Immunizations recommended for life should be up to date, especially those for children and boosters of tetanus for adults.
- ❑ Courses or boosters of diphtheria, hepatitis A, typhoid, and yellow fever are usually advised.
- ❑ Vaccines sometimes advised are: BCG, cholera, hepatitis B, meningococcal A and C, and rabies.
- ❑ A yellow fever certificate is required if aged over 1 year old and entering from an infected country.

Malaria Advice

- ❑ Malaria is a serious and sometimes fatal disease transmitted by mosquitoes. You cannot be vaccinated against malaria.

MALARIA PRECAUTIONS

- ❑ Malaria precautions are essential in all areas all year round with peak cases from July to September. Avoid mosquito bites by covering up with clothing such as long sleeves and long trousers especially after sunset, using insect repellents on exposed skin and, when necessary, sleeping under a mosquito net.
- ❑ Check with your doctor or nurse about suitable antimalarial tablets.
- ❑ Prompt investigation of fever is essential.

GERMANY

General Advice

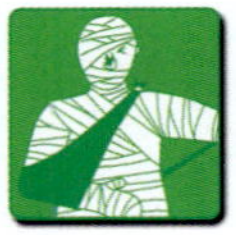
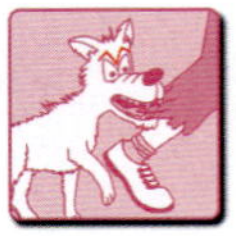

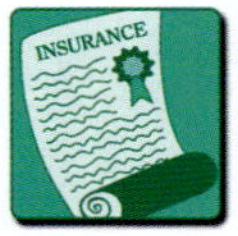

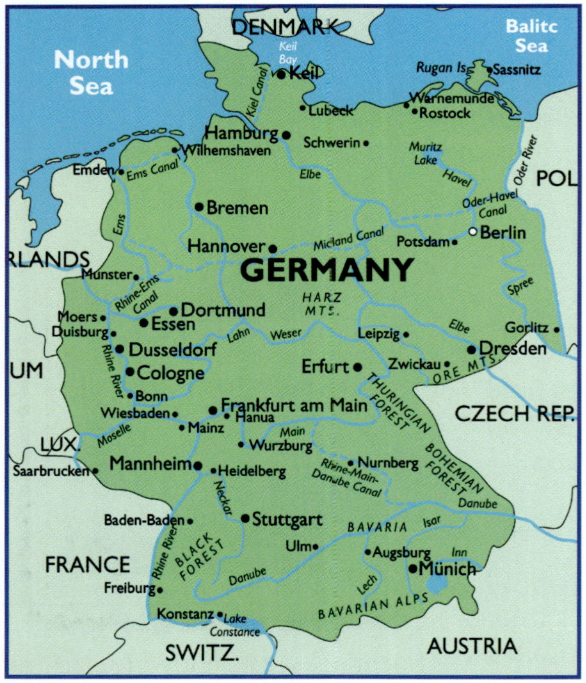

Immunization Advice

- ❑ Immunizations recommended for life should be up to date, especially those for children.
- ❑ Vaccines sometimes advised are: hepatitis B, rabies, tick-borne encephalitis.
- ❑ No certificate of vaccination for yellow fever is required.

Malaria Advice

- ❑ Malaria is not normally present.

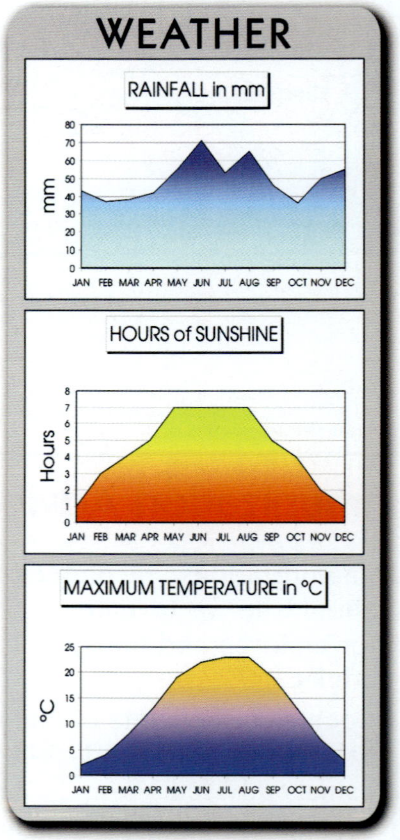

—Weather in Berlin—

GHANA

General Advice

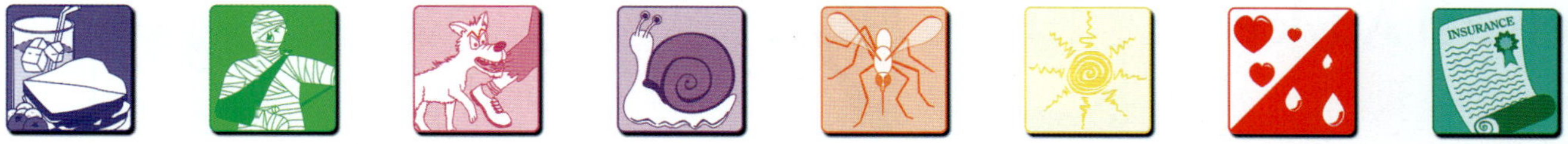

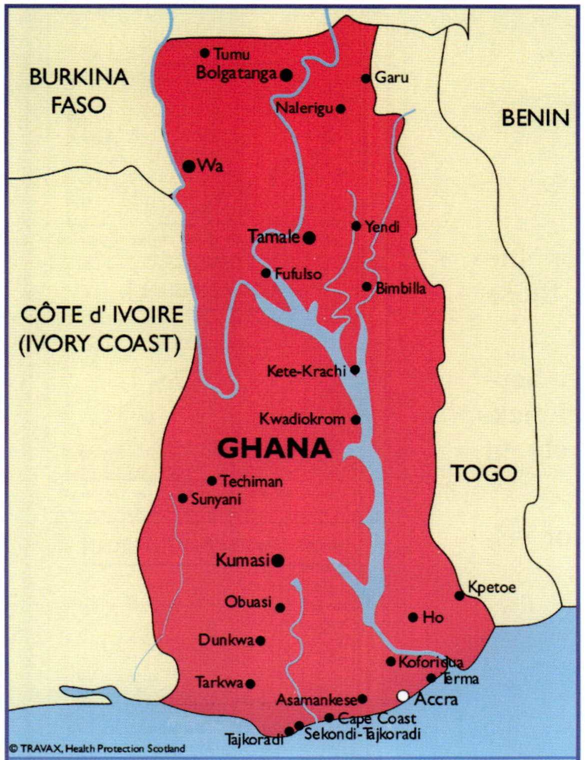

High risk antimalarials usually advised

Surrounding countries with malaria risk

This map is only intended as a guide since mosquitoes do not respect boundaries and the risk areas shown may not be exact. **Reproduced with permission from Fitfortravel, Health Protection Scotland's Travel website www.fitfortravel.nhs.uk.**

Immunization Advice

- ❑ Immunizations recommended for life should be up to date, especially those for children and boosters of tetanus for adults.
- ❑ Courses or boosters of diphtheria, hepatitis A, typhoid, and yellow fever are usually advised.
- ❑ Vaccines sometimes advised are: BCG, cholera, hepatitis B, meningococcal A and C, and rabies.
- ❑ A yellow fever certificate is required from all travelers aged over 9 months old.

Malaria Advice

- ❑ Malaria is a serious and sometimes fatal disease transmitted by mosquitoes. You cannot be vaccinated against malaria.

MALARIA PRECAUTIONS

- ❑ Malaria precautions are essential in all areas all year round. Avoid mosquito bites by covering up with clothing such as long sleeves and long trousers especially after sunset, using insect repellents on exposed skin and, when necessary, sleeping under a mosquito net.
- ❑ Check with your doctor or nurse about suitable anti-malarial tablets.
- ❑ Prompt investigation of fever is essential.

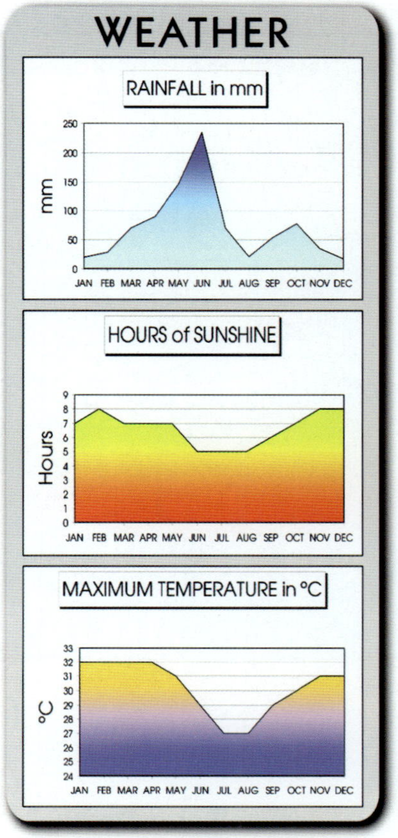

GREECE

General Advice

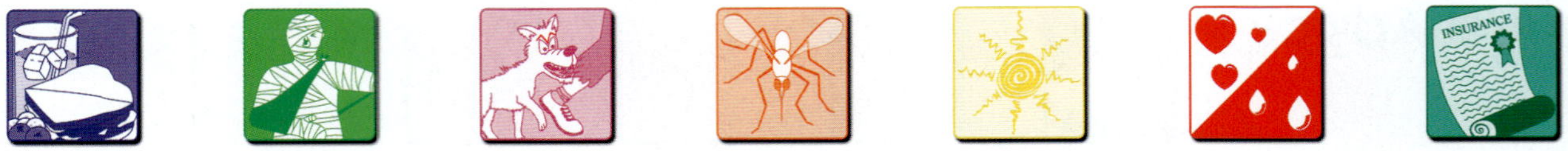

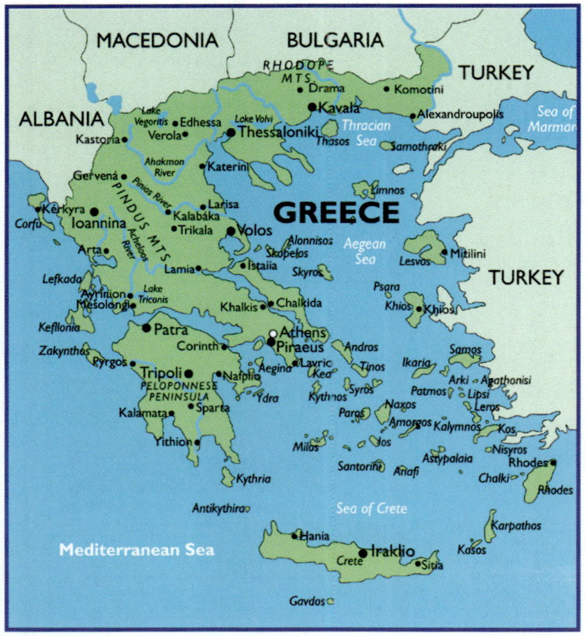

Immunization Advice

- ❑ Immunizations recommended for life should be up to date, especially those for children.
- ❑ Vaccines sometimes advised are: hepatitis A, hepatitis B, rabies, and tick-borne encephalitis which is rarely in Thessaloniki.
- ❑ No certificate of vaccination for for yellow fever is required.

Malaria Advice

- ❑ Malaria is not normally present.

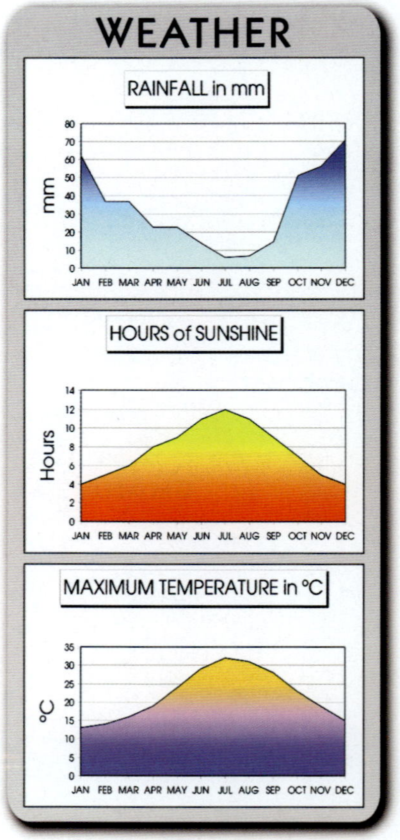

GRENADA

General Advice

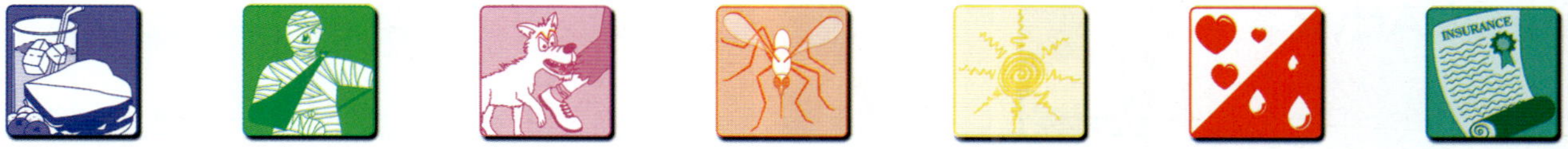

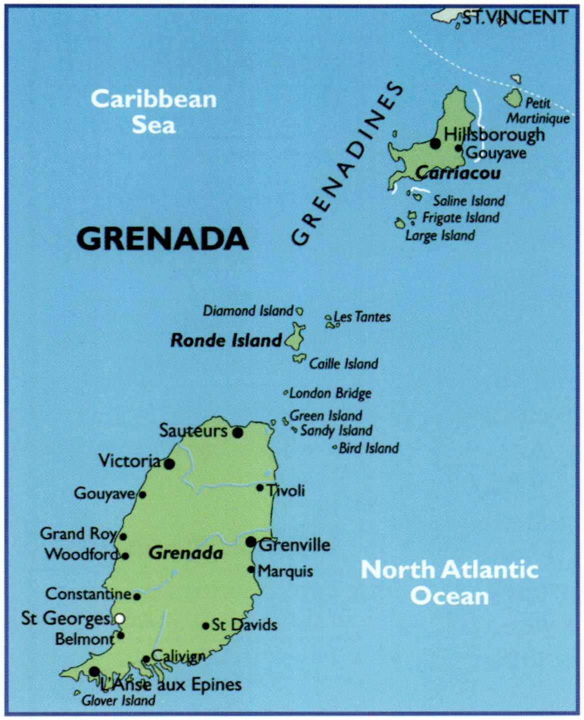

Immunization Advice

- ❑ Immunizations recommended for life should be up to date, especially those for children and boosters of tetanus for adults.
- ❑ Vaccines sometimes advised are: hepatitis A, hepatitis B, rabies.
- ❑ A yellow fever certificate is required if aged over 1 year old and entering from an infected country.

Malaria Advice

- ❑ Malaria is not normally present.

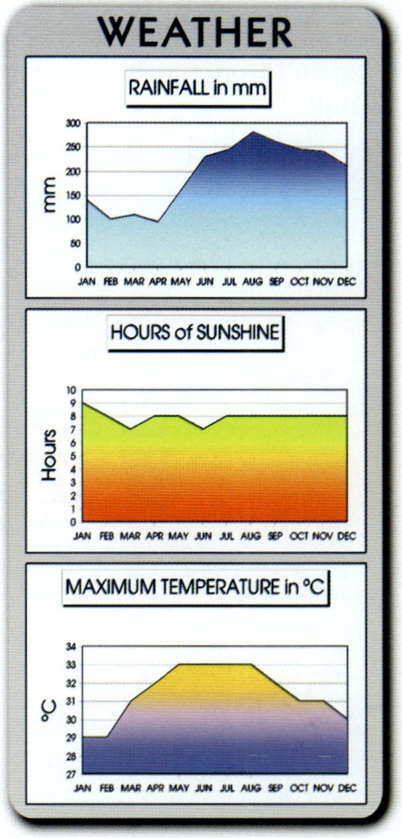

GUATEMALA

General Advice

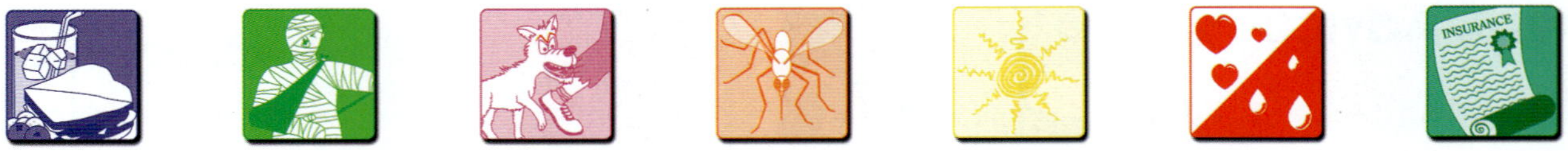

Immunization Advice

- ❑ Immunizations recommended for life should be up to date, especially those for children and boosters of tetanus for adults.
- ❑ Courses or boosters of hepatitis A are usually advised.
- ❑ Vaccines sometimes advised are: BCG, hepatitis B, rabies, typhoid.
- ❑ A yellow fever certificate is required if aged over 1 year old and entering from an infected country.

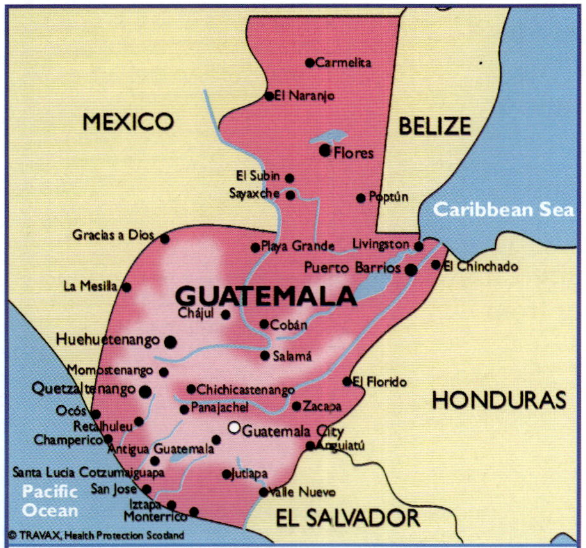

Low to no risk antimalarials not usually advised	**Variable risk** antimalarials usually advised	Surrounding countries with malaria risk

This map is only intended as a guide since mosquitoes do not respect boundaries and the risk areas shown may not be exact. **Reproduced with permission from Fitfortravel, Health Protection Scotland's Travel website www.fitfortravel.nhs.uk.**

Malaria Advice

- ❑ Malaria is a serious and sometimes fatal disease transmitted by mosquitoes. You cannot be vaccinated against malaria.

MALARIA PRECAUTIONS

- ❑ Malaria precautions are essential in most areas below 1500m all year round. Risk is minimal in Guatemala City, Antigua and lake Atitlan. Avoid mosquito bites by covering up with clothing such as long sleeves and long trousers especially after sunset, using insect repellents on exposed skin and, when necessary, sleeping under a mosquito net.
- ❑ Check with your doctor or nurse about suitable antimalarial tablets.
- ❑ Prompt investigation of fever is essential.

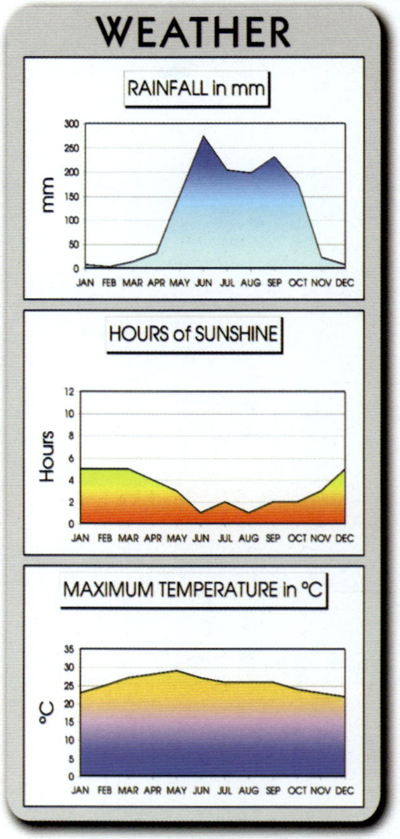

GUYANA

General Advice

Immunization Advice

- ❑ Immunizations recommended for life should be up to date, especially those for children and boosters of tetanus for adults.
- ❑ Courses or boosters of hepatitis A and yellow fever are usually advised.
- ❑ Vaccines sometimes advised are: BCG, hepatitis B, rabies, typhoid.
- ❑ A yellow fever certificate is required if entering from an infected country except Argentina, Paraguay, Suriname, and Trinidad and Tobago.

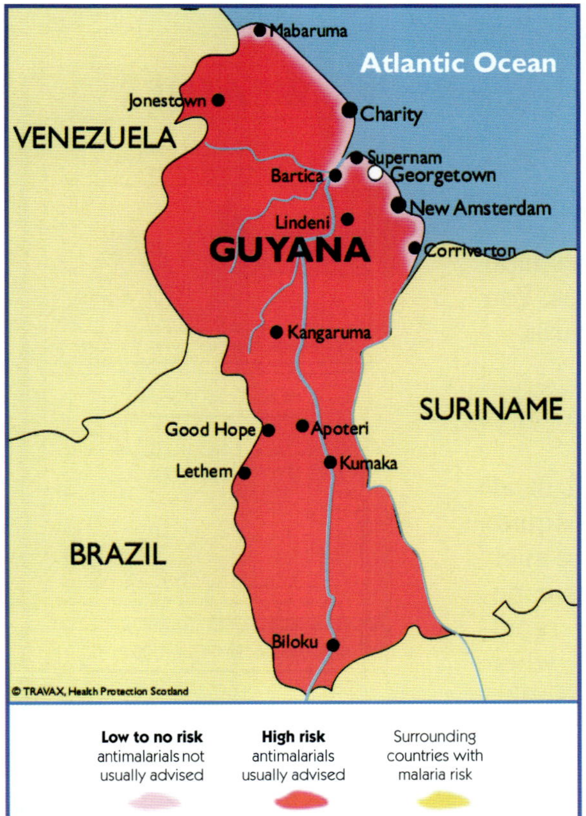

This map is only intended as a guide since mosquitoes do not respect boundaries and the risk areas shown may not be exact. **Reproduced with permission from Fitfortravel, Health Protection Scotland's Travel website www.fitfortravel.nhs.uk.**

Malaria Advice

- ❑ Malaria is a serious and sometimes fatal disease transmitted by mosquitoes. You cannot be vaccinated against malaria.

MALARIA PRECAUTIONS

- ❑ Malaria precautions are essential especially in rural interior areas, all year round. Risk is minimal along coastal areas including Georgetown. Avoid mosquito bites by covering up with clothing such as long sleeves and long trousers especially after sunset, using insect repellents on exposed skin and, when necessary, sleeping under a mosquito net.
- ❑ Check with your doctor or nurse about suitable antimalarial tablets.
- ❑ Prompt investigation of fever is essential.

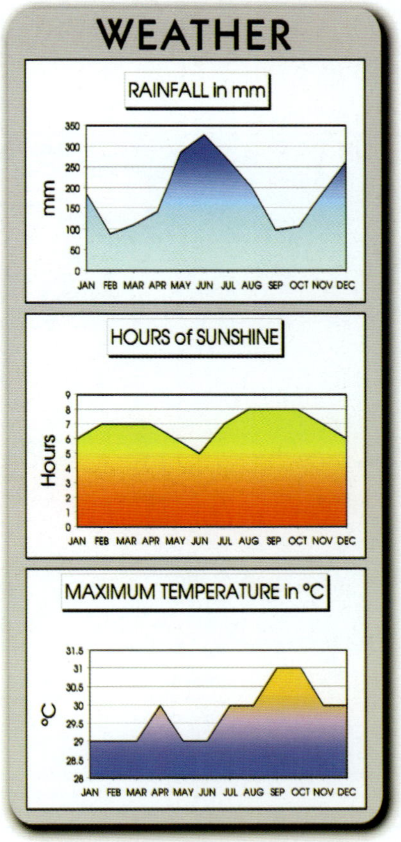

HAITI

General Advice

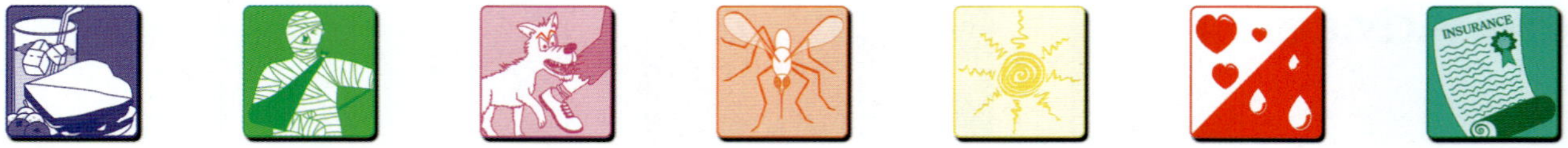

Immunization Advice

❑ Immunizations recommended for life should be up to date, especially those for children and boosters of tetanus for adults.

❑ Courses or boosters of diphtheria, hepatitis A, and typhoid are usually advised.

❑ Vaccines sometimes advised are: BCG, cholera, hepatitis B, rabies.

❑ A yellow fever certificate is required if entering from an infected country.

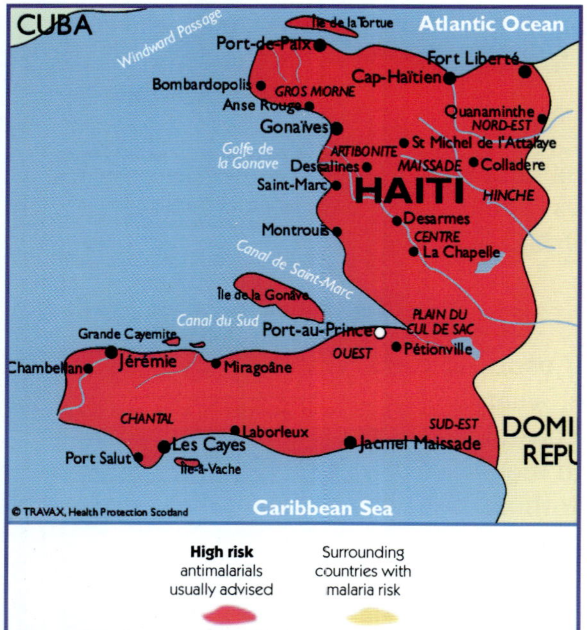

This map is only intended as a guide since mosquitoes do not respect boundaries and the risk areas shown may not be exact. **Reproduced with permission from Fitfortravel, Health Protection Scotland's Travel website www.fitfortravel.nhs.uk.**

Malaria Advice

❑ Malaria is a serious and sometimes fatal disease transmitted by mosquitoes. You cannot be vaccinated against malaria.

MALARIA PRECAUTIONS

❑ Malaria precautions are essential in all areas, all year round. Avoid mosquito bites by covering up with clothing such as long sleeves and long trousers especially after sunset, using insect repellents on exposed skin and, when necessary, sleeping under a mosquito net.

❑ Check with your doctor or nurse about suitable antimalarial tablets.

❑ Prompt investigation of fever is essential.

WEATHER

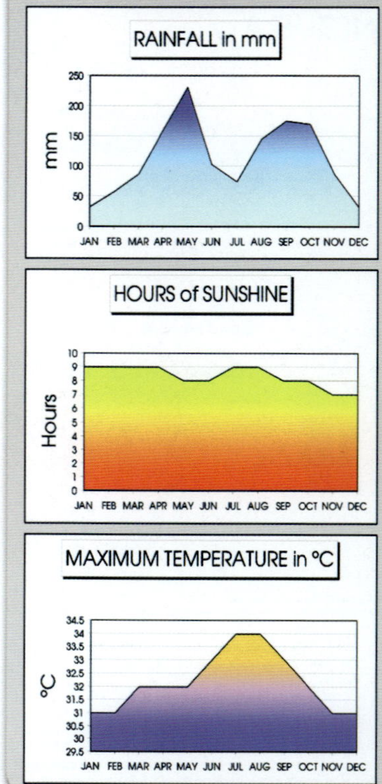

HONDURAS

General Advice

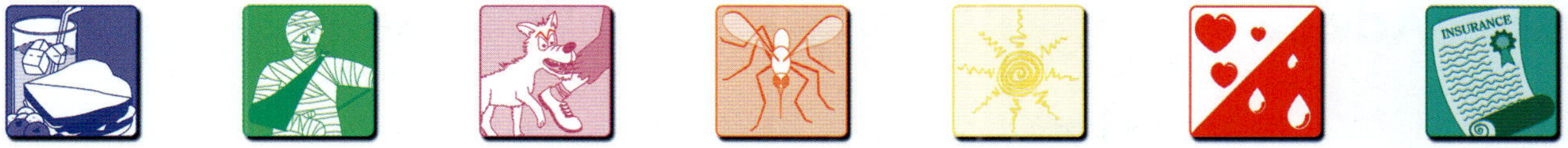

Immunization Advice

- ❑ Immunizations recommended for life should be up to date, especially those for children and boosters of tetanus for adults.
- ❑ Courses or boosters of hepatitis A and typhoid are usually advised.
- ❑ Vaccines sometimes advised are: BCG, hepatitis B, rabies.

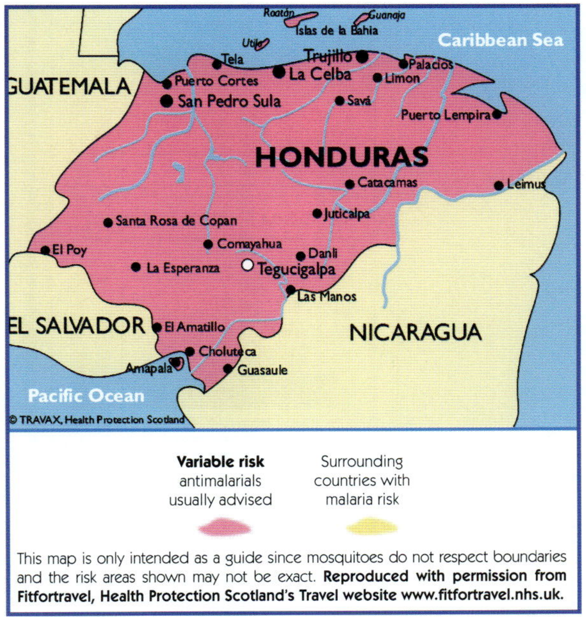

- ❑ A yellow fever certificate is required if aged over 1 year old and entering from an infected country.

Malaria Advice

- ❑ Malaria is a serious and sometimes fatal disease transmitted by mosquitoes. You cannot be vaccinated against malaria.

MALARIA PRECAUTIONS

- ❑ Malaria precautions are essential in all areas, all year round. Risk is highest in Colon and Gracias a Dios Departments and is moderate in Atlantida and Olancho. Avoid mosquito bites by covering up with clothing such as long sleeves and long trousers especially after sunset, using insect repellents on exposed skin and, when necessary, sleeping under a mosquito net.
- ❑ Check with your doctor or nurse about suitable antimalarial tablets.
- ❑ Prompt investigation of fever is essential.

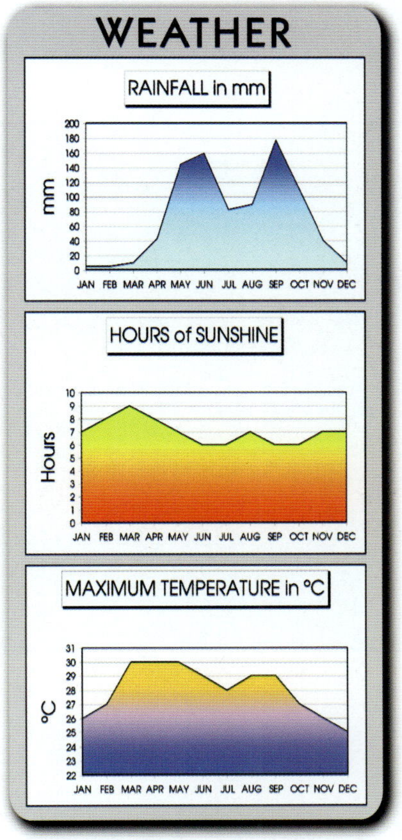

HONG KONG

General Advice

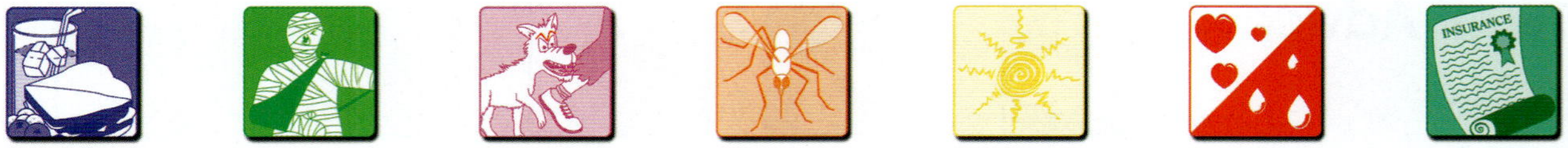

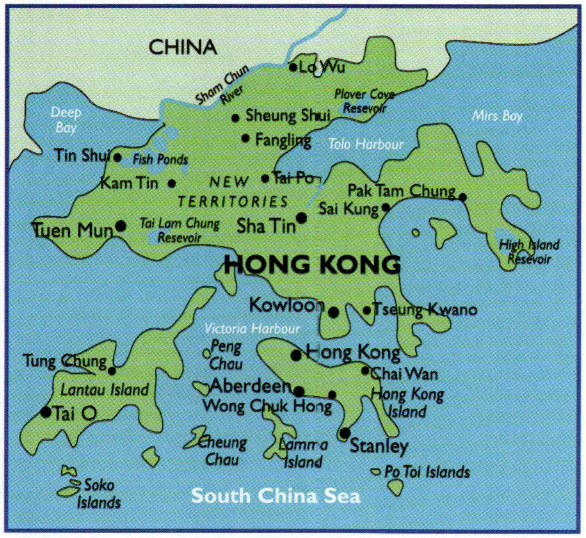

Immunization Advice

- ❑ Immunizations recommended for life should be up to date, especially those for children and boosters of tetanus for adults.
- ❑ Vaccines sometimes advised are: BCG, hepatitis A, hepatitis B, rabies.
- ❑ No certificate of vaccination for yellow fever is required.

Malaria Advice

- ❑ Malaria is not normally present.

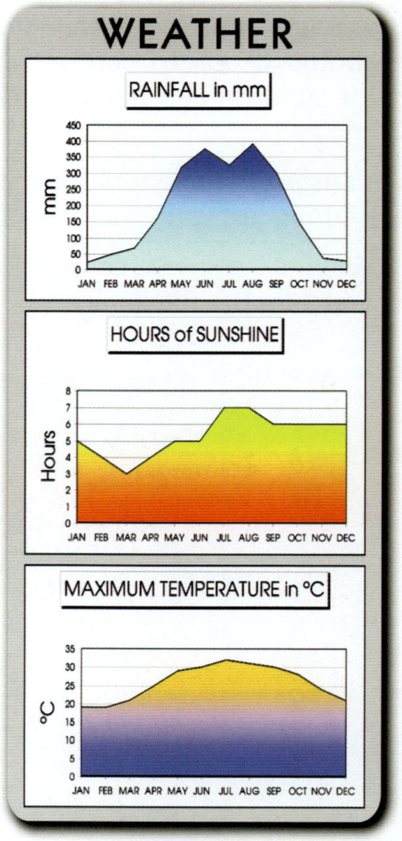

INDIA

General Advice

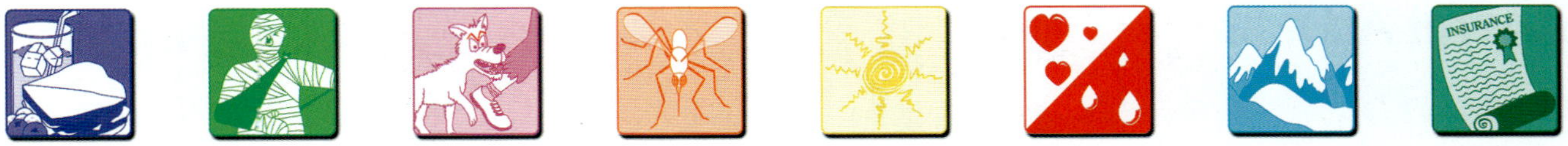

Immunization Advice

- ❑ Immunizations recommended for life should be up to date, especially those for children and boosters of tetanus for adults.
- ❑ Courses or boosters of diphtheria, hepatitis A, poliomyelitis, and typhoid are usually advised.
- ❑ Vaccines sometimes advised are: BCG, cholera, hepatitis B, Japanese encephalitis, rabies.
- ❑ A yellow fever certificate is required if entering from an infected country. (India may consider additional countries to be yellow fever infected; check with an online resource).

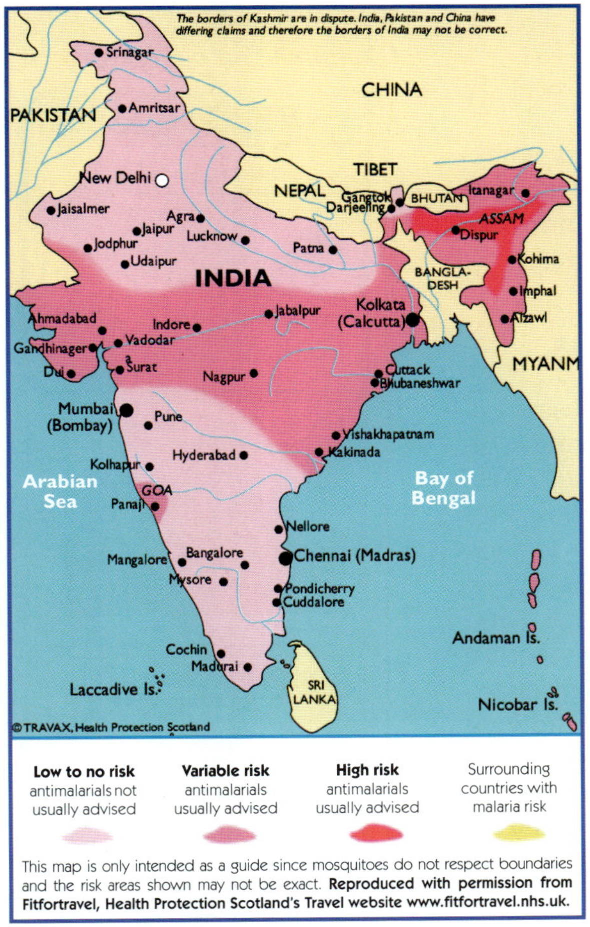

Malaria Advice

- ❑ Malaria is a serious and sometimes fatal disease transmitted by mosquitoes. You cannot be vaccinated against malaria.

MALARIA PRECAUTIONS

- ❑ Malaria precautions are essential in all areas below 2000 m all year round. The highest risk is in the eastern state of Assam. Avoid mosquito bites by covering up with clothing such as long sleeves and long trousers especially after sunset, using insect repellents on exposed skin and, when necessary, sleeping under a mosquito net.
- ❑ Check with your doctor or nurse about suitable antimalarial tablets.
- ❑ Prompt investigation of fever is essential.

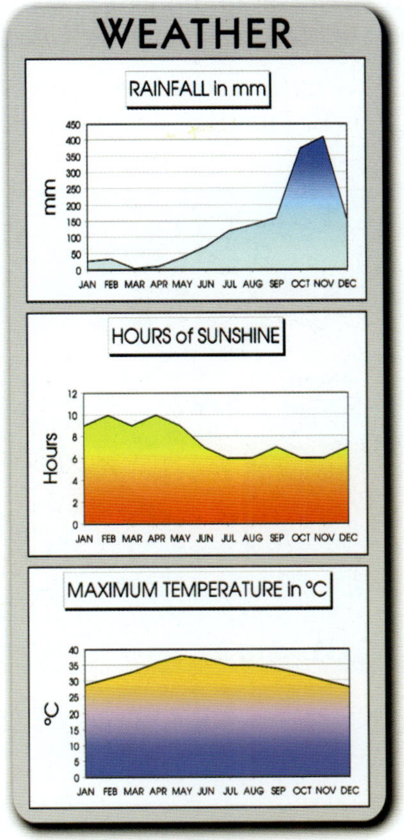

—Weather in Chennai—

INDONESIA (Bali and Lombok)

General Advice

Immunization Advice

- ❑ Immunizations recommended for life should be up to date, especially those for children and boosters of tetanus for adults.
- ❑ Courses or boosters of diphtheria, hepatitis A, and typhoid are usually advised.
- ❑ Vaccines sometimes advised are: BCG, cholera, hepatitis B, Japanese encephalitis, rabies.

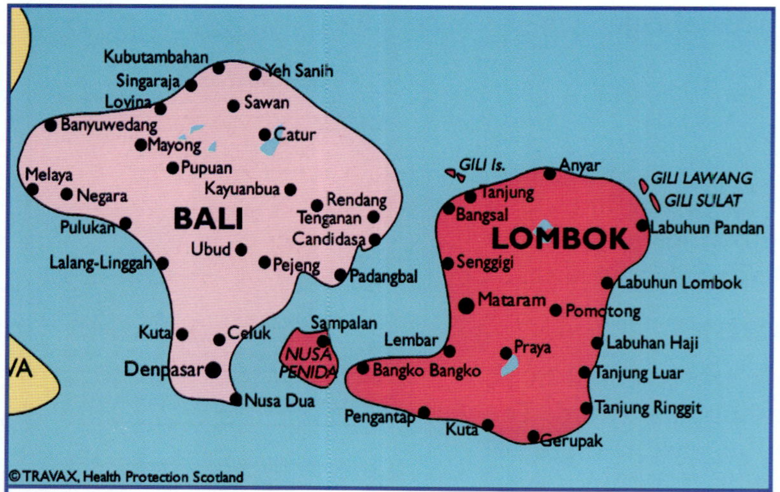

Low to no risk antimalarials not usually advised — **High risk** antimalarials usually advised — Surrounding countries with malaria risk

This map is only intended as a guide since mosquitoes do not respect boundaries and the risk areas shown may not be exact. **Reproduced with permission from Fitfortravel, Health Protection Scotland's Travel website www.fitfortravel.nhs.uk.**

- ❑ A yellow fever certificate is required if aged over 9 months old and entering from an infected country.

Malaria Advice

- ❑ Malaria is a serious and sometimes fatal disease transmitted by mosquitoes. You cannot be vaccinated against malaria.

MALARIA PRECAUTIONS

- ❑ Malaria precautions are essential in most areas all year round. The risk is minimal in all big cities and tourist resorts of Bali and Java but higher in nearby islands that may be visited on excursions including Lombok and West Papua. Avoid mosquito bites by covering up with clothing such as long sleeves and long trousers especially after sunset, using insect repellents on exposed skin and, when necessary, sleeping under a mosquito net.
- ❑ Check with your doctor or nurse about suitable antimalarial tablets.
- ❑ Prompt investigation of fever is essential.

(*Continued on next page*.)

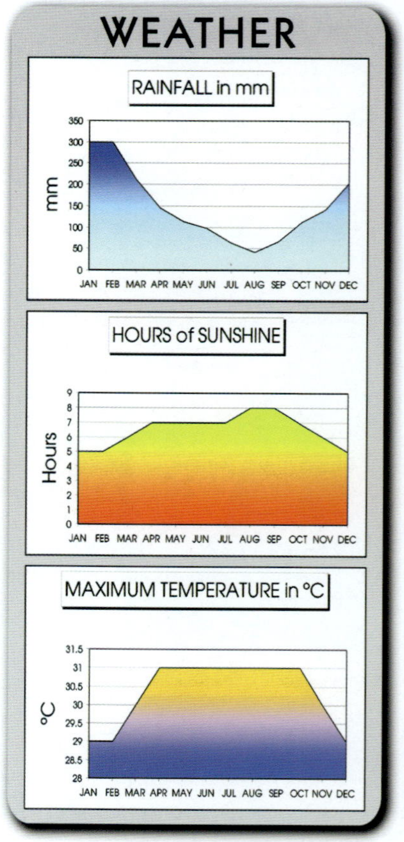

—Weather in Jakarta—

INDONESIA—con't (Kalimantan, Java, East & Sumatra)

General Advice

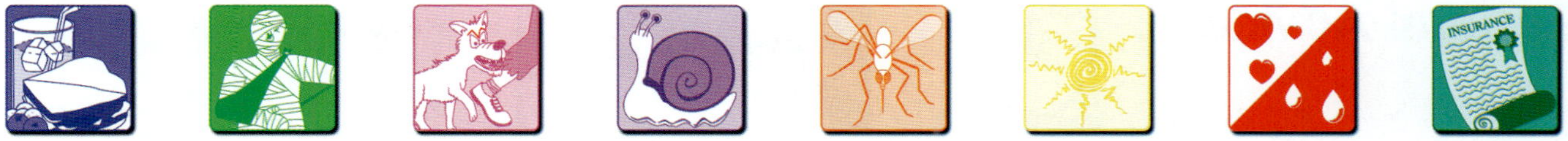

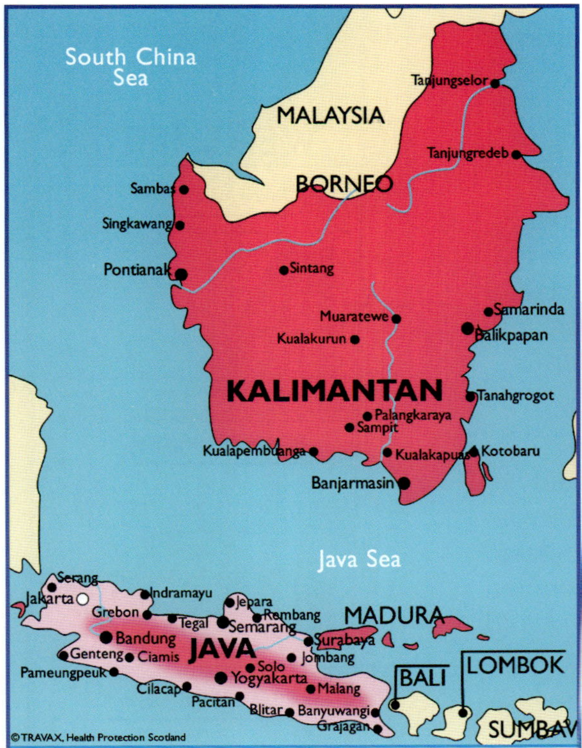

Low to no risk	High risk	Surrounding
antimalarials not usually advised	antimalarials usually advised	countries with malaria risk

This map is only intended as a guide since mosquitoes do not respect boundaries and the risk areas shown may not be exact. **Reproduced with permission from Fitfortravel, Health Protection Scotland's Travel website www.fitfortravel.nhs.uk.**

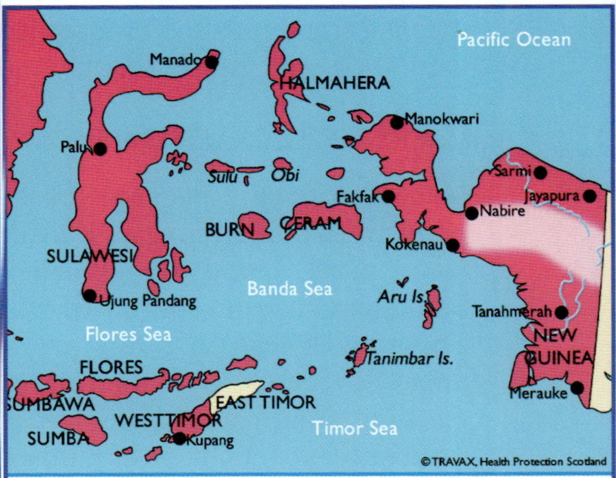

Low to no risk	High risk	Surrounding
antimalarials not usually advised	antimalarials usually advised	countries with malaria risk

This map is only intended as a guide since mosquitoes do not respect boundaries and the risk areas shown may not be exact. **Reproduced with permission from Fitfortravel, Health Protection Scotland's Travel website www.fitfortravel.nhs.uk.**

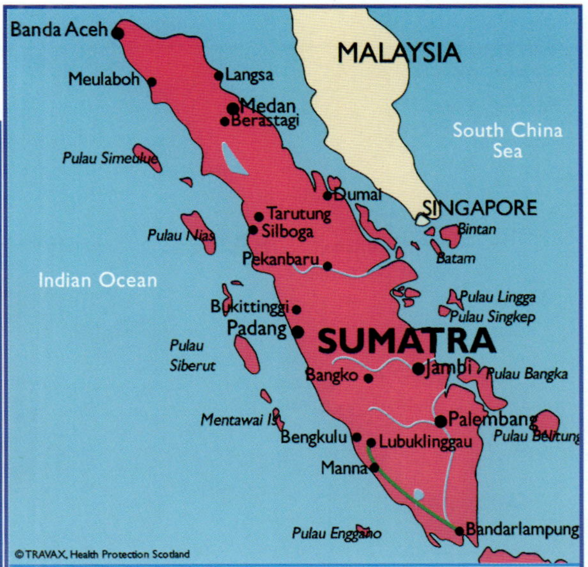

High risk	Surrounding
antimalarials usually advised (except in major cities)	countries with malaria risk

This map is only intended as a guide since mosquitoes do not respect boundaries and the risk areas shown may not be exact. **Reproduced with permission from Fitfortravel, Health Protection Scotland's Travel website www.fitfortravel.nhs.uk.**

IRAN

General Advice

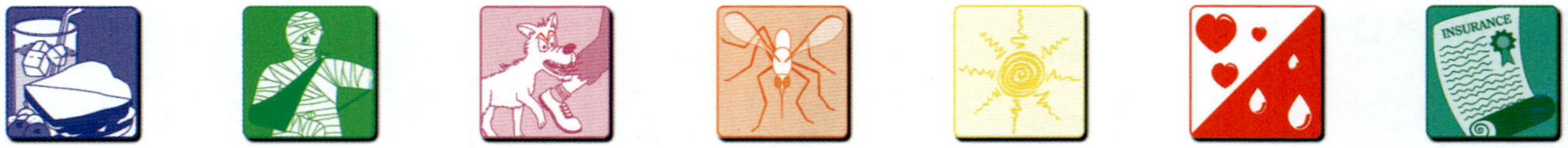

Immunization Advice

- ❑ Immunizations recommended for life should be up to date, especially those for children and boosters of tetanus for adults.
- ❑ Courses or boosters of diphtheria and hepatitis A are usually advised.
- ❑ Vaccines sometimes advised are: cholera, hepatitis B, rabies, typhoid.
- ❑ A yellow fever certificate is required if entering from an infected country.
- ❑ Prompt investigation of fever is essential.

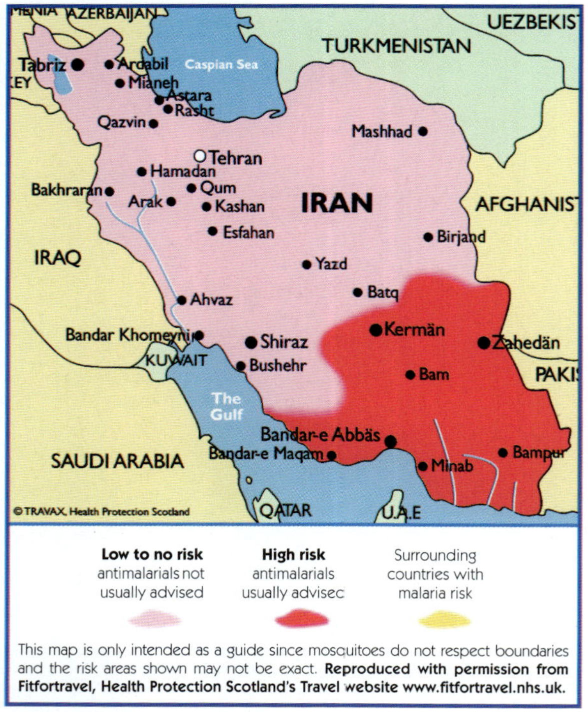

Malaria Advice

- ❑ Malaria is a serious and sometimes fatal disease transmitted by mosquitoes. You cannot be vaccinated against malaria.

MALARIA PRECAUTIONS

- ❑ Malaria precautions are essential in rural areas of Hormozgan, Kerman (tropical part), and southern Sistan-Baluchestan, from March to November. The risk is less in other areas. Avoid mosquito bites by covering up with clothing such as long sleeves and long trousers especially after sunset, using insect repellents on exposed skin and, when necessary, sleeping under a mosquito net.
- ❑ Check with your doctor or nurse about suitable antimalarial tablets.

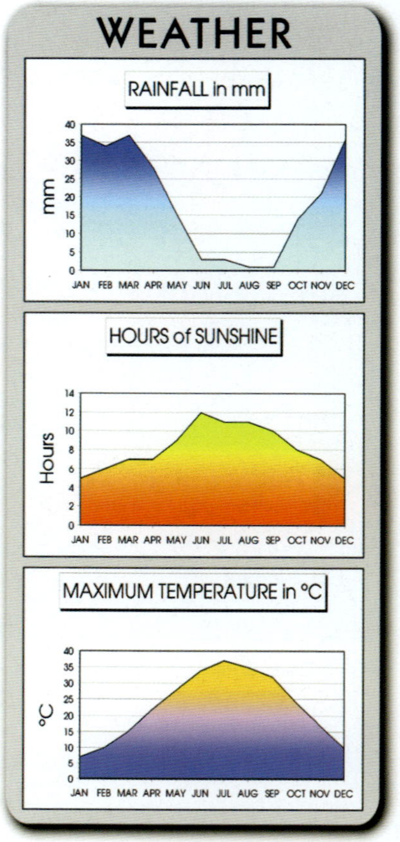

IRAQ

General Advice

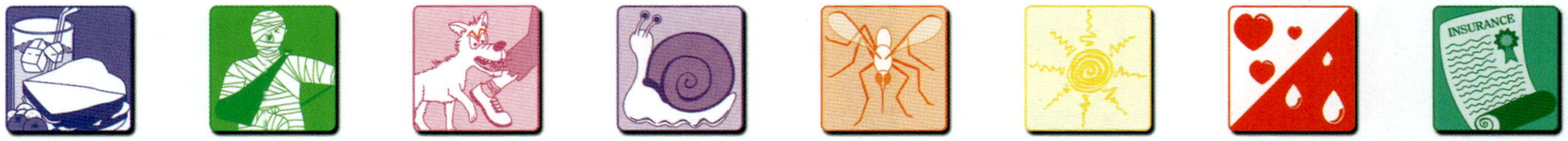

Immunization Advice

- ❑ Immunizations recommended for life should be up to date, especially those for children and boosters of tetanus for adults.
- ❑ Courses or boosters of diphtheria, hepatitis A, and typhoid are usually advised.
- ❑ Vaccines sometimes advised are: BCG, cholera, hepatitis B, rabies.
- ❑ A yellow fever certificate is required if entering from an infected country.
- ❑ Prompt investigation of fever is essential.

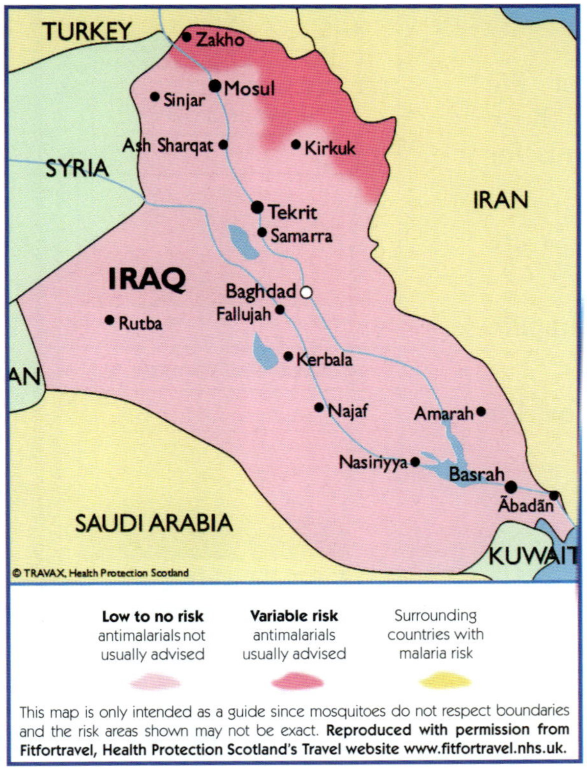

Malaria Advice

- ❑ Malaria is a serious and sometimes fatal disease transmitted by mosquitoes. You cannot be vaccinated against malaria.

MALARIA PRECAUTIONS

- ❑ Malaria precautions are essential in northern areas of Duhok, Erbil, and Sulaimniya provinces, below 1500 m from May to November. Avoid mosquito bites by covering up with clothing such as long sleeves and long trousers especially after sunset, using insect repellents on exposed skin and, when necessary, sleeping under a mosquito net.
- ❑ Check with your doctor or nurse about suitable antimalarial tablets.

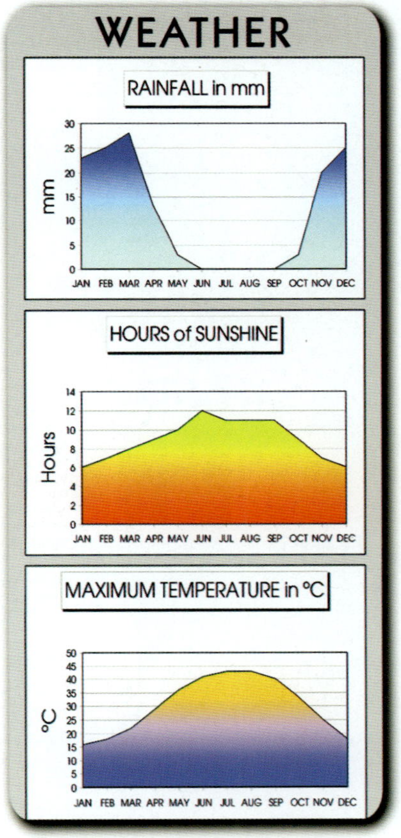

ISRAEL

General Advice

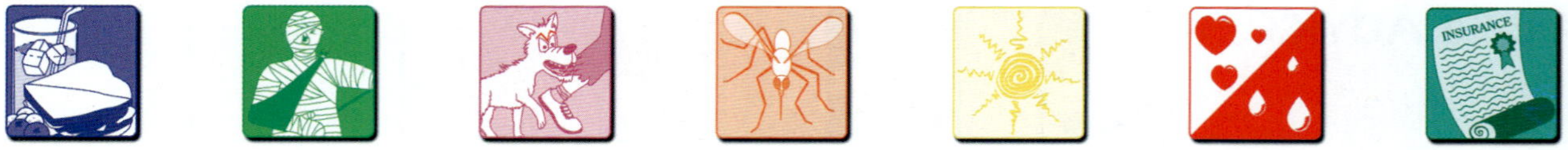

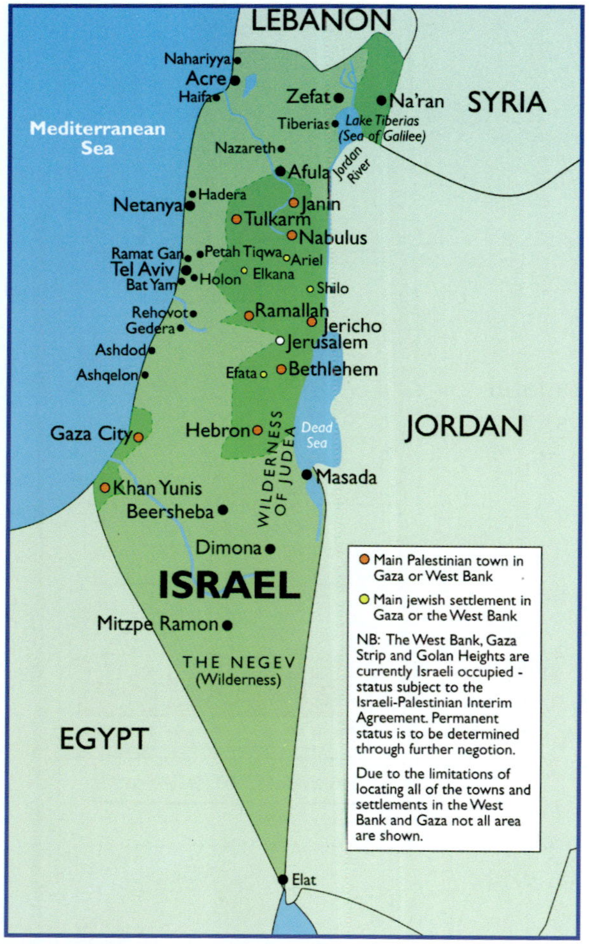

Immunization Advice

- ❑ Immunizations recommended for life should be up to date, especially those for children and boosters of tetanus for adults.
- ❑ Courses or boosters of hepatitis A are usually advised.
- ❑ Vaccines sometimes advised are: hepatitis B, rabies.
- ❑ No certificate of vaccination for for yellow fever is required.

Malaria Advice

- ❑ Malaria is not normally present.

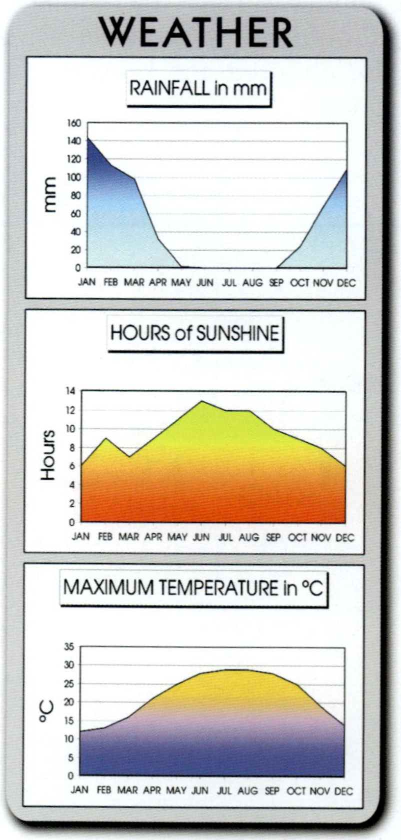

—Weather in Jerusalem—

JAMAICA

General Advice

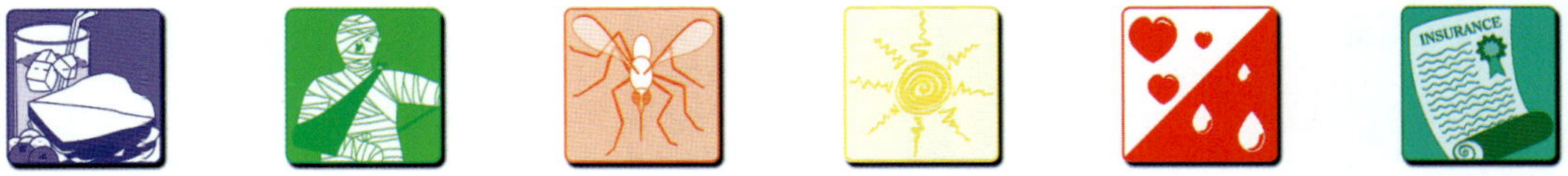

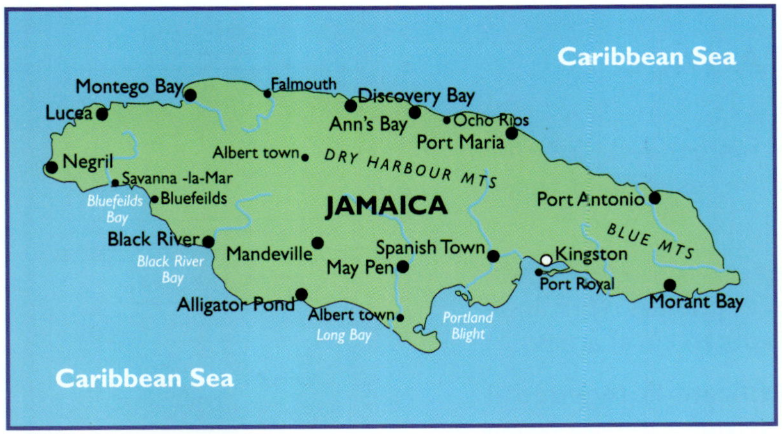

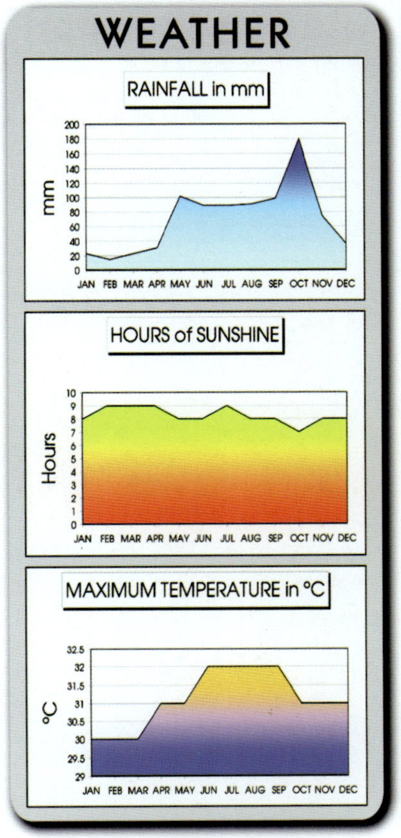

Immunization Advice

- ❑ Immunizations recommended for life should be up to date, especially those for children and boosters of tetanus for adults.
- ❑ Courses or boosters of hepatitis A are usually advised.
- ❑ Vaccines sometimes advised are: hepatitis B.
- ❑ A yellow fever certificate is required if aged over 1 year old and entering from an infected country.

Malaria Advice

- ❑ Malaria is not normally present.

General Advice

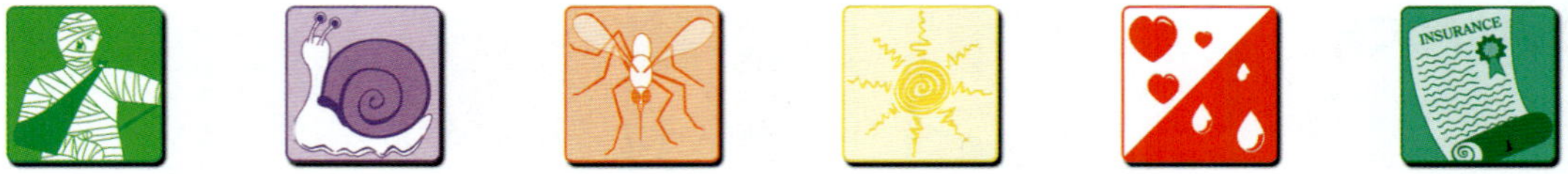

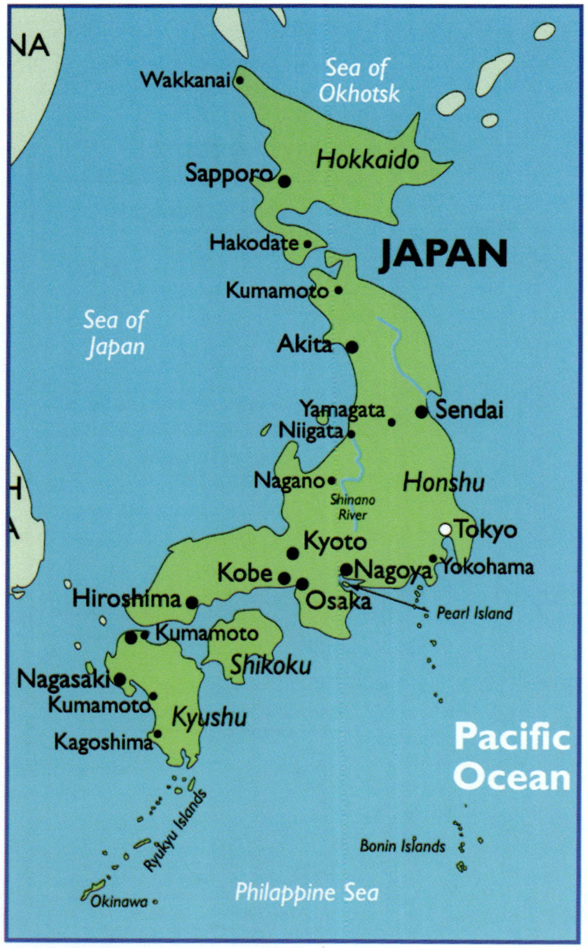

Immunization Advice

- ❑ Immunizations recommended for life should be up to date, especially those for children.
- ❑ Vaccines sometimes advised are: hepatitis B, Japanese encephalitis (for long stays or frequent visits to rural areas).
- ❑ A yellow fever certificate is required if aged over 1 year old and entering Japan within 6 days of an overnight stay or longer in an infected country.
- ❑ No certificate of vaccination for for yellow fever is required.

Malaria Advice

- ❑ Malaria is not normally present.

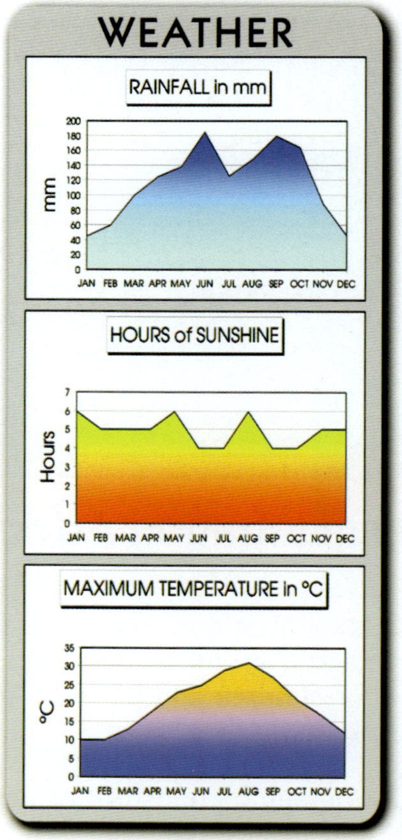

—Weather in Tokyo—

JORDAN

General Advice

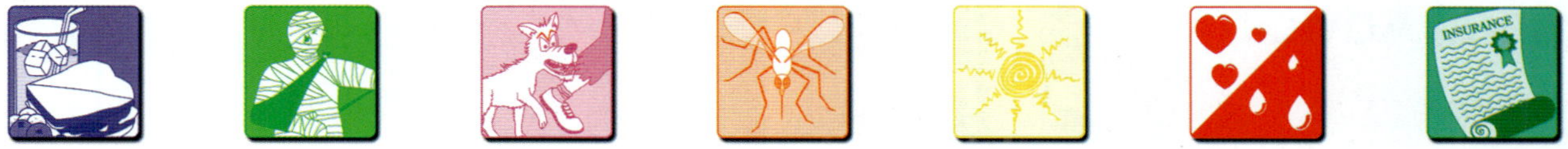

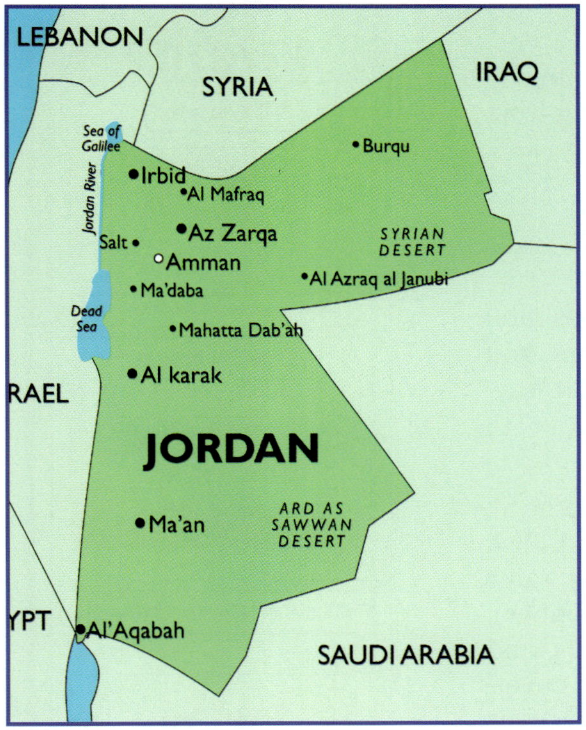

Immunization Advice

- ❑ Immunizations recommended for life should be up to date, especially those for children and boosters of tetanus for adults.
- ❑ Courses or boosters of hepatitis A are usually advised.
- ❑ Vaccines sometimes advised are: hepatitis B, rabies, typhoid.
- ❑ A yellow fever certificate is required if aged over 1 year old and entering from an infected country.

Malaria Advice

- ❑ Malaria is not normally present.

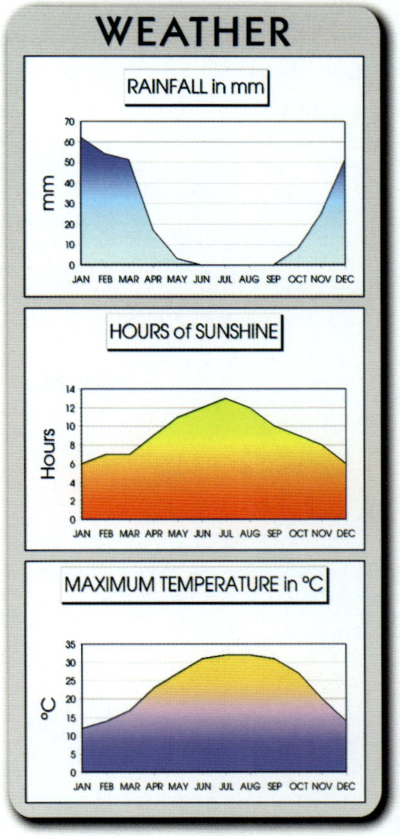

KENYA

General Advice

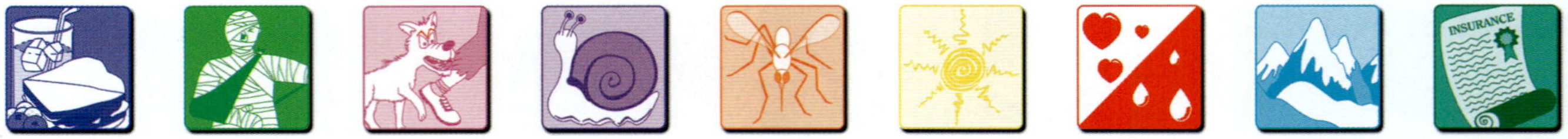

Immunization Advice

- ❑ Immunizations recommended for life should be up to date, especially those for children and boosters of tetanus for adults.

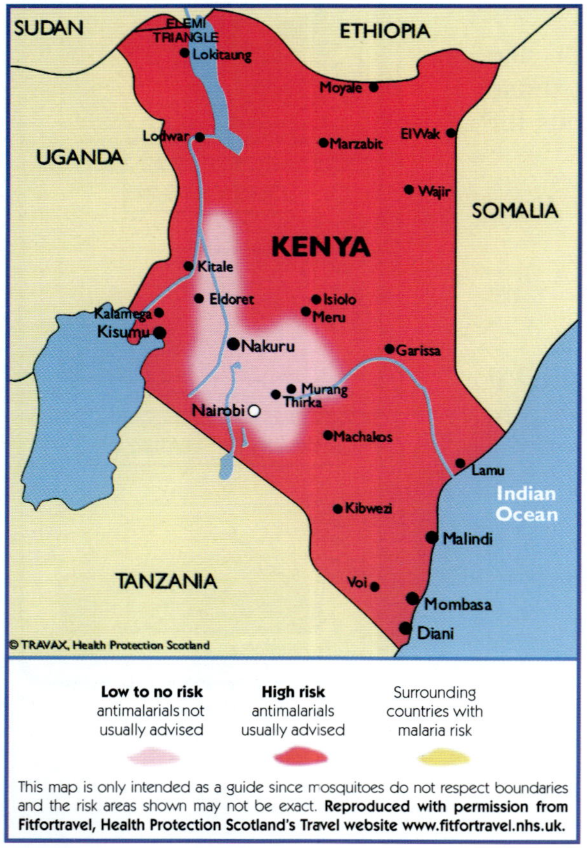

This map is only intended as a guide since mosquitoes do not respect boundaries and the risk areas shown may not be exact. **Reproduced with permission from Fitfortravel, Health Protection Scotland's Travel website www.fitfortravel.nhs.uk.**

- ❑ Courses or boosters of diphtheria, hepatitis A, and typhoid are usually advised.
- ❑ Vaccines sometimes advised are: BCG, cholera, hepatitis B, meningococcal A and C, rabies, yellow fever (see yellow fever map).
- ❑ A yellow fever certificate is required if aged over 1 year old and entering from an infected country.

Malaria Advice

- ❑ Malaria is a serious and sometimes fatal disease transmitted by mosquitoes. You cannot be vaccinated against malaria.

MALARIA PRECAUTIONS

- ❑ Malaria precautions are essential in all areas below 2500 m all year round. Risk is highest during and after the rains (April–June and November–December). Risk is minimal in the highlands and Nairobi. Avoid mosquito bites by covering up with clothing such as long sleeves and long trousers especially after sunset, using insect repellents on exposed skin and, when necessary, sleeping under a mosquito net.
- ❑ Check with your doctor or nurse about suitable antimalarial tablets.
- ❑ Prompt investigation of fever is essential.

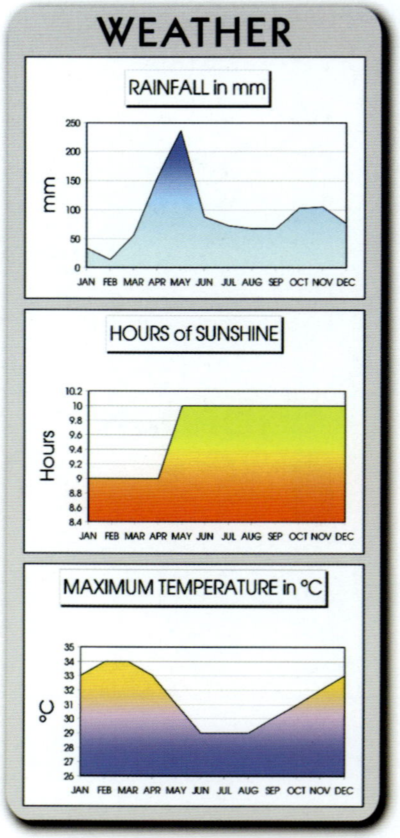

—Weather in Mombasa—

DEMOCRATIC REPUBLIC OF NORTH KOREA

General Advice

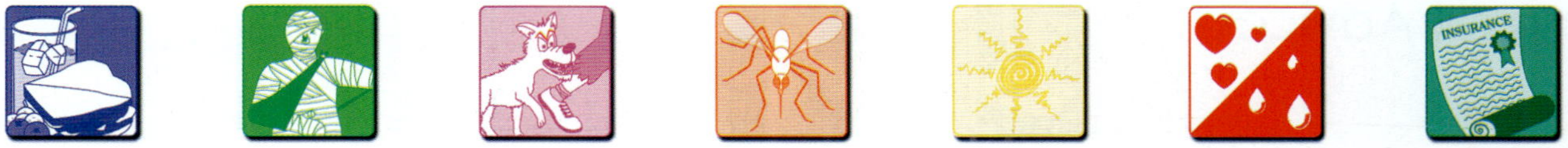

Immunization Advice

- ❑ Immunizations recommended for life should be up to date, especially those for children and boosters of tetanus for adults.
- ❑ Courses or boosters of diphtheria, hepatitis A, and typhoid are usually advised.
- ❑ Vaccines sometimes advised are: BCG, hepatitis B, Japanese encephalitis, rabies.
- ❑ A yellow fever certificate is required if aged over 1 year old and entering from an infected country.

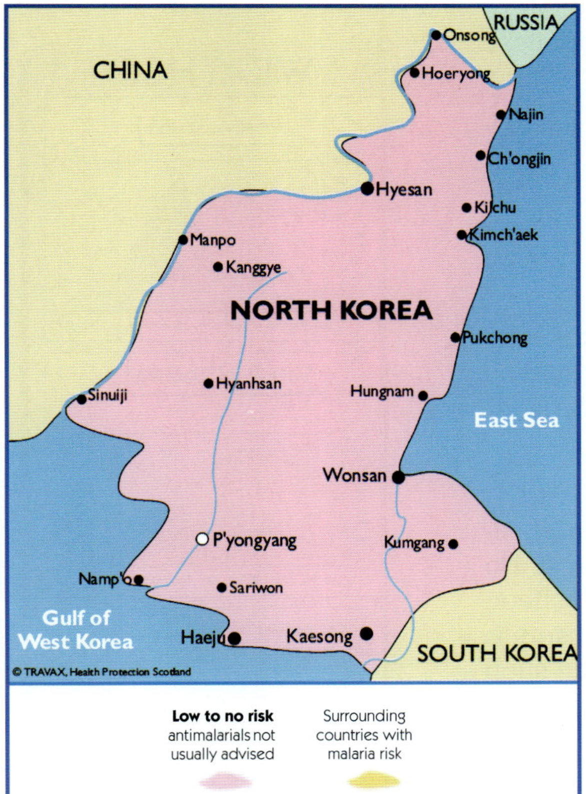

This map is only intended as a guide since mosquitoes do not respect boundaries and the risk areas shown may not be exact. **Reproduced with permission from Fitfortravel, Health Protection Scotland's Travel website www.fitfortravel.nhs.uk.**

Malaria Advice

- ❑ Malaria is a serious and sometimes fatal disease transmitted by mosquitoes. You cannot be vaccinated against malaria.

MALARIA PRECAUTIONS

- ❑ Malaria precautions are essential in some southern areas all year round. Avoid mosquito bites by covering up with clothing such as long sleeves and long trousers especially after sunset, using insect repellents on exposed skin and, when necessary, sleeping under a mosquito net.
- ❑ Antimalarial tablets are not normally recommended.
- ❑ Prompt investigation of fever is essential.

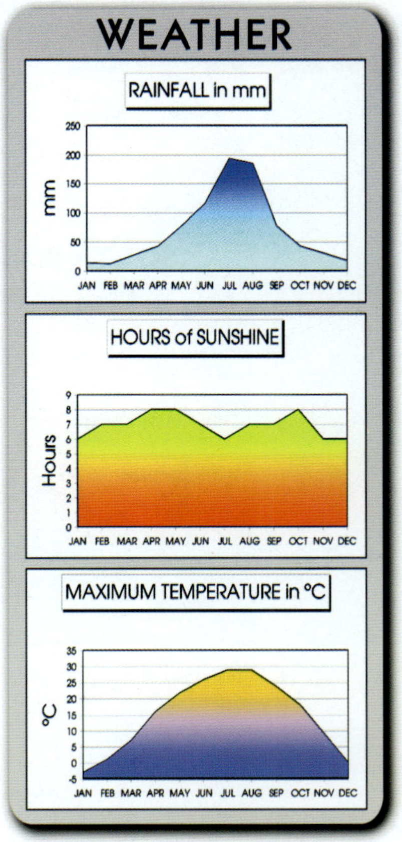

REPUBLIC OF SOUTH KOREA

General Advice

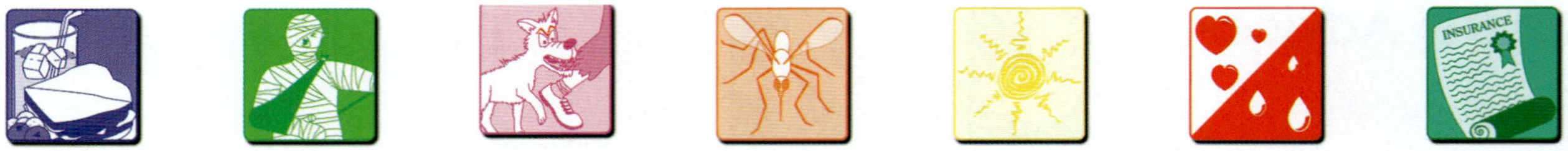

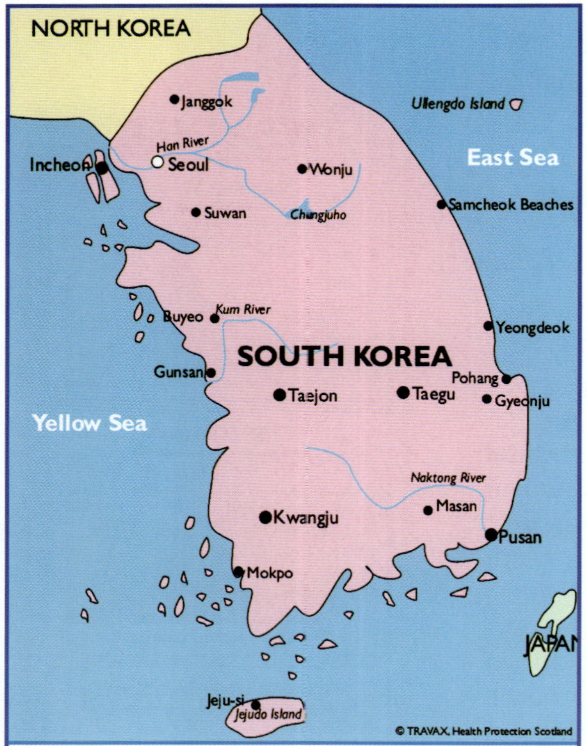

Low to no risk antimalarials not usually advised

Surrounding countries with malaria risk

This map is only intended as a guide since mosquitoes do not respect boundaries and the risk areas shown may not be exact. **Reproduced with permission from Fitfortravel, Health Protection Scotland's Travel website www.fitfortravel.nhs.uk.**

Immunization Advice

- ❑ Immunizations recommended for life should be up to date, especially those for children.
- ❑ Vaccines sometimes advised are: BCG; hepatitis A, hepatitis B, Japanese encephalitis, rabies, typhoid.
- ❑ No certificate of vaccination for for yellow fever is required.

Malaria Advice

- ❑ Malaria is a serious and sometimes fatal disease transmitted by mosquitoes. You cannot be vaccinated against malaria.

MALARIA PRECAUTIONS

- ❑ Malaria precautions are essential in some northern areas of Gangwon Do and Kyunggi Do provinces and Incheon City all year round. Avoid mosquito bites by covering up with clothing such as long sleeves and long trousers especially after sunset, using insect repellents on exposed skin and, when necessary, sleeping under a mosquito net.
- ❑ Antimalarial tablets are not normally recommended.
- ❑ Prompt investigation of fever is essential.

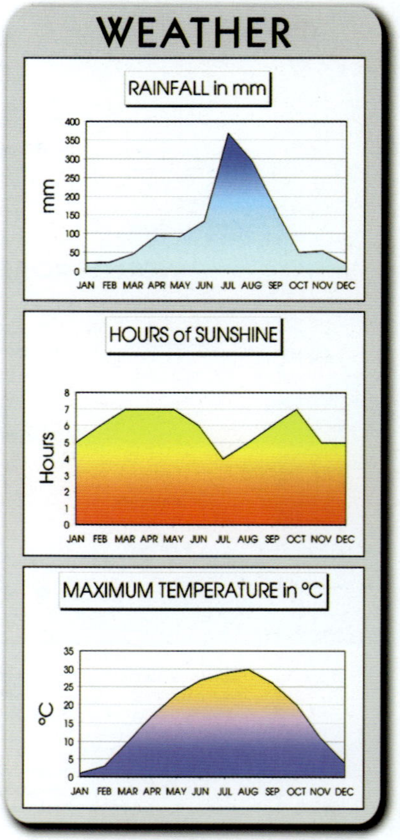

LAOS PEOPLE'S DEMOCRATIC REPUBLIC

General Advice

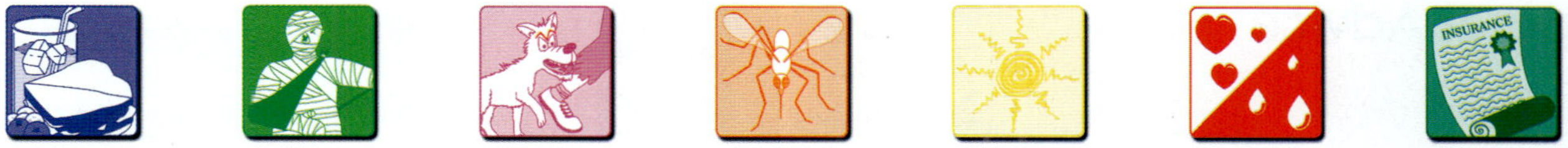

Immunization Advice

- ❑ Immunizations recommended for life should be up to date, especially those for children and boosters of tetanus for adults.
- ❑ Courses or boosters of diphtheria, hepatitis A, and typhoid are usually advised.
- ❑ Vaccines sometimes advised are: BCG, cholera, hepatitis B, Japanese encephalitis, rabies.
- ❑ A yellow fever certificate is required if entering from an infected country.

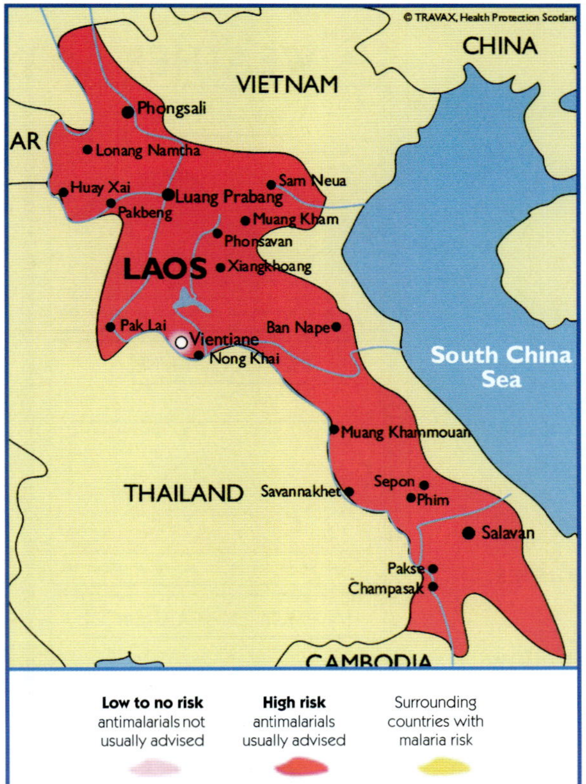

This map is only intended as a guide since mosquitoes do not respect boundaries and the risk areas shown may not be exact. **Reproduced with permission from Fitfortravel, Health Protection Scotland's Travel website www.fitfortravel.nhs.uk.**

Malaria Advice

- ❑ Malaria is a serious and sometimes fatal disease transmitted by mosquitoes. You cannot be vaccinated against malaria.

MALARIA PRECAUTIONS

- ❑ Malaria precautions are essential in all areas all year round. The risk is minimal in Vientiane. Avoid mosquito bites by covering up with clothing such as long sleeves and long trousers especially after sunset, using insect repellents on exposed skin and, when necessary, sleeping under a mosquito net.
- ❑ Check with your doctor or nurse about suitable antimalarial tablets.
- ❑ Prompt investigation of fever is essential.

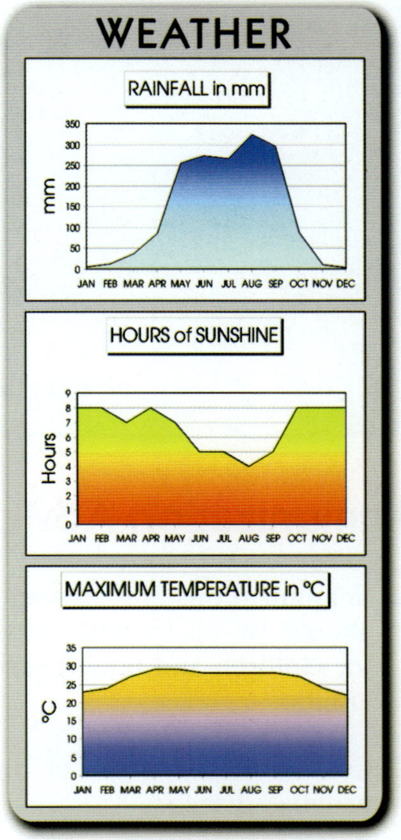

LATVIA

General Advice

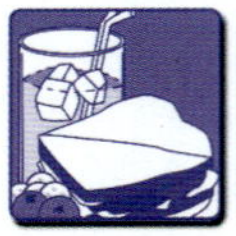

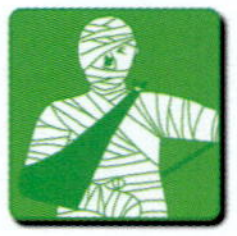

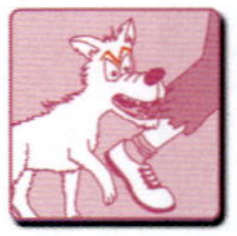

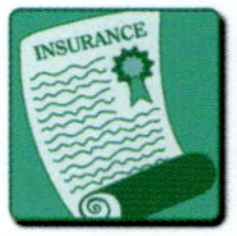

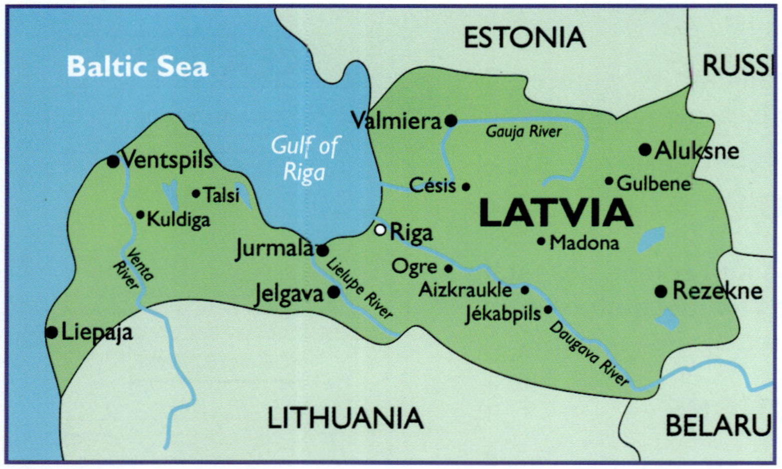

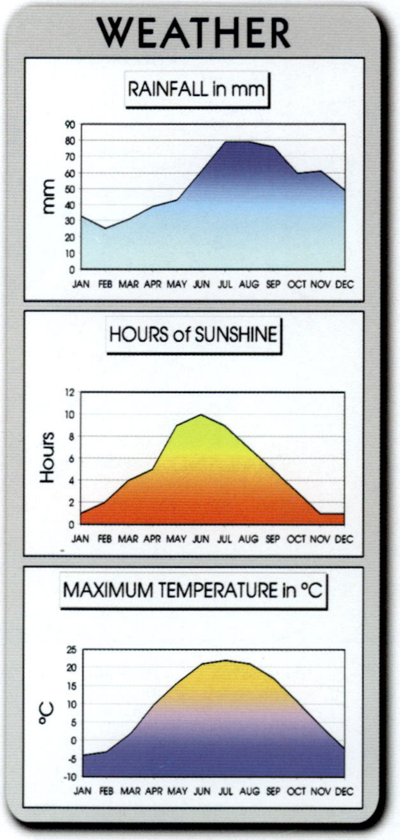

Immunization Advice

- ❑ Immunizations recommended for life should be up to date, especially those for children and boosters of tetanus for adults.
- ❑ Courses or boosters of diphtheria are usually advised.
- ❑ Vaccines sometimes advised are: BCG, hepatitis A, hepatitis B, rabies, tick-borne encephalitis.
- ❑ No certificate of vaccination for yellow fever is required.

Malaria Advice

- ❑ Malaria is not normally present.

LITHUANIA

General Advice

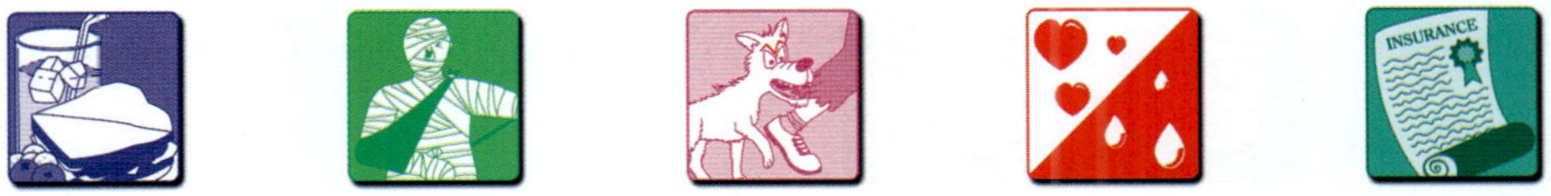

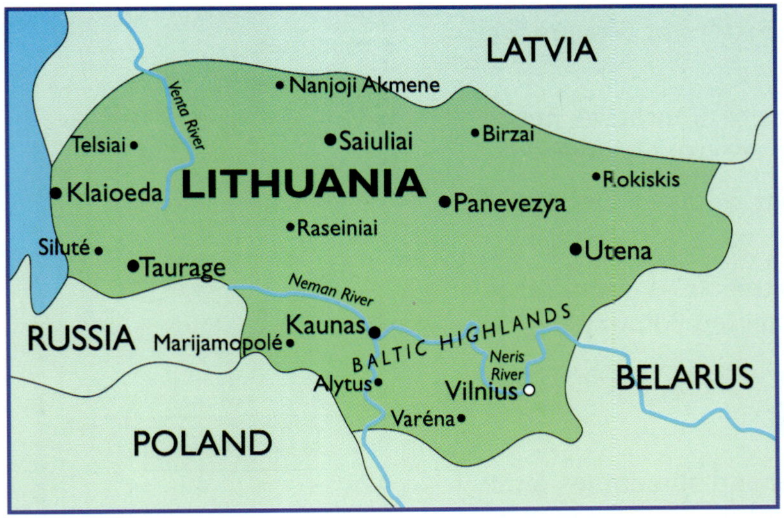

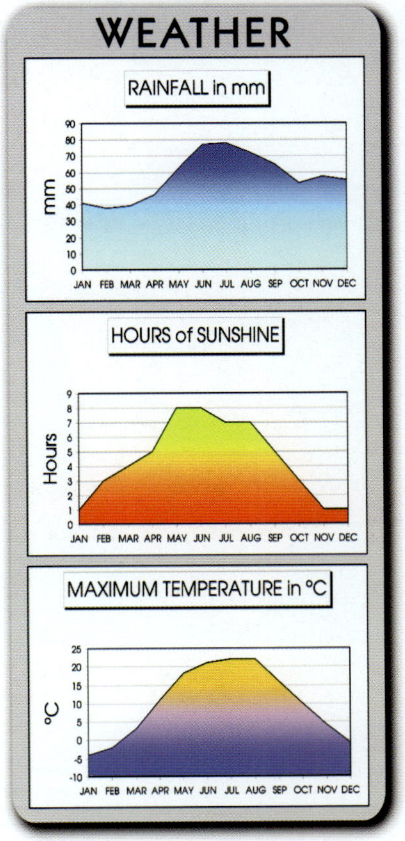

Immunization Advice

- ❑ Immunizations recommended for life should be up to date, especially those for children and boosters of tetanus for adults.
- ❑ Vaccines sometimes advised are: BCG, hepatitis A, hepatitis B, rabies, tick-borne encephalitis.
- ❑ No certificate of vaccination for yellow fever is required.

Malaria Advice

- ❑ Malaria is not normally present.

MADAGASCAR

General Advice

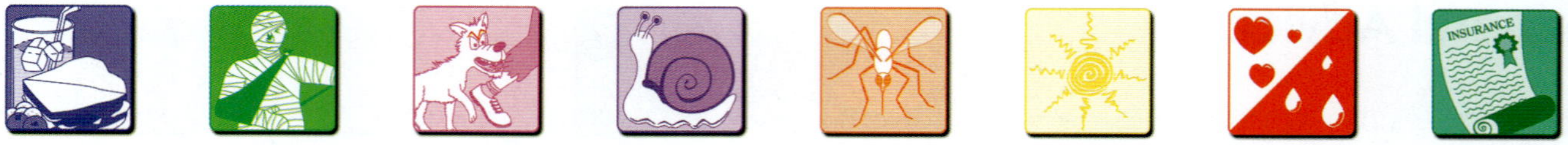

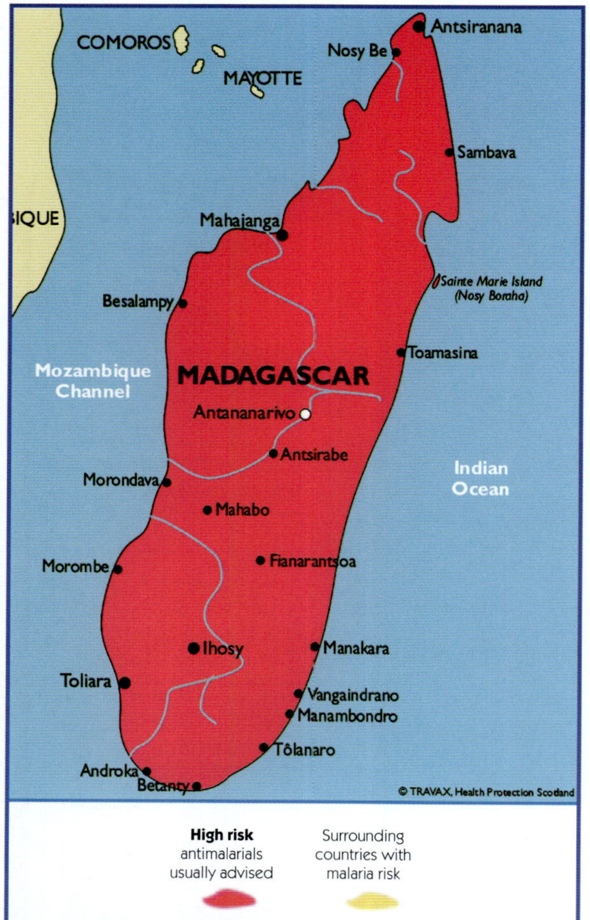

This map is only intended as a guide since mosquitoes do not respect boundaries and the risk areas shown may not be exact. **Reproduced with permission from Fitfortravel, Health Protection Scotland's Travel website www.fitfortravel.nhs.uk.**

Immunization Advice

- ❑ Immunizations recommended for life should be up to date, especially those for children and boosters of tetanus for adults.
- ❑ Courses or boosters of diphtheria, hepatitis A, and typhoid are usually advised.
- ❑ Vaccines sometimes advised are: BCG, hepatitis B, rabies.
- ❑ A yellow fever certificate is required if entering from an infected country.

Malaria Advice

- ❑ Malaria is a serious and sometimes fatal disease transmitted by mosquitoes. You cannot be vaccinated against malaria.

MALARIA PRECAUTIONS

- ❑ Malaria precautions are essential in all areas all year round. Avoid mosquito bites by covering up with clothing such as long sleeves and long trousers especially after sunset, using insect repellents on exposed skin and, when necessary, sleeping under a mosquito net.
- ❑ Check with your doctor or nurse about suitable antimalarial tablets.
- ❑ Prompt investigation of fever is essential.

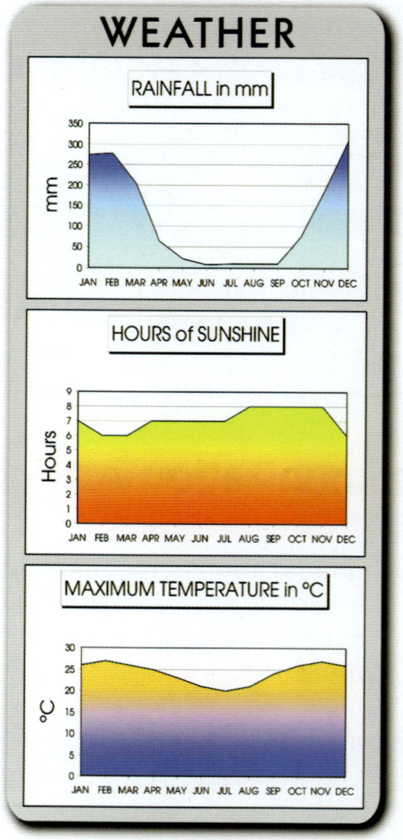

MALAWI

General Advice

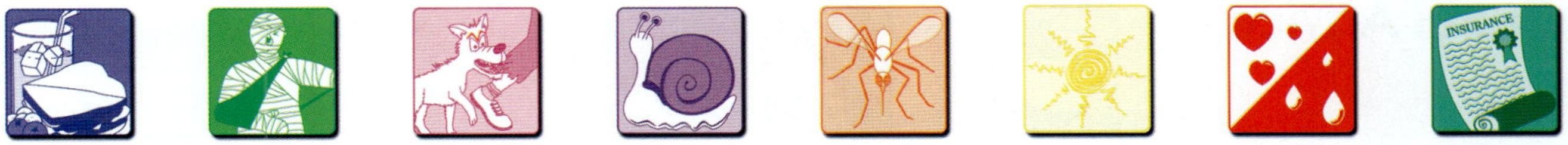

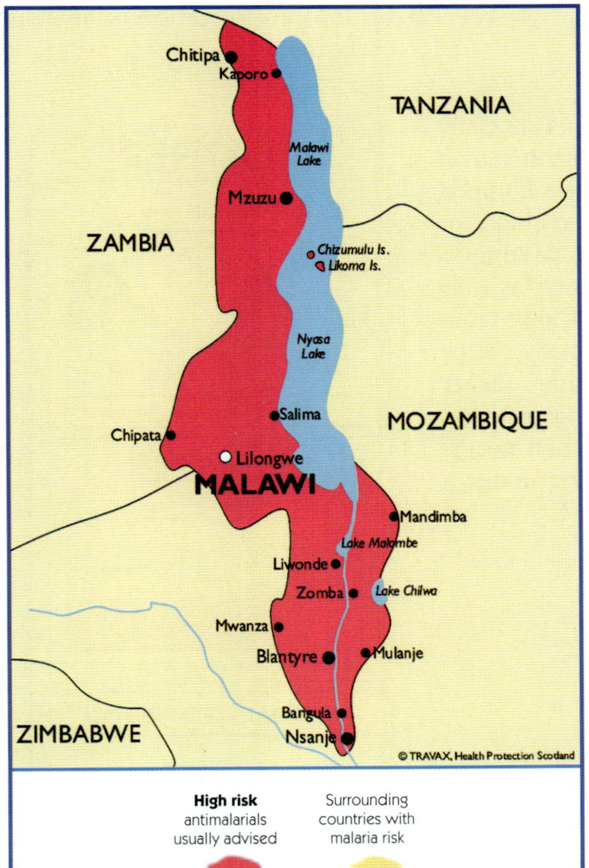

This map is only intended as a guide since mosquitoes do not respect boundaries and the risk areas shown may not be exact. **Reproduced with permission from Fitfortravel, Health Protection Scotland's Travel website www.fitfortravel.nhs.uk.**

Immunization Advice

❑ Immunizations recommended for life should be up to date, especially those for children and boosters of tetanus for adults.

❑ Courses or boosters of hepatitis A and typhoid are usually advised.

❑ Vaccines sometimes advised are: BCG, cholera, hepatitis B, rabies.

❑ A yellow fever certificate is required if aged over 1 year old and entering from an infected country.

Malaria Advice

❑ Malaria is a serious and sometimes fatal disease transmitted by mosquitoes. You cannot be vaccinated against malaria.

MALARIA PRECAUTIONS

❑ Malaria precautions are essential in all areas all year round. Avoid mosquito bites by covering up with clothing such as long sleeves and long trousers especially after sunset, using insect repellents on exposed skin and, when necessary, sleeping under a mosquito net.

❑ Check with your doctor or nurse about suitable antimalarial tablets.

❑ Prompt investigation of fever is essential.

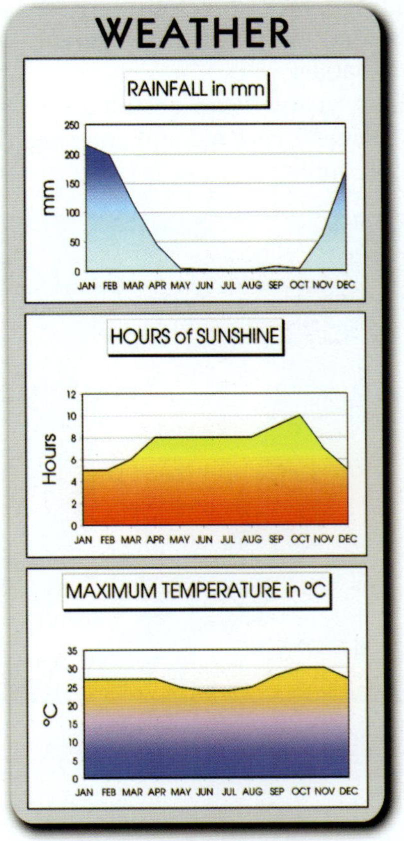

MALAYSIA

General Advice

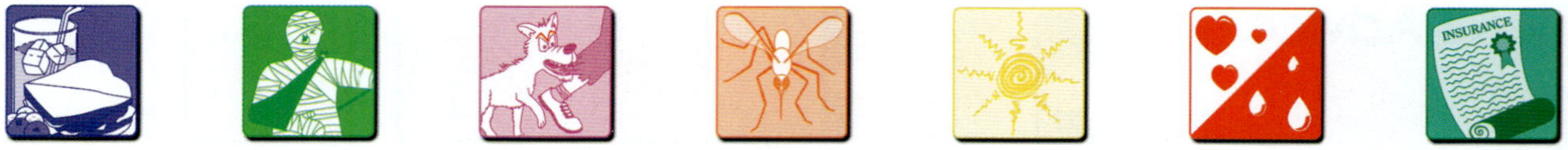

Immunization Advice

- ❑ Immunizations recommended for life should be up to date, especially those for children and boosters of tetanus for adults.
- ❑ Courses or boosters of diphtheria, hepatitis A, and typhoid are usually advised.
- ❑ Vaccines sometimes advised are: BCG, cholera, hepatitis B, Japanese encephalitis, rabies.
- ❑ A yellow fever certificate is required if aged over 1 year old and entering from an infected country.

Malaria Advice

- ❑ Malaria is a serious and sometimes fatal disease transmitted by mosquitoes. You cannot be vaccinated against malaria.

MALARIA PRECAUTIONS

- ❑ Malaria precautions are essential in all areas, especially deep hinterland, all year round. There is a risk in Taman Negara National Park. The risk is low in Kuala Lumpur, other urban areas, coastal areas, most islands, and for those transitting across Peninsula Malaysia. Avoid mosquito bites by covering up with clothing such as long sleeves and long trousers especially after sunset, using insect repellents on exposed skin and, when necessary, sleeping under a mosquito net.
- ❑ Check with your doctor or nurse about suitable antimalarial tablets.
- ❑ Prompt investigation of fever is essential.

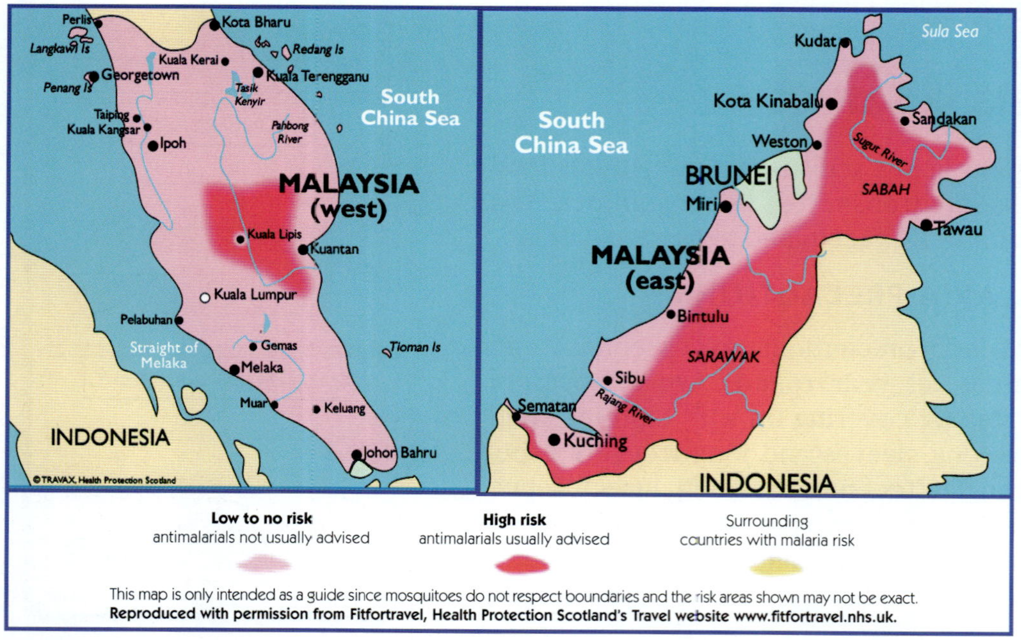

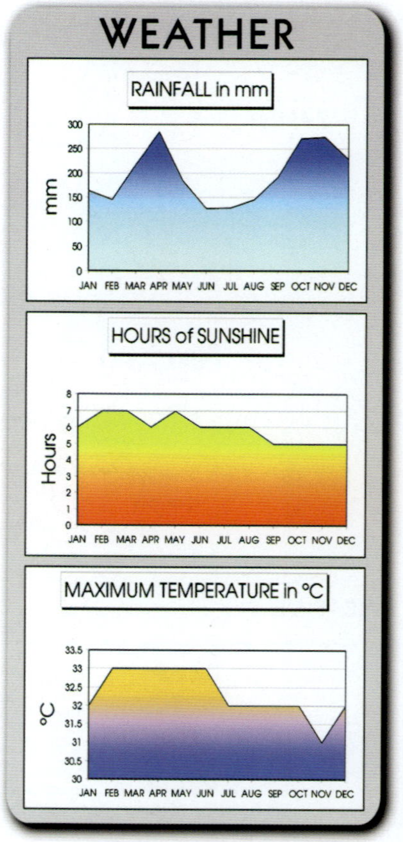

MALI

General Advice

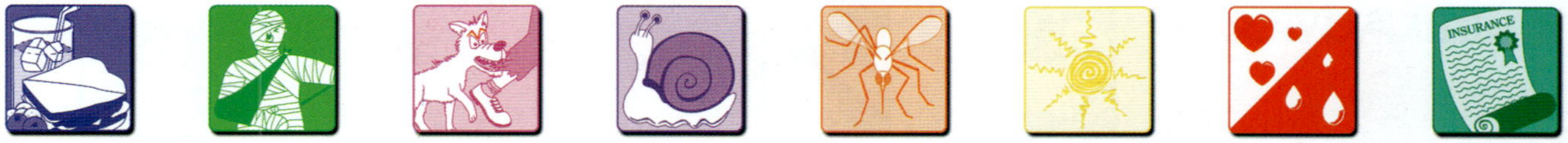

Immunization Advice

- ❑ Immunizations recommended for life should be up to date, especially those for children and boosters of tetanus for adults.

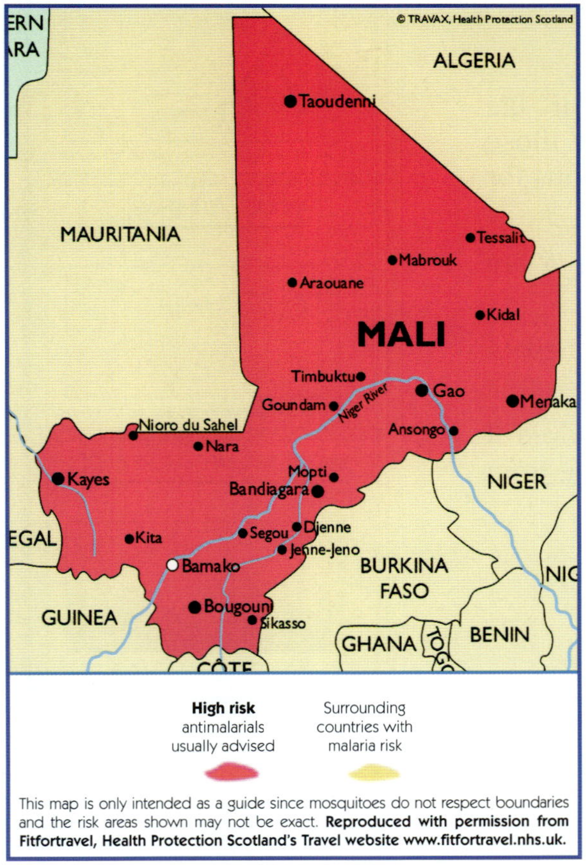

- ❑ Courses or boosters of diphtheria, hepatitis A, poliomyelitis, typhoid, and yellow fever are usually advised.
- ❑ Vaccines sometimes advised are: BCG, cholera, hepatitis B, meningococcal A and C, rabies.
- ❑ A yellow fever certificate is required for all travelers aged over 1 year.

Malaria Advice

- ❑ Malaria is a serious and sometimes fatal disease transmitted by mosquitoes. You cannot be vaccinated against malaria.

MALARIA PRECAUTIONS

- ❑ Malaria precautions are essential in all areas all year round. Avoid mosquito bites by covering up with clothing such as long sleeves and long trousers especially after sunset, using insect repellents on exposed skin and, when necessary, sleeping under a mosquito net.
- ❑ Check with your doctor or nurse about suitable antimalarial tablets.
- ❑ Prompt investigation of fever is essential.

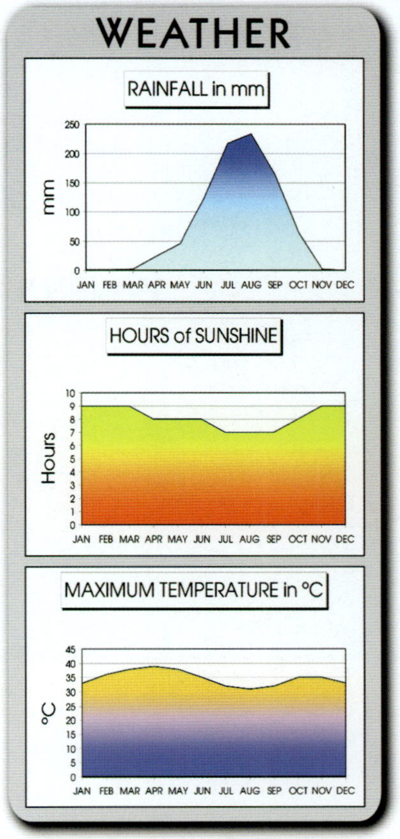

MAURITIUS

General Advice

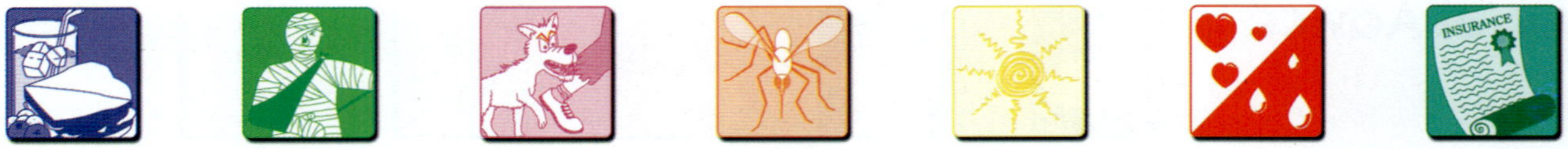

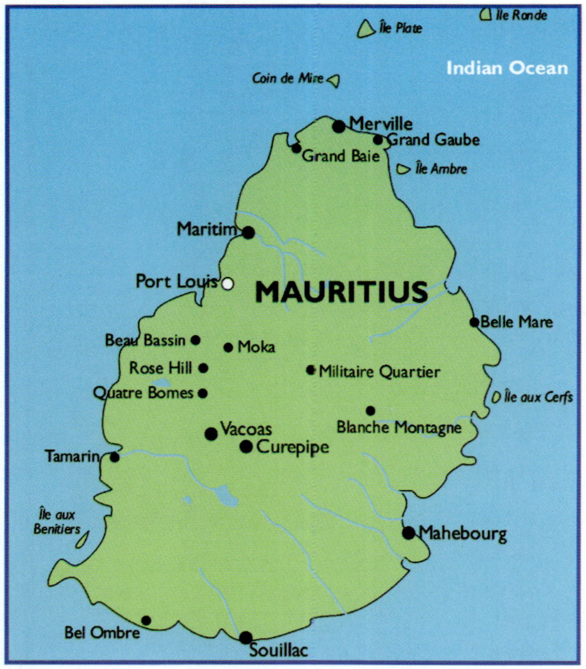

Immunization Advice

- ❑ Immunizations recommended for life should be up to date, especially those for children and boosters of tetanus for adults.
- ❑ Courses or boosters of hepatitis A are usually advised.
- ❑ Vaccines sometimes advised are: hepatitis B, rabies.
- ❑ A yellow fever certificate is required if aged over 1 year old and entering from an infected country.

Malaria Advice

- ❑ Malaria is not normally present.

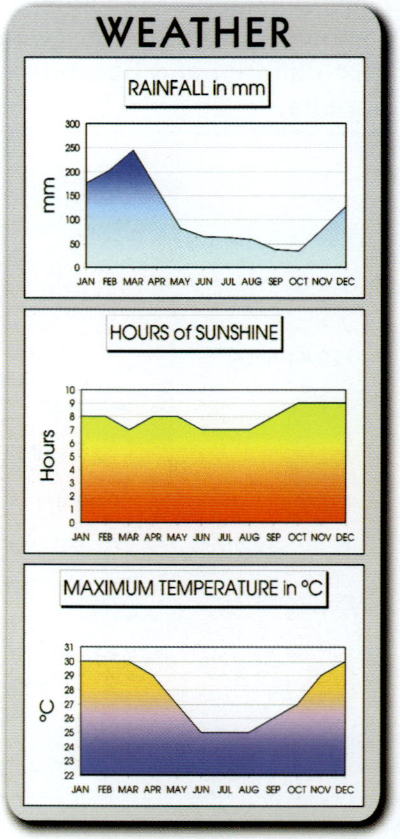

MEXICO

General Advice

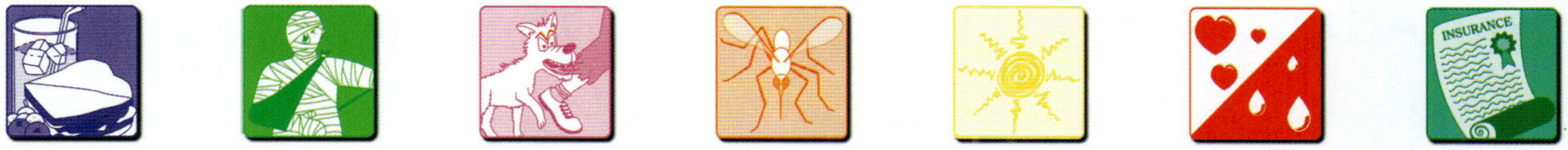

Immunization Advice

- ❑ Immunizations recommended for life should be up to date, especially those for children and boosters of tetanus for adults.
- ❑ Courses or boosters of hepatitis A and typhoid are usually advised.
- ❑ Vaccines sometimes advised are: hepatitis B, rabies.
- ❑ No certificate of vaccination for yellow fever is required.

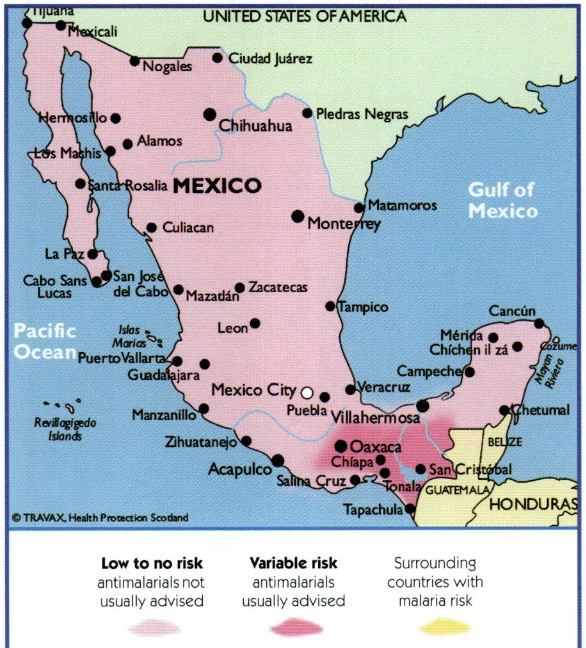

This map is only intended as a guide since mosquitoes do not respect boundaries and the risk areas shown may not be exact. **Reproduced with permission from Fitfortravel, Health Protection Scotland's Travel website www.fitfortravel.nhs.uk.**

Malaria Advice

- ❑ Malaria is a serious and sometimes fatal disease transmitted by mosquitoes. You cannot be vaccinated against malaria.

MALARIA PRECAUTIONS

- ❑ Malaria precautions are essential in rural areas especially in Chiapas and Oaxana, all year round. There is minimal malaria in other areas including popular tourist resort such as Mexico City, Acapulco, and Cancun (see malaria map for risk areas). Avoid mosquito bites by covering up with clothing such as long sleeves and long trousers especially after sunset, using insect repellents on exposed skin and, when necessary, sleeping under a mosquito net.
- ❑ Check with your doctor or nurse about suitable antimalarial tablets.
- ❑ Prompt investigation of fever is essential.

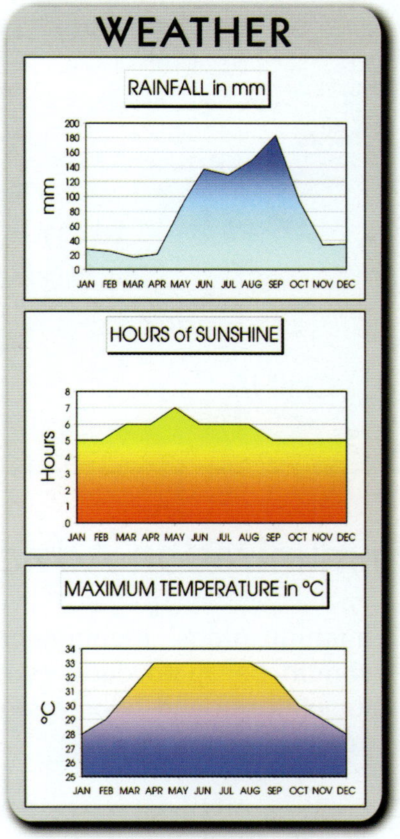

—Weather in Cancun—

MONGOLIA

General Advice

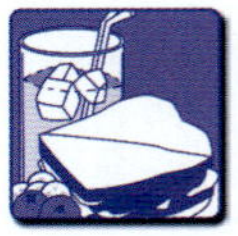
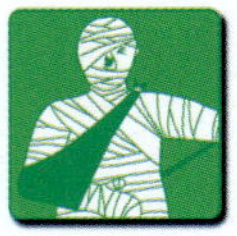
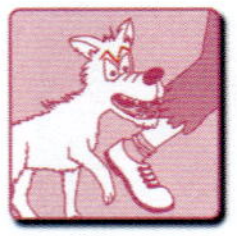

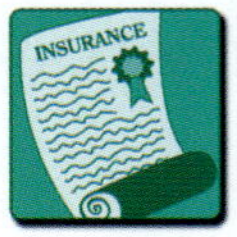

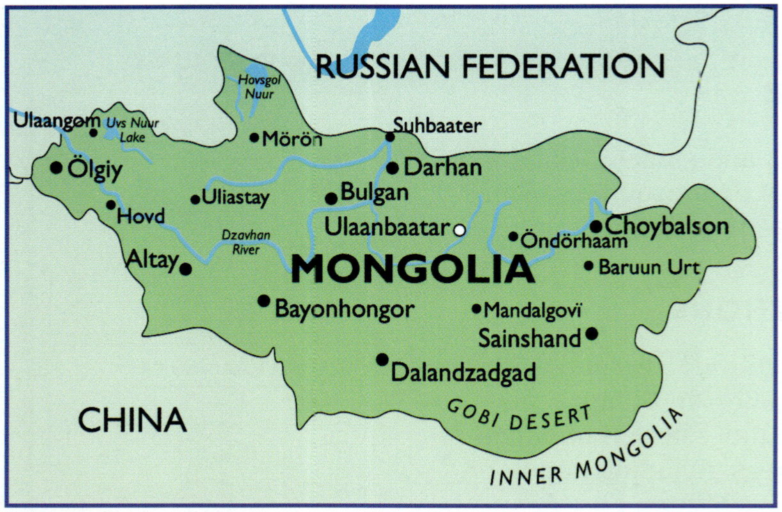

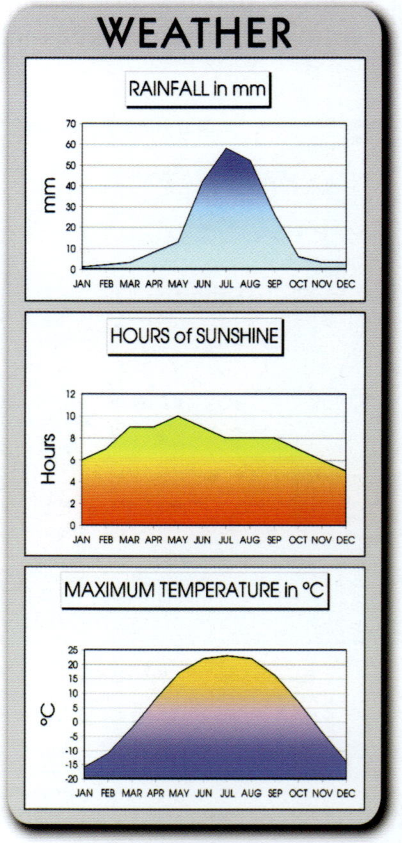

Immunization Advice

- ❑ Immunizations recommended for life should be up to date, especially those for children and boosters of tetanus for adults.
- ❑ Courses or boosters of hepatitis A are usually advised.
- ❑ Vaccines sometimes advised are: BCG, hepatitis B, rabies, tick-borne encephalitis, typhoid.
- ❑ No certificate of vaccination for yellow fever is required.

Malaria Advice

- ❑ Malaria is not normally present.

MOROCCO

General Advice

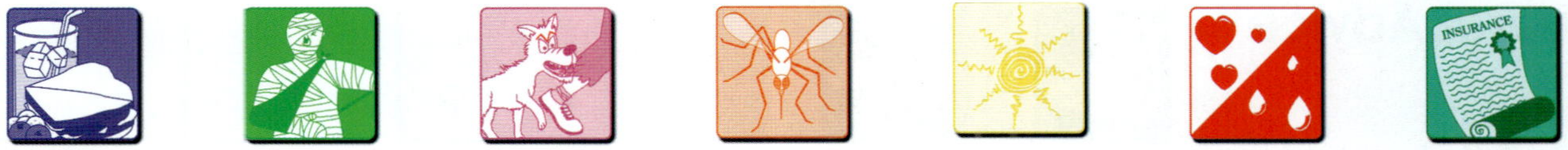

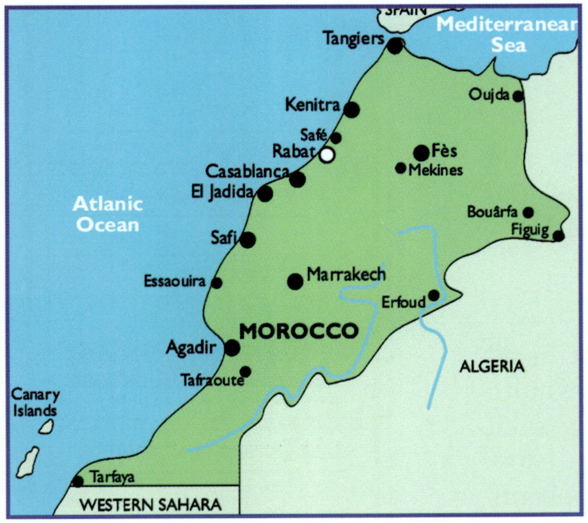

Immunization Advice

- ❑ Immunizations recommended for life should be up to date, especially those for children and boosters of tetanus for adults.
- ❑ Courses or boosters of hepatitis A and typhoid are usually advised.
- ❑ Vaccines sometimes advised are: BCG, hepatitis B, rabies.
- ❑ No certificate of vaccination for yellow fever is required.

Malaria Advice

- ❑ Malaria is not normally present.

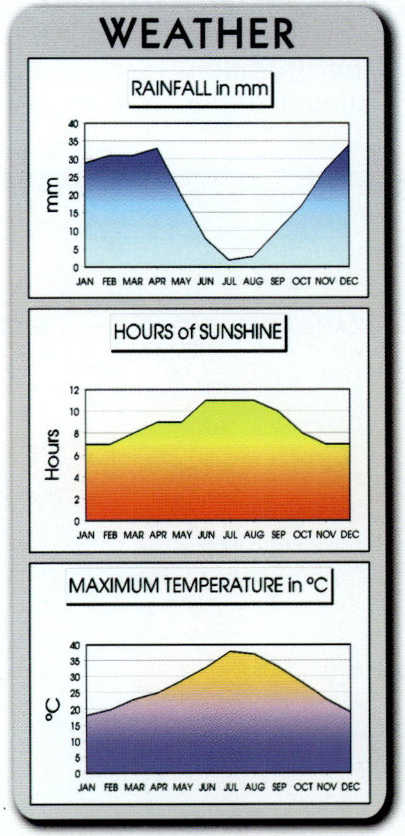

—Weather in Marrakech—

MOZAMBIQUE

General Advice

Immunization Advice

- ❑ Immunizations recommended for life should be up to date, especially those for children and boosters of tetanus for adults.
- ❑ Courses or boosters of hepatitis A and typhoid are usually advised.
- ❑ Vaccines sometimes advised are: BCG, cholera, hepatitis B, rabies.
- ❑ A yellow fever certificate is required if aged over 1 year old and entering from an infected country.

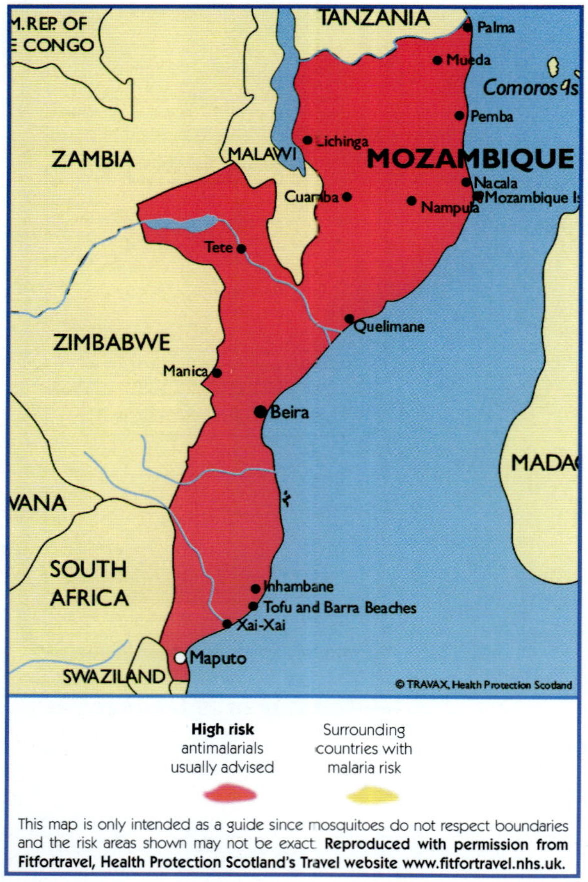

Malaria Advice

- ❑ Malaria is a serious and sometimes fatal disease transmitted by mosquitoes. You cannot be vaccinated against malaria.

MALARIA PRECAUTIONS

- ❑ Malaria precautions are essential in all areas all year round. Avoid mosquito bites by covering up with clothing such as long sleeves and long trousers especially after sunset, using insect repellents on exposed skin and, when necessary, sleeping under a mosquito net.
- ❑ Check with your doctor or nurse about suitable antimalarial tablets.
- ❑ Prompt investigation of fever is essential.

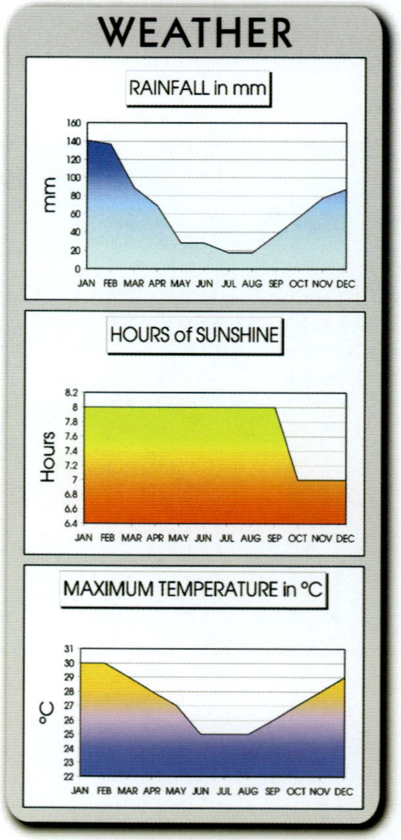

MYANMAR

General Advice

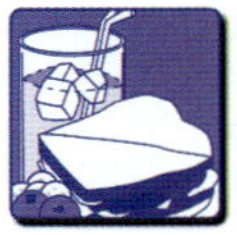
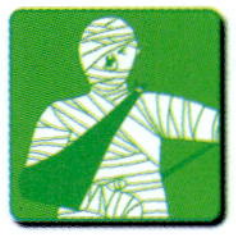
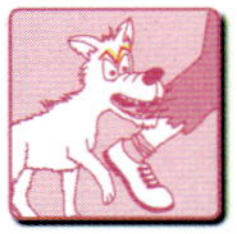
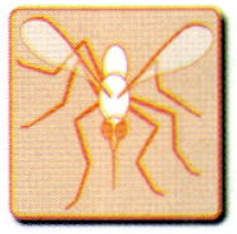
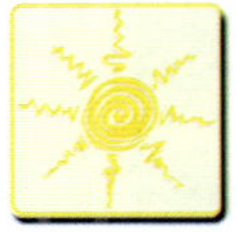

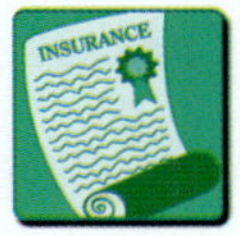

Immunization Advice

- ❑ Immunizations recommended for life should be up to date, especially those for children and boosters of tetanus for adults.
- ❑ Courses or boosters of diphtheria, hepatitis A, and typhoid are usually advised.
- ❑ Vaccines sometimes advised are: BCG, cholera, hepatitis B, Japanese encephalitis, rabies.
- ❑ A yellow fever certificate is required if entering from an infected country. Nationals and residents of Myanmar are required to possess certificates of vaccination on departure to a yellow fever infected area.

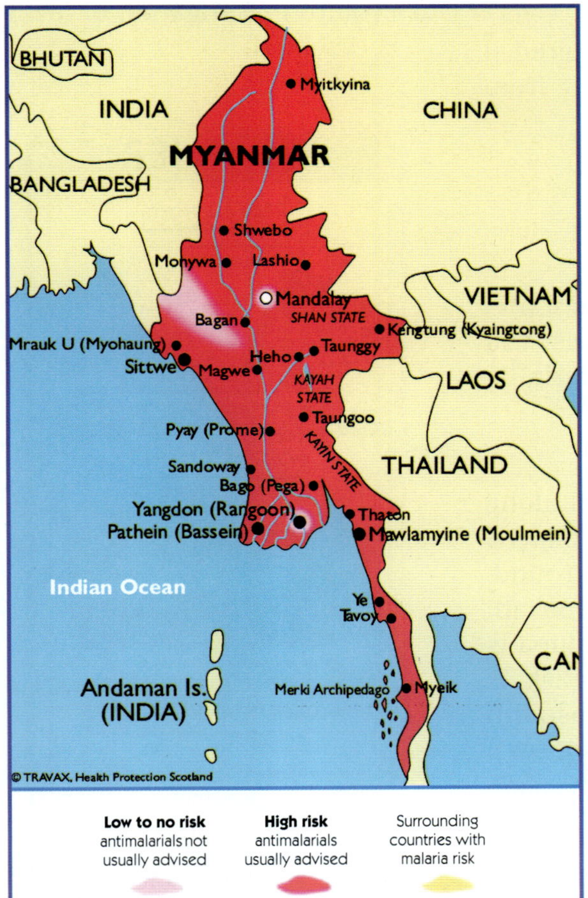

This map is only intended as a guide since mosquitoes do not respect boundaries and the risk areas shown may not be exact. **Reproduced with permission from Fitfortravel, Health Protection Scotland's Travel website www.fitfortravel.nhs.uk.**

Malaria Advice

- ❑ Malaria is a serious and sometimes fatal disease transmitted by mosquitoes. You cannot be vaccinated against malaria.

MALARIA PRECAUTIONS

- ❑ Malaria precautions are essential in all areas below 1000 m all year round. Risk is highest in Kayin and eastern Shan states. The risk is less in Yangon and Mandalay. Avoid mosquito bites by covering up with clothing such as long sleeves and long trousers especially after sunset, using insect repellents on exposed skin and, when necessary, sleeping under a mosquito net.
- ❑ Check with your doctor or nurse about suitable antimalarial tablets.
- ❑ Prompt investigation of fever is essential.

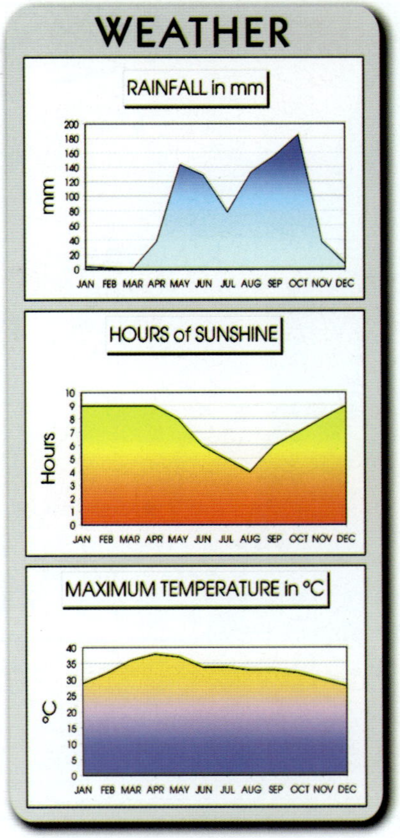

NAMIBIA

General Advice

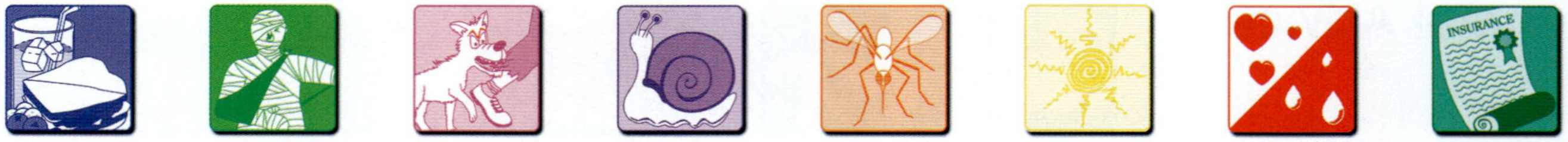

Immunization Advice

- ❑ Immunizations recommended for life should be up to date, especially those for children and boosters of tetanus for adults.

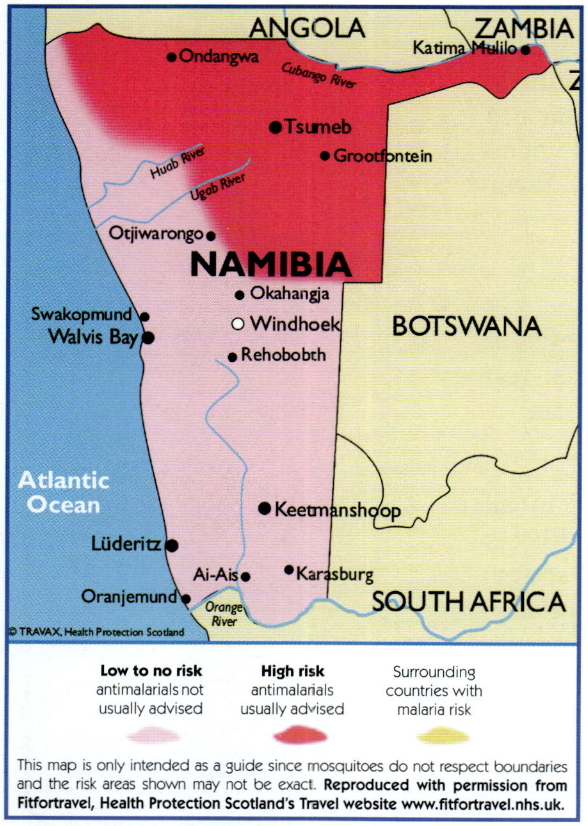

- ❑ Courses or boosters of hepatitis A and typhoid are usually advised.
- ❑ Vaccines sometimes advised are: BCG, cholera, hepatitis B, rabies.
- ❑ A yellow fever certificate is required if aged over 1 year old and entering from an infected country.

Malaria Advice

- ❑ Malaria is a serious and sometimes fatal disease transmitted by mosquitoes. You cannot be vaccinated against malaria.

MALARIA PRECAUTIONS

- ❑ Malaria precautions are essential along the Kunene river and in Caprivi and Kavango regions all year round. Risk in Ohangwena, Omaheke, Omusati, Oshana, Oshikoto, and Otijozondjupa is high from November to June. Risk is lower in all other areas. Avoid mosquito bites by covering up with clothing such as long sleeves and long trousers especially after sunset, using insect repellents on exposed skin and, when necessary, sleeping under a mosquito net.
- ❑ Check with your doctor or nurse about suitable antimalarial tablets.
- ❑ Prompt investigation of fever is essential.

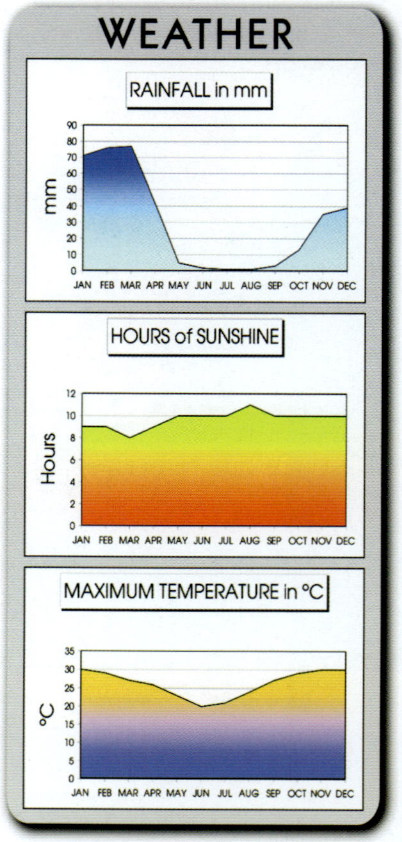

NEPAL

General Advice

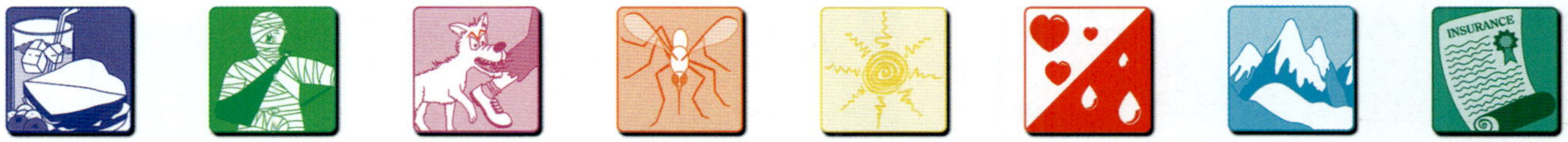

Immunization Advice

- ❑ Immunizations recommended for life should be up to date, especially those for children and boosters of tetanus for adults.
- ❑ Courses or boosters of diphtheria, hepatitis A, poliomyelitis, and typhoid are usually advised.

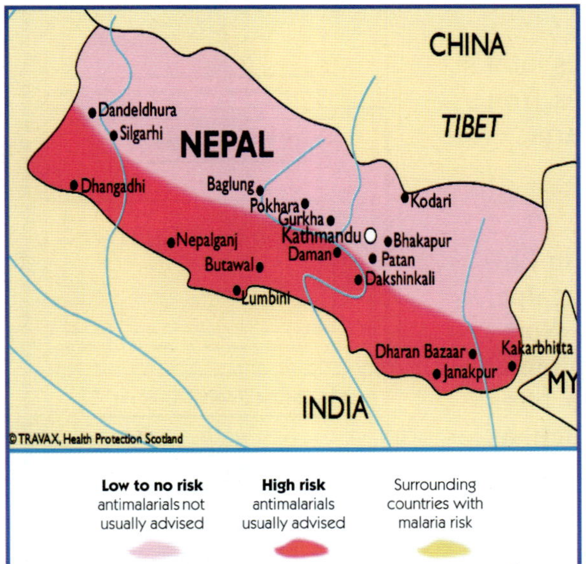

This map is only intended as a guide since mosquitoes do not respect boundaries and the risk areas shown may not be exact. **Reproduced with permission from Fitfortravel, Health Protection Scotland's Travel website www.fitfortravel.nhs.uk.**

- ❑ Vaccines sometimes advised are: BCG, cholera, hepatitis B, Japanese encephalitis, rabies.
- ❑ A yellow fever certificate is required if entering from an infected country.

Malaria Advice

- ❑ Malaria is a serious and sometimes fatal disease transmitted by mosquitoes. You cannot be vaccinated against malaria.

MALARIA PRECAUTIONS

- ❑ Malaria precautions are essential in all low lying areas. Risk is confined to low lying southern plains of Bara, Dhanukha, Kapilvastu, Mahotari, Parsa, Rautahat, Rupendehi, and Sarlahi, all year round. Avoid mosquito bites by covering up with clothing such as long sleeves and long trousers especially after sunset, using insect repellents on exposed skin and, when necessary, sleeping under a mosquito net.
- ❑ Check with your doctor or nurse about suitable antimalarial tablets.
- ❑ Prompt investigation of fever is essential.

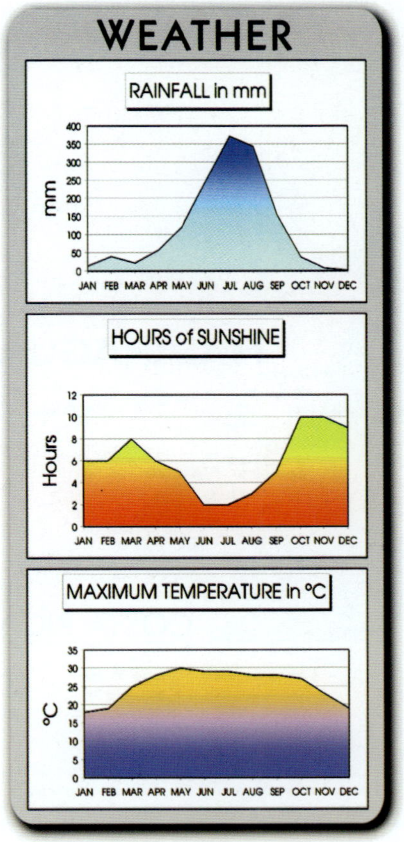

NICARAGUA

General Advice

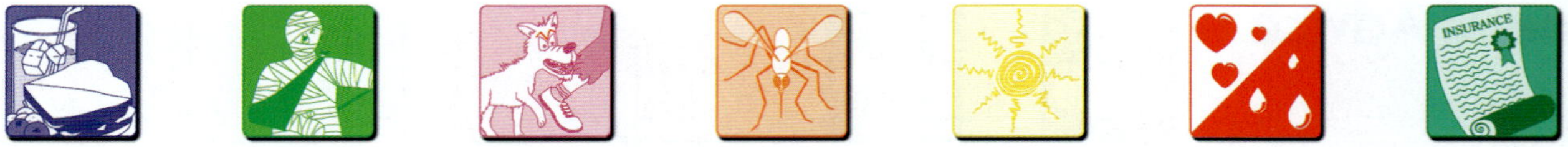

Immunization Advice

- ❑ Immunizations recommended for life should be up to date, especially those for children and boosters of tetanus for adults.
- ❑ Courses or boosters of hepatitis A and typhoid are usually advised.
- ❑ Vaccines sometimes advised are: BCG, hepatitis B, rabies.
- ❑ A yellow fever certificate is required if aged over 1 year old and entering from an infected country.

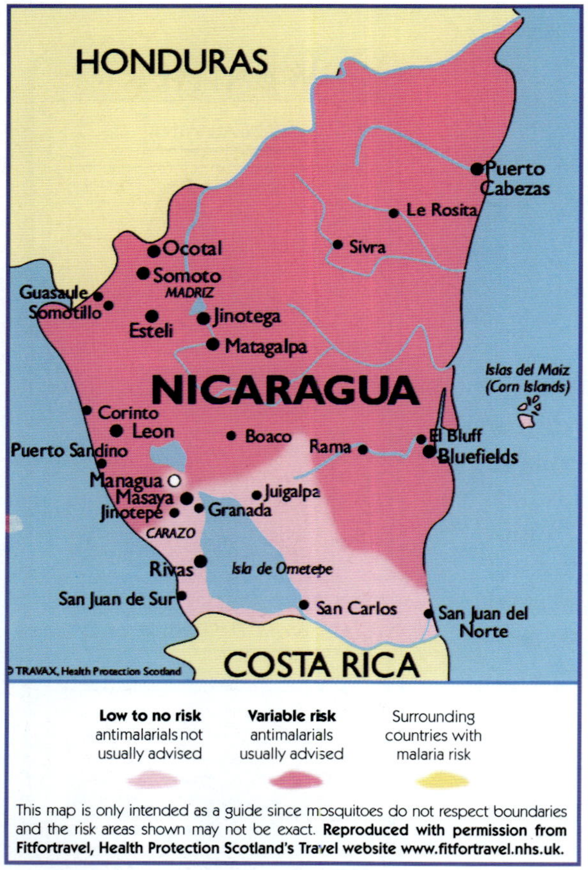

Malaria Advice

- ❑ Malaria is a serious and sometimes fatal disease transmitted by mosquitoes. You cannot be vaccinated against malaria.

MALARIA PRECAUTIONS

- ❑ Malaria precautions are essential in Chinandega, Leon, Managua, Matagalpa, Regions Autonoma del Atlantico Norte and Sur, all year round. There is minimal risk in Managua. Avoid mosquito bites by covering up with clothing such as long sleeves and long trousers especially after sunset, using insect repellents on exposed skin and, when necessary, sleeping under a mosquito net.
- ❑ Check with your doctor or nurse about suitable antimalarial tablets.
- ❑ Prompt investigation of fever is essential.

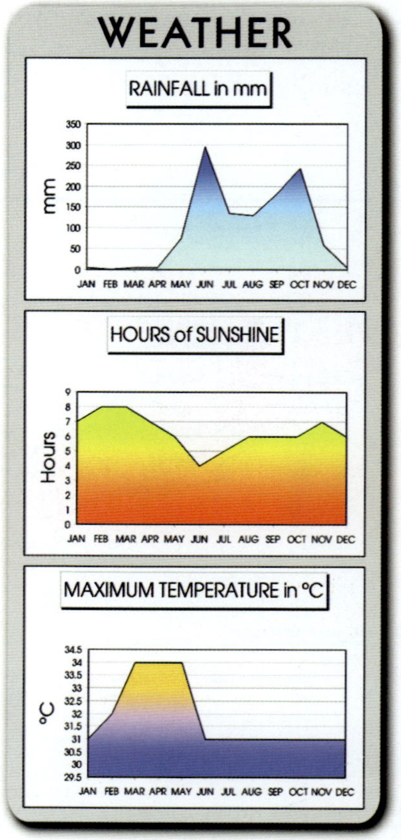

NIGER

General Advice

Immunization Advice

- ❑ Immunizations recommended for life should be up to date, especially those for children and boosters of tetanus for adults.
- ❑ Courses or boosters of diphtheria, hepatitis A, poliomyelitis, typhoid, and yellow fever are usually advised.
- ❑ Vaccines sometimes advised are: BCG, cholera, hepatitis B, meningococcal A and C, rabies.
- ❑ A yellow fever certificate is mandatory as a condition of entry for all travelers aged over 1 year and is recommended for those leaving Niger.

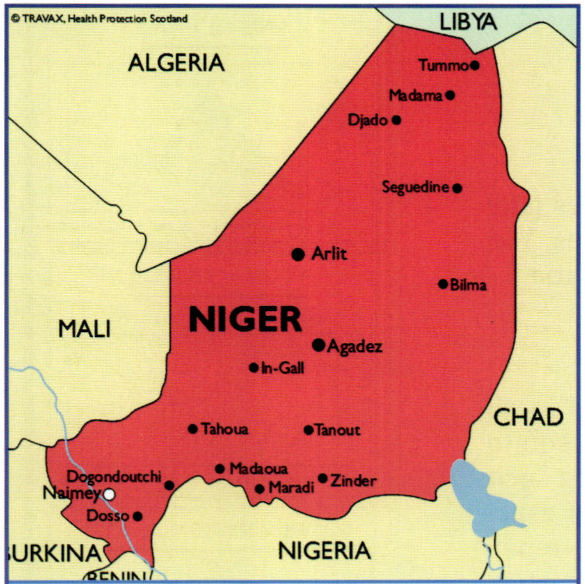

High risk antimalarials usually advised

Surrounding countries with malaria risk

This map is only intended as a guide since mosquitoes do not respect boundaries and the risk areas shown may not be exact. **Reproduced with permission from Fitfortravel, Health Protection Scotland's Travel website www.fitfortravel.nhs.uk.**

Malaria Advice

- ❑ Malaria is a serious and sometimes fatal disease transmitted by mosquitoes. You cannot be vaccinated against malaria.

MALARIA PRECAUTIONS

- ❑ Malaria precautions are essential in all areas all year round. Avoid mosquito bites by covering up with clothing such as long sleeves and long trousers especially after sunset, using insect repellents on exposed skin and, when necessary, sleeping under a mosquito net.
- ❑ Check with your doctor or nurse about suitable antimalarial tablets.
- ❑ Prompt investigation of fever is essential.

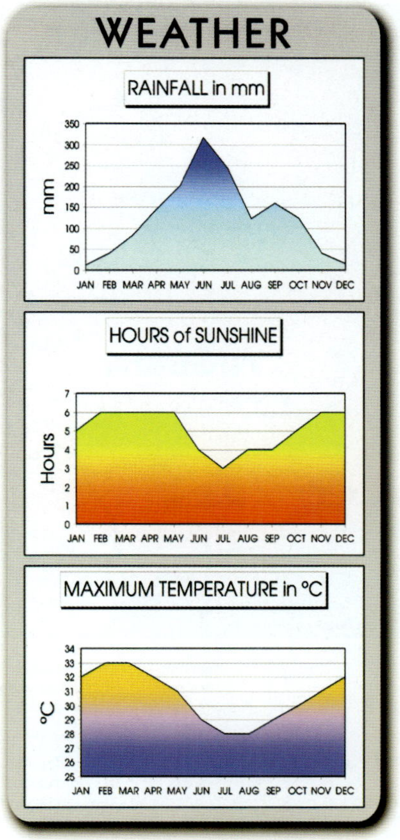

NIGERIA

General Advice

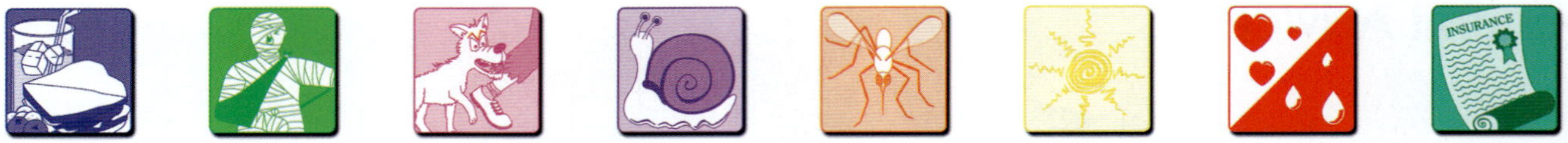

Immunization Advice

- ❑ Immunizations recommended for life should be up to date, especially those for children and boosters of tetanus for adults.

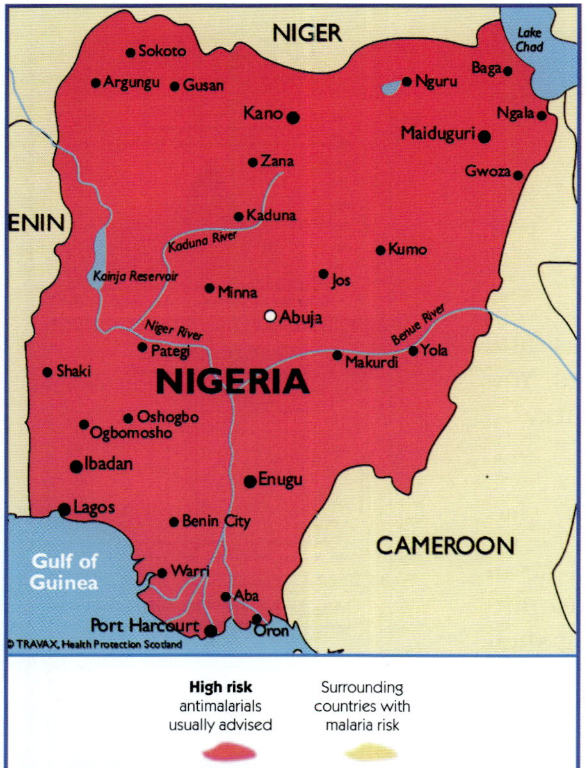

This map is only intended as a guide since mosquitoes do not respect boundaries and the risk areas shown may not be exact. **Reproduced with permission from Fitfortravel, Health Protection Scotland's Travel website www.fitfortravel.nhs.uk.**

- ❑ Courses or boosters of diphtheria, hepatitis A, poliomyelitis, typhoid, and yellow fever are usually advised.
- ❑ Vaccines sometimes advised are: BCG, cholera, hepatitis B, meningococcal A and C, rabies.
- ❑ A yellow fever certificate is required if aged over 1 year old and entering from an infected country.

Malaria Advice

- ❑ Malaria is a serious and sometimes fatal disease transmitted by mosquitoes. You cannot be vaccinated against malaria.

MALARIA PRECAUTIONS

- ❑ Malaria precautions are essential in all areas all year round. Avoid mosquito bites by covering up with clothing such as long sleeves and long trousers especially after sunset, using insect repellents on exposed skin and, when necessary, sleeping under a mosquito net.
- ❑ Check with your doctor or nurse about suitable antimalarial tablets.
- ❑ Prompt investigation of fever is essential.

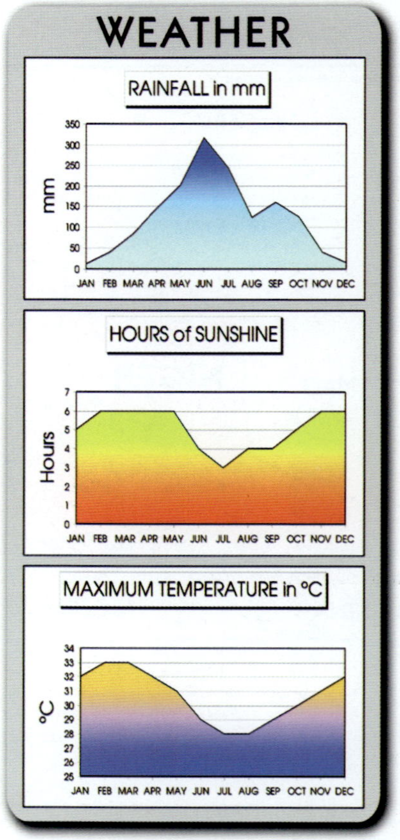

NORWAY

General Advice

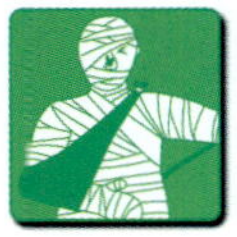

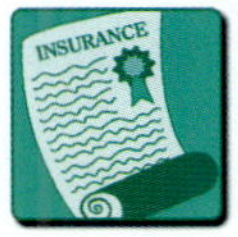

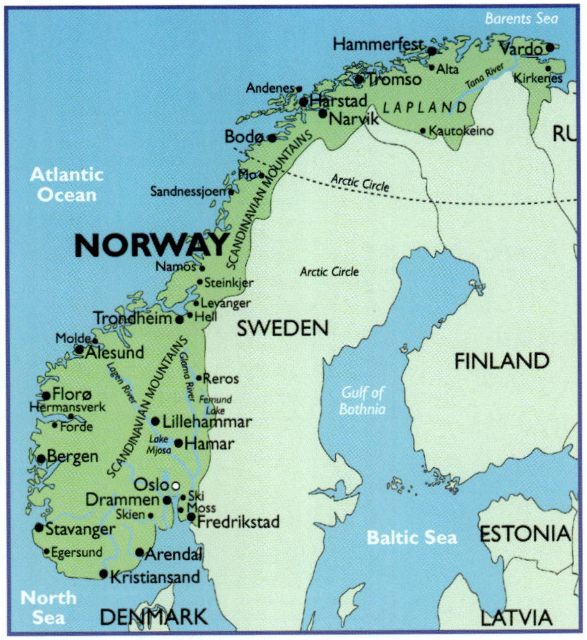

Immunization Advice

- ❑ Immunizations recommended for life should be up to date, especially those for children.
- ❑ Vaccines sometimes advised are: tick-borne encephalitis.
- ❑ Rabies is not normally present but any animal or bat bite must be carefully assessed.
- ❑ No certificate of vaccination for yellow fever is required.

Malaria Advice

- ❑ Malaria is not normally present.

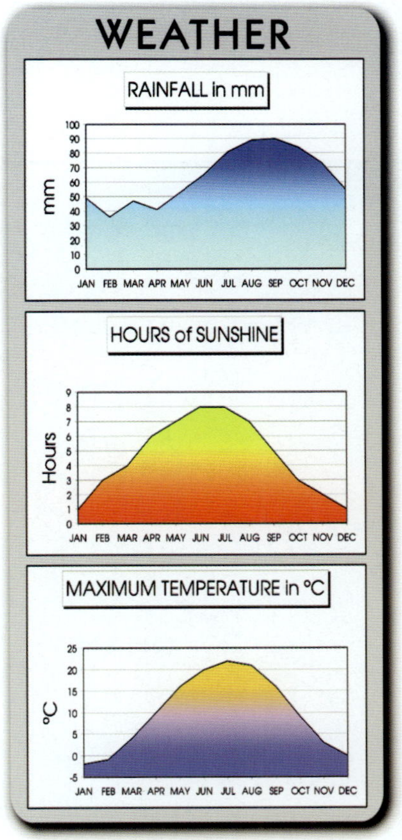

OMAN

General Advice

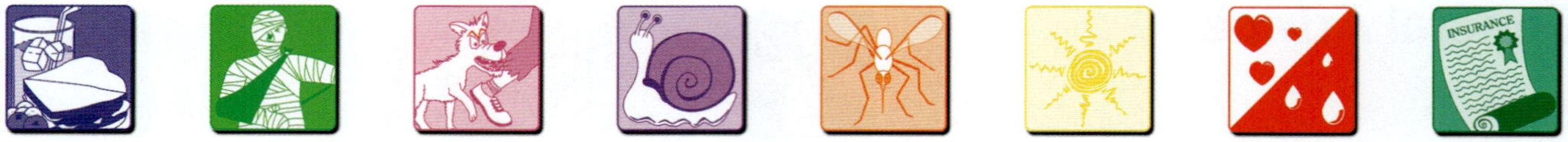

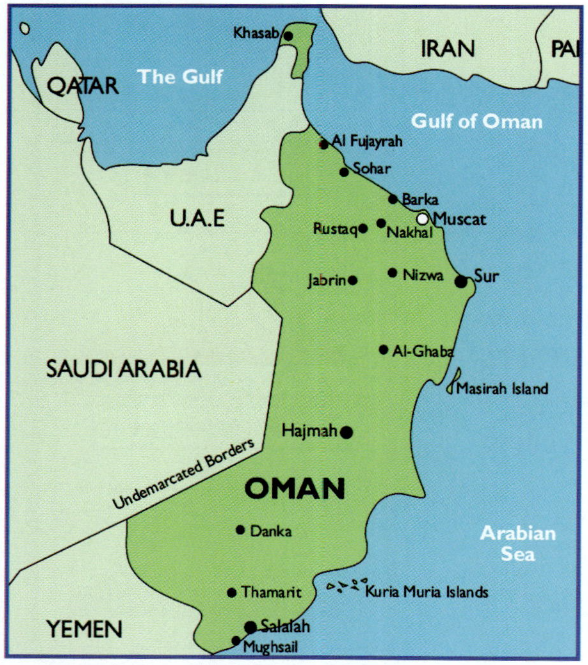

Immunization Advice

- ❑ Immunizations recommended for life should be up to date, especially those for children and boosters of tetanus for adults.
- ❑ Courses or boosters of hepatitis A are usually advised.
- ❑ Vaccines sometimes advised are: hepatitis B, rabies, typhoid.
- ❑ A yellow fever certificate is required if entering from an infected country.

Malaria Advice

- ❑ Malaria is not normally present.

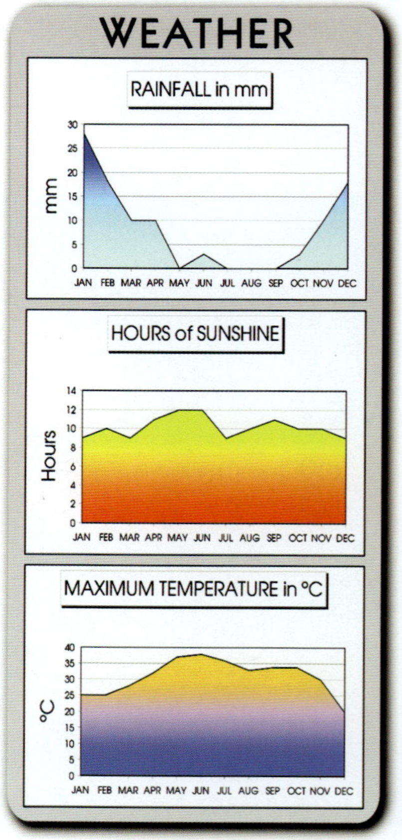

PAKISTAN

General Advice

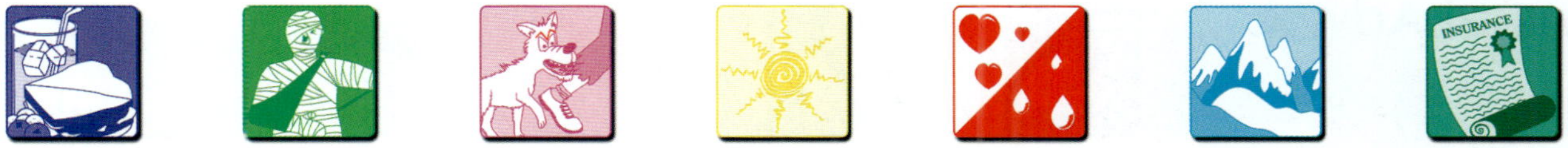

Immunization Advice

- ❑ Immunizations recommended for life should be up to date, especially those for children and boosters of tetanus for adults.

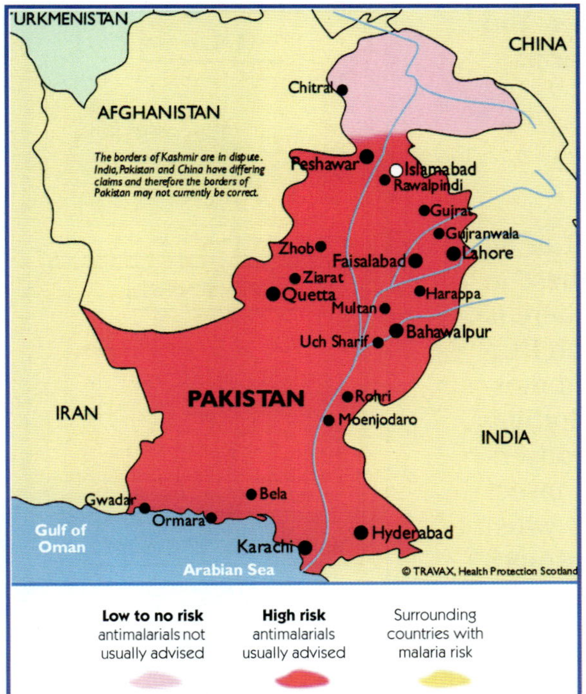

This map is only intended as a guide since mosquitoes do not respect boundaries and the risk areas shown may not be exact. **Reproduced with permission from Fitfortravel, Health Protection Scotland's Travel website www.fitfortravel.nhs.uk.**

- ❑ Courses or boosters of diphtheria, hepatitis A, poliomyelitis, and typhoid are usually advised.
- ❑ Vaccines sometimes advised are: BCG, cholera, hepatitis B, Japanese encephalitis, rabies.
- ❑ A yellow fever certificate is required if entering from an infected country (infants under 6 months of age are exempt if their mother's vaccination certificate shows that she was vaccinated before the birth of the child).

Malaria Advice

- ❑ Malaria is a serious and sometimes fatal disease transmitted by mosquitoes. You cannot be vaccinated against malaria.

MALARIA PRECAUTIONS

- ❑ Malaria precautions are essential in all areas below 2000 m all year round. Avoid mosquito bites by covering up with clothing such as long sleeves and long trousers especially after sunset, using insect repellents on exposed skin and, when necessary, sleeping under a mosquito net.
- ❑ Check with your doctor or nurse about suitable antimalarial tablets.
- ❑ Prompt investigation of fever is essential.

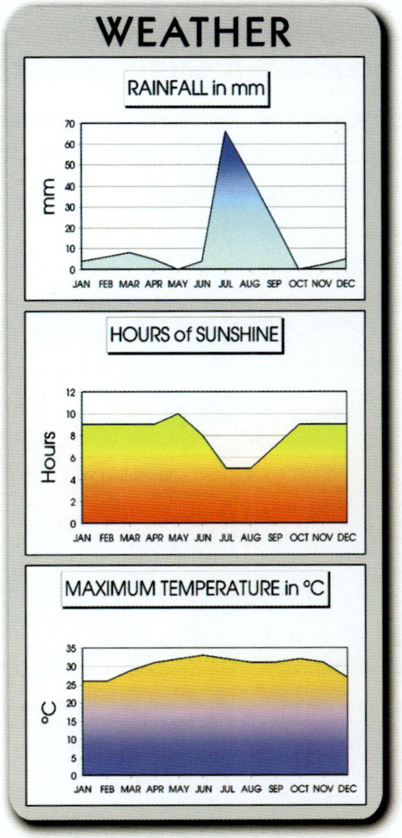

—Weather in Karachi—

PANAMA

General Advice

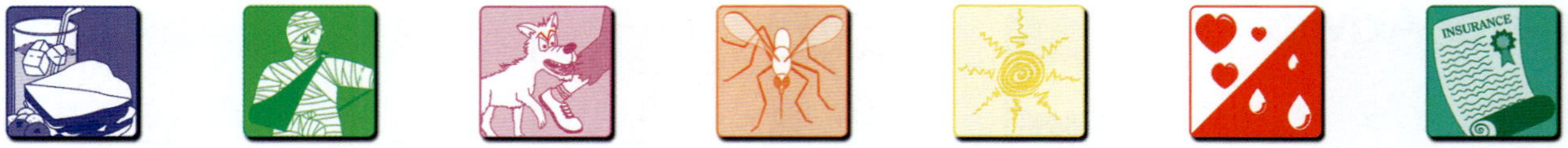

Immunization Advice

- ❑ Immunizations recommended for life should be up to date, especially those for children and boosters of tetanus for adults.
- ❑ Courses or boosters of hepatitis A and typhoid are usually advised.
- ❑ Vaccines sometimes advised are: BCG, hepatitis B, rabies, yellow fever (see yellow fever map).
- ❑ A yellow fever certificate is required if entering from an infected country.

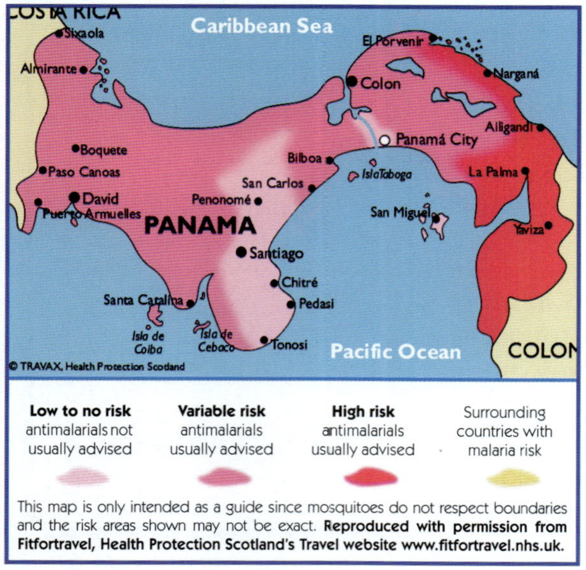

Malaria Advice

- ❑ Malaria is a serious and sometimes fatal disease transmitted by mosquitoes. You cannot be vaccinated against malaria.

MALARIA PRECAUTIONS

- ❑ Malaria precautions are essential in all areas all year round. Risk is highest in Darien and San Blas provinces. There is low to no risk in the Canal Zone and Panama City (see malaria map). Avoid mosquito bites by covering up with clothing such as long sleeves and long trousers especially after sunset, using insect repellents on exposed skin and, when necessary, sleeping under a mosquito net.
- ❑ Check with your doctor or nurse about suitable antimalarial tablets.
- ❑ Prompt investigation of fever is essential.

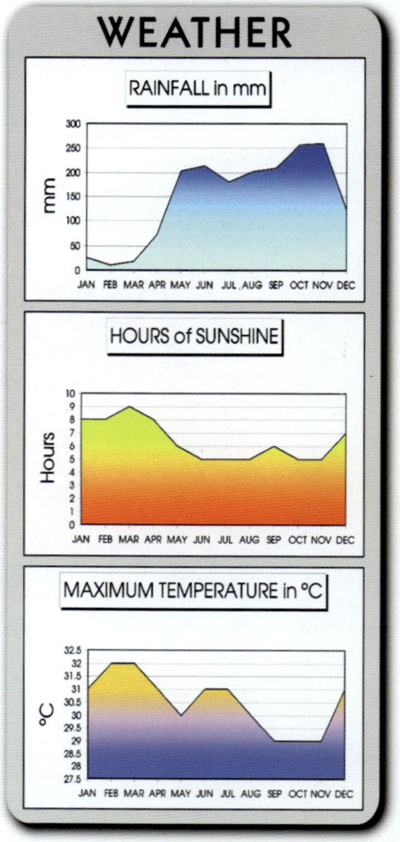

PAPUA NEW GUINEA

General Advice

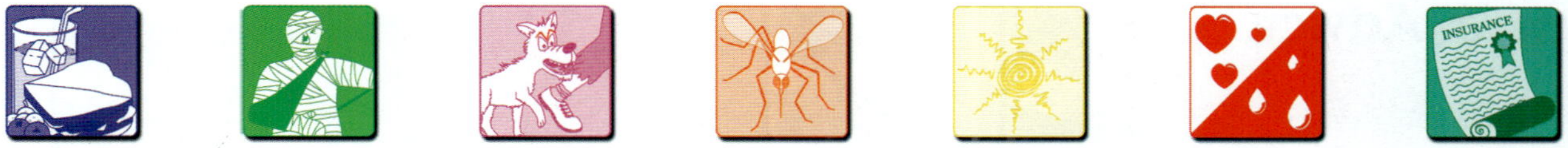

Immunization Advice

- ❑ Immunizations recommended for life should be up to date, especially those for children and boosters of tetanus for adults.
- ❑ Courses or boosters of diphtheria, hepatitis A, and typhoid are usually advised.
- ❑ Vaccines sometimes advised are: BCG, cholera, hepatitis B, Japanese encephalitis, rabies.
- ❑ A yellow fever certificate is required if aged over 1 year old and entering from an infected country.

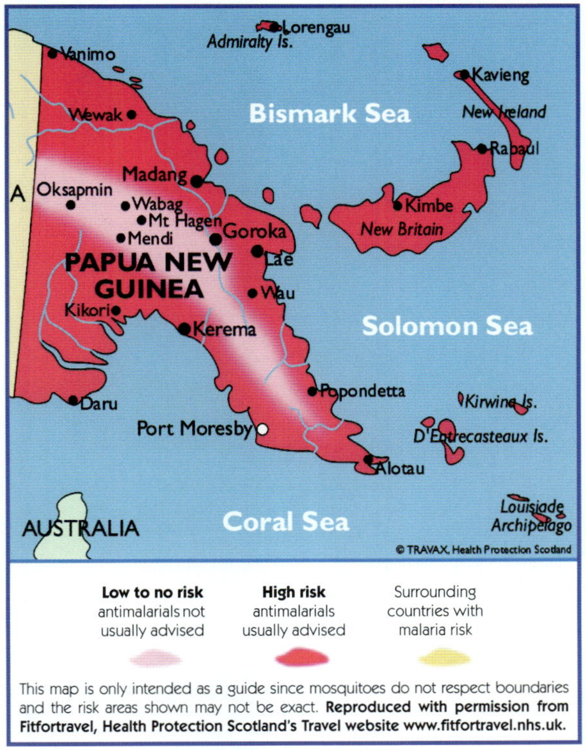

Malaria Advice

- ❑ Malaria is a serious and sometimes fatal disease transmitted by mosquitoes. You cannot be vaccinated against malaria.

MALARIA PRECAUTION

- ❑ Malaria precautions are essential in all areas below 1800 m all year round. Avoid mosquito bites by covering up with clothing such as long sleeves and long trousers especially after sunset, using insect repellents on exposed skin and, when necessary, sleeping under a mosquito net.
- ❑ Check with your doctor or nurse about suitable antimalarial tablets.
- ❑ Prompt investigation of fever is essential.

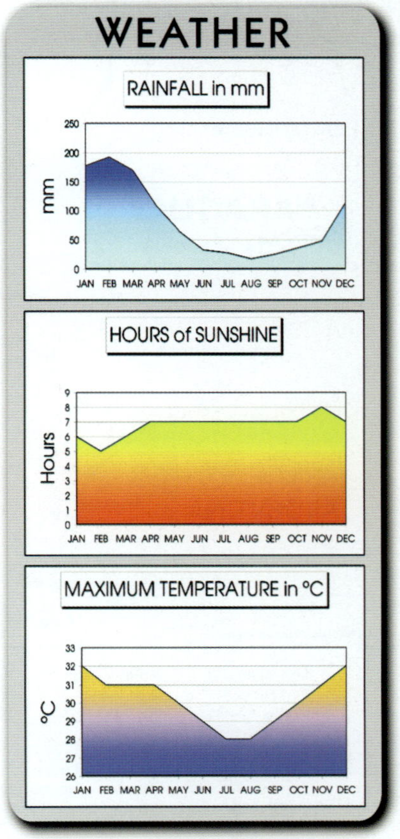

PARAGUAY

General Advice

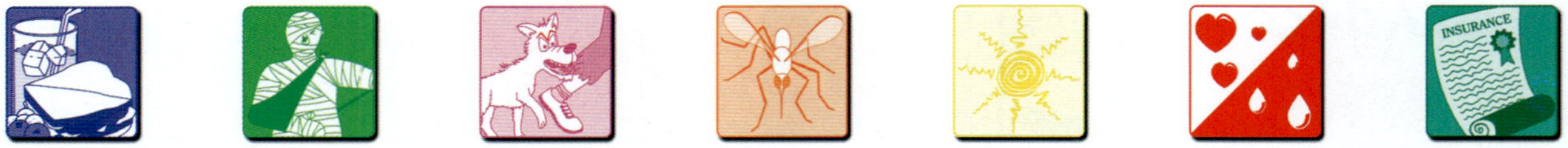

Immunization Advice

- ❑ Immunizations recommended for life should be up to date, especially those for children and boosters of tetanus for adults.

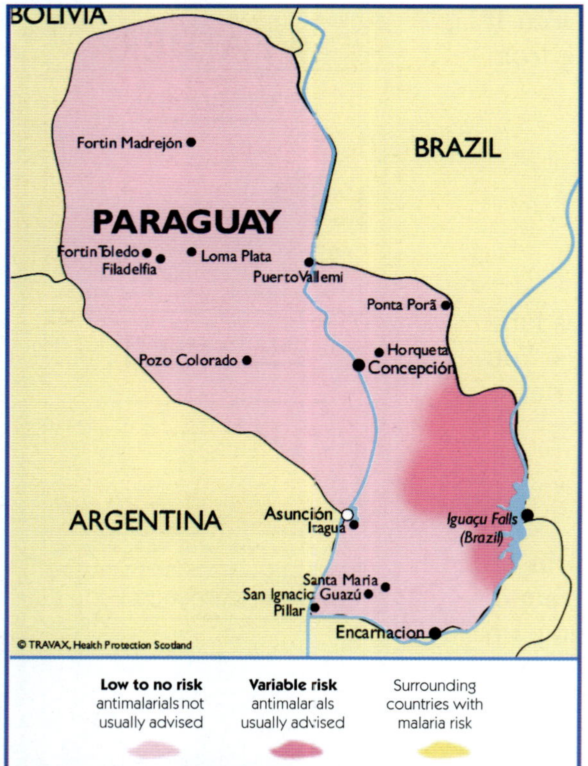

This map is only intended as a guide since mosquitoes do not respect boundaries and the risk areas shown may not be exact. **Reproduced with permission from Fitfortravel, Health Protection Scotland's Travel website www.fitfortravel.nhs.uk.**

- ❑ Courses or boosters of diphtheria, hepatitis A, and yellow fever are usually advised.
- ❑ Vaccines sometimes advised are: BCG, hepatitis B, rabies, typhoid.
- ❑ A yellow fever certificate is required if aged over 1 year old and entering from an infected country.

Malaria Advice

- ❑ Malaria is a serious and sometimes fatal disease transmitted by mosquitoes. You cannot be vaccinated against malaria.

MALARIA PRECAUTIONS

- ❑ Malaria precautions are essential in Alto Parana, Caaguaza, and Canindeyu departments, all year round. The risk is less in other areas. Avoid mosquito bites by covering up with clothing such as long sleeves and long trousers especially after sunset, using insect repellents on exposed skin and, when necessary, sleeping under a mosquito net.
- ❑ Check with your doctor or nurse about suitable antimalarial tablets.
- ❑ Prompt investigation of fever is essential.

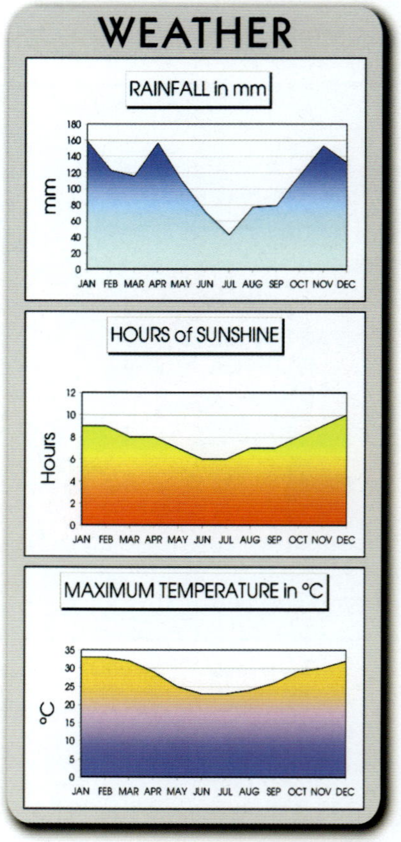

PERU

General Advice

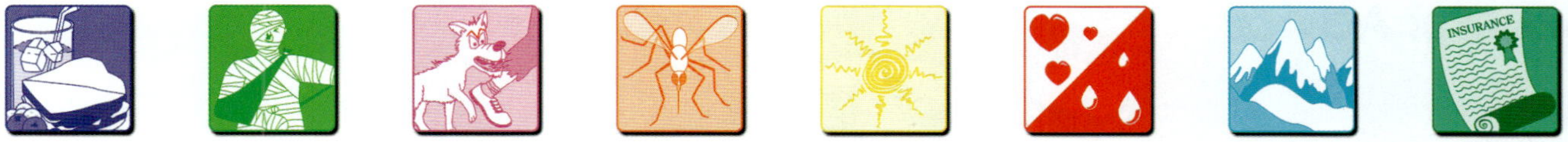

Immunization Advice

- ❑ Immunizations recommended for life should be up to date, especially those for children and boosters of tetanus for adults.
- ❑ Courses or boosters of hepatitis A and typhoid are usually advised.
- ❑ Vaccines sometimes advised are: BCG, hepatitis B, rabies, yellow fever (see yellow fever map).
- ❑ No certificate of vaccination for yellow fever is required.

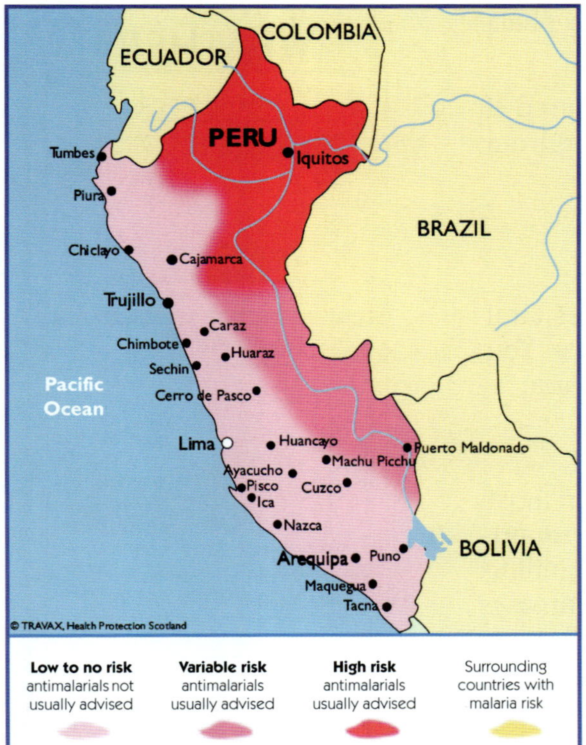

This map is only intended as a guide since mosquitoes do not respect boundaries and the risk areas shown may not be exact. **Reproduced with permission from Fitfortravel, Health Protection Scotland's Travel website www.fitfortravel.nhs.uk.**

Malaria Advice

- ❑ Malaria is a serious and sometimes fatal disease transmitted by mosquitoes. You cannot be vaccinated against malaria.

MALARIA PRECAUTIONS

- ❑ Malaria precautions are essential in most areas below 2000 m. The risk is highest in the Amazon basin and especially in Loreto district. Risk is lower in other areas and low to no risk west of the Andes. There is no risk at altitude and along the Inca trail including Cuzco, Maccu Piccu, and Lake Titicaca (see map). Avoid mosquito bites by covering up with clothing such as long sleeves and long trousers especially after sunset, using insect repellents on exposed skin and, when necessary, sleeping under a mosquito net.
- ❑ Check with your doctor or nurse about suitable antimalarial tablets.
- ❑ Prompt investigation of fever is essential.

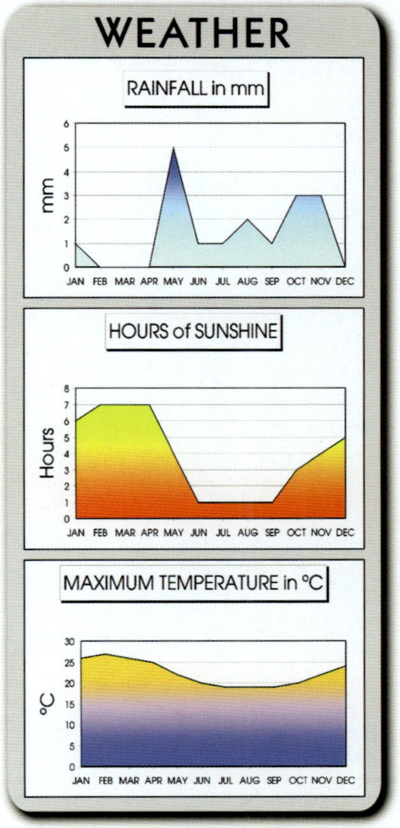

PHILIPPINES

General Advice

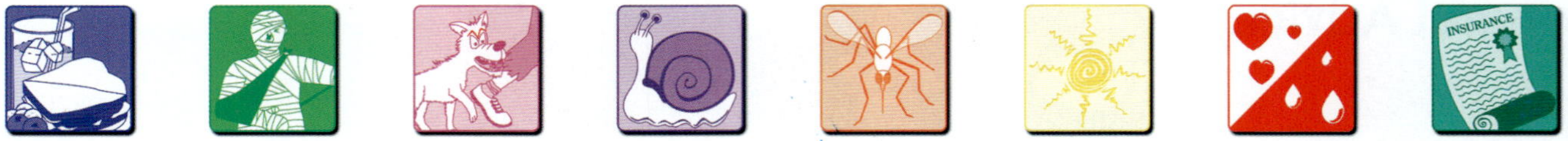

Immunization Advice

- ❑ Immunizations recommended for life should be up to date, especially those for children and boosters of tetanus for adults.
- ❑ Courses or boosters of diphtheria, hepatitis A, and typhoid are usually advised.
- ❑ Vaccines sometimes advised are: BCG, cholera, hepatitis B, Japanese encephalitis, rabies.
- ❑ A yellow fever certificate is required if aged over 1 year old and entering from an infected country.

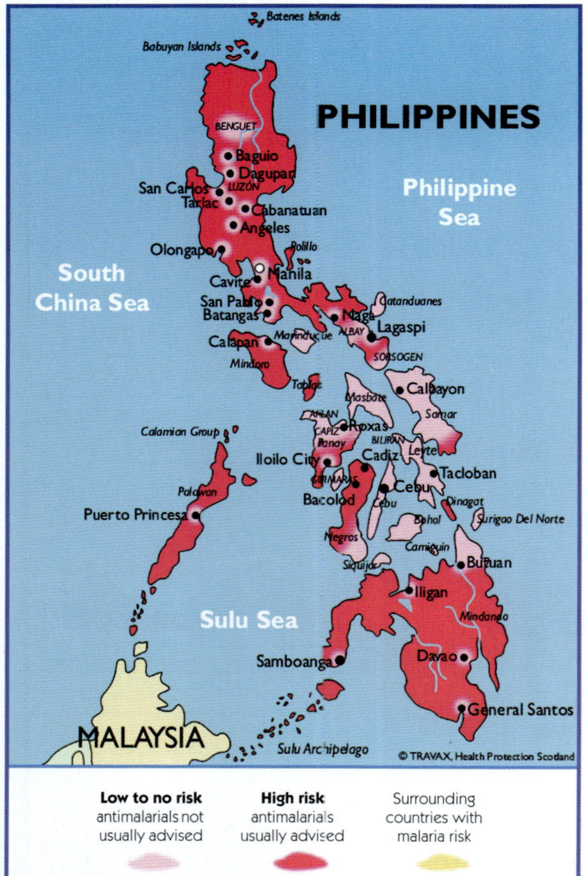

This map is only intended as a guide since mosquitoes do not respect boundaries and the risk areas shown may not be exact. **Reproduced with permission from Fitfortravel, Health Protection Scotland's Travel website www.fitfortravel.nhs.uk.**

Malaria Advice

- ❑ Malaria is a serious and sometimes fatal disease transmitted by mosquitoes. You cannot be vaccinated against malaria.

MALARIA PRECAUTIONS

- ❑ Malaria precautions are essential in most rural areas below 600 m all year round. There is no risk in urban areas including Manila (see malaria map for risk areas). Avoid mosquito bites by covering up with clothing such as long sleeves and long trousers especially after sunset, using insect repellents on exposed skin and, when necessary, sleeping under a mosquito net.
- ❑ Check with your doctor or nurse about suitable antimalarial tablets.
- ❑ Prompt investigation of fever is essential.

WEATHER

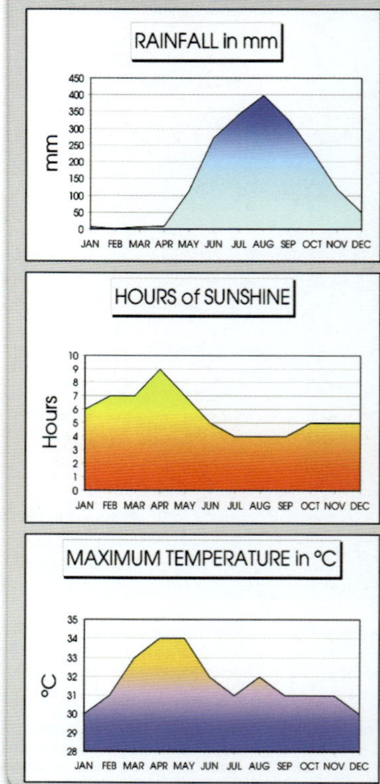

POLAND

General Advice

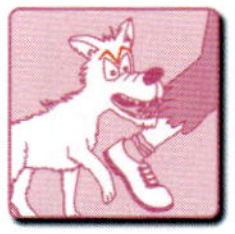

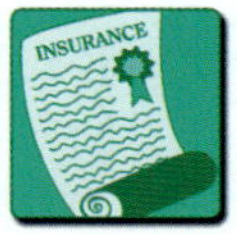

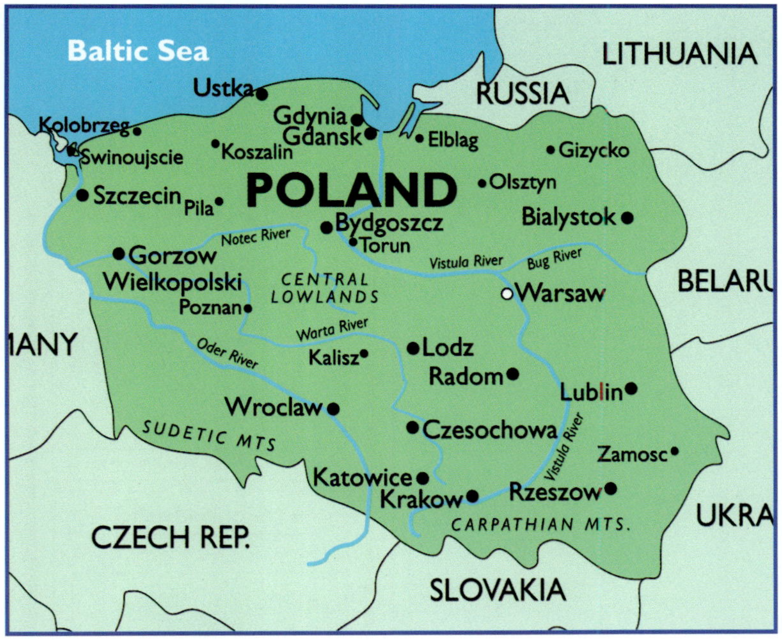

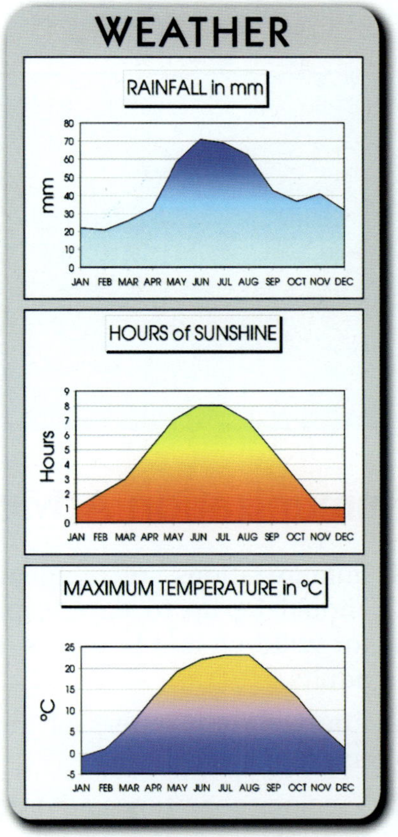

Immunization Advice

- Immunizations recommended for life should be up to date, especially those for children and boosters of tetanus for adults.
- Vaccines sometimes advised are: hepatitis A, hepatitis B, rabies, tick-borne encephalitis.
- No certificate of vaccination for yellow fever is required.

Malaria Advice

- Malaria is not normally present.

PUERTO RICO

General Advice

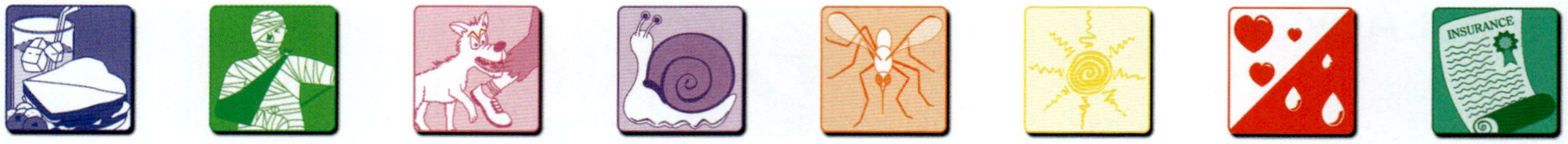

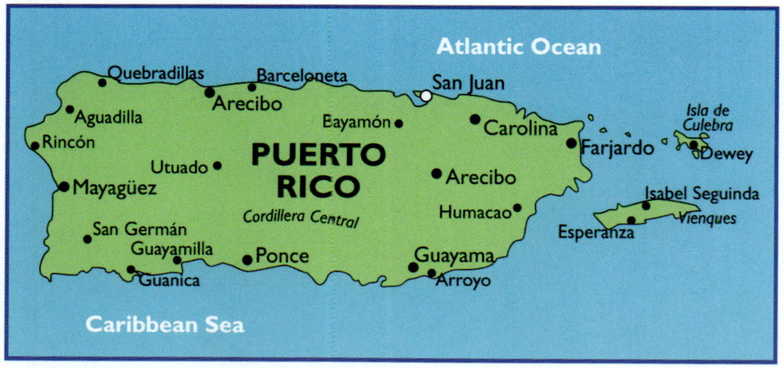

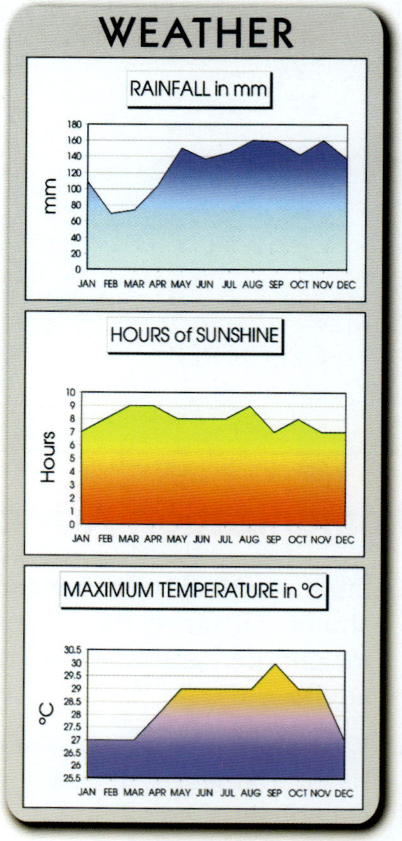

Immunization Advice

- ❑ Immunizations recommended for life should be up to date, especially those for children and boosters of tetanus for adults.
- ❑ Courses or boosters of hepatitis A are usually advised.
- ❑ Vaccines sometimes advised are: hepatitis B, rabies.
- ❑ No certificate of vaccination for yellow fever is required.

Malaria Advice

- ❑ Malaria is not normally present.

QATAR

General Advice

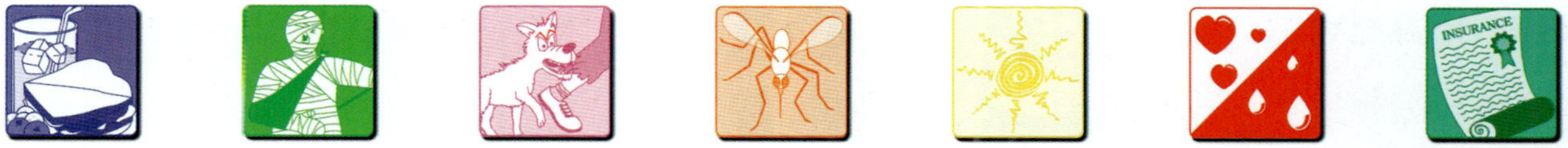

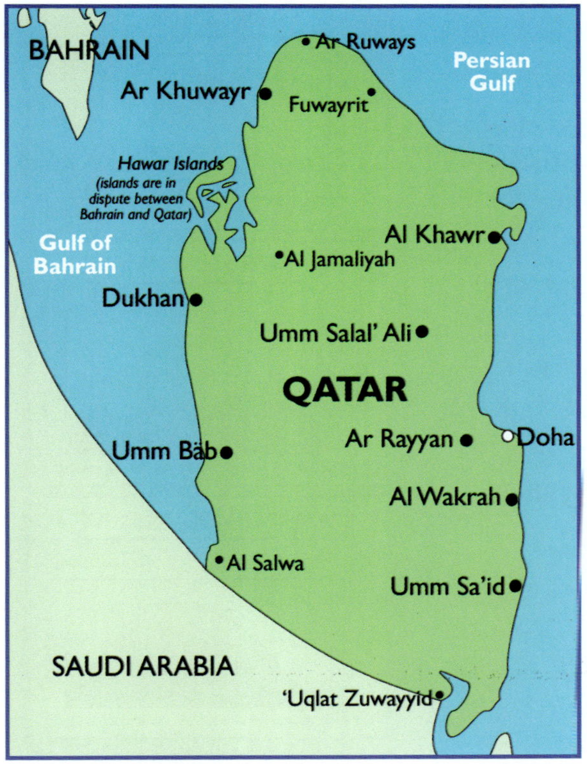

Immunization Advice

- ❑ Immunizations recommended for life should be up to date, especially those for children and boosters of tetanus for adults.
- ❑ Courses or boosters of hepatitis A are usually advised. Vaccines sometimes advised are: BCG, hepatitis B, rabies, typhoid.
- ❑ No certificate of vaccination for yellow fever is required.

Malaria Advice

- ❑ Malaria is not normally present.

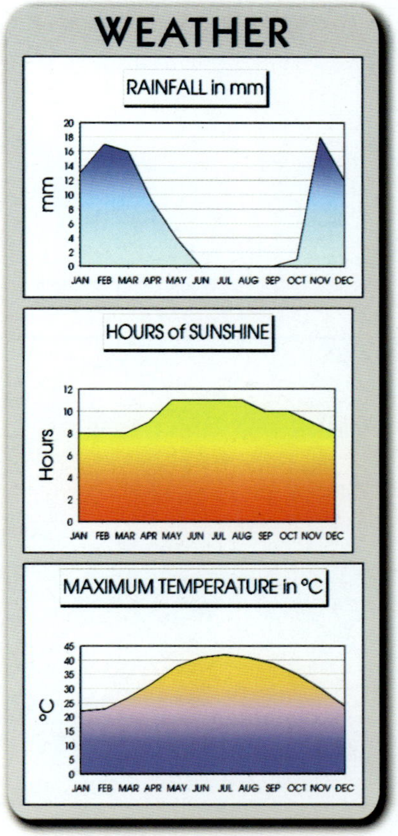

ROMANIA

General Advice

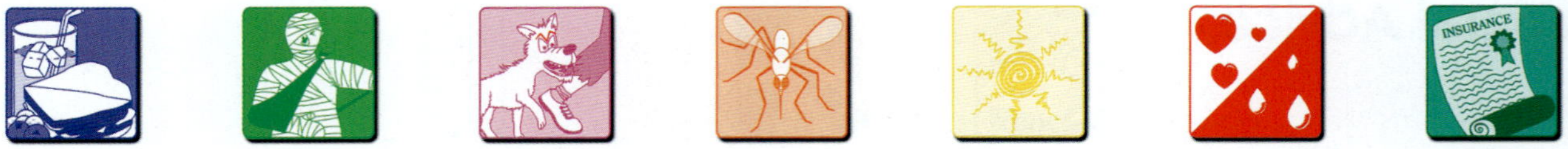

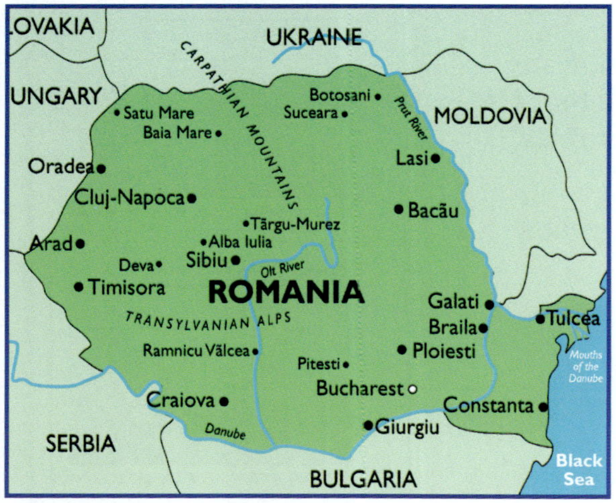

Immunization Advice

- ❑ Immunizations recommended for life should be up to date, especially those for children and boosters of tetanus for adults.
- ❑ Courses or boosters of hepatitis A are usually advised.
- ❑ Vaccines sometimes advised are: BCG, hepatitis B, rabies, tick-borne encephalitis, typhoid.
- ❑ No certificate of vaccination for yellow fever is required.

Malaria Advice

- ❑ Malaria is not normally present.

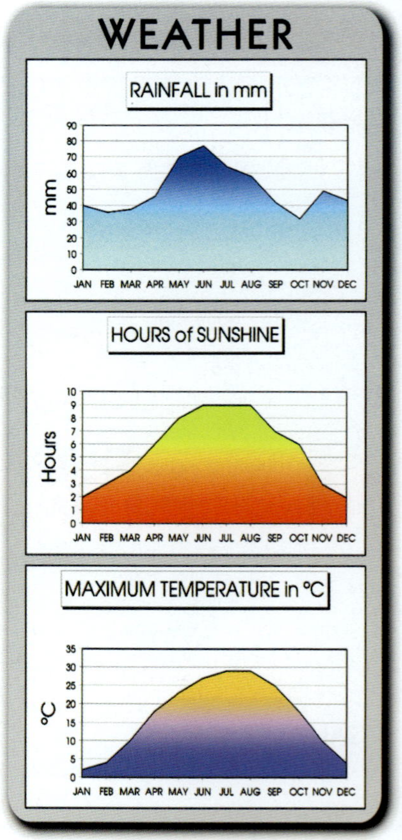

RUSSIAN FEDERATION

General Advice

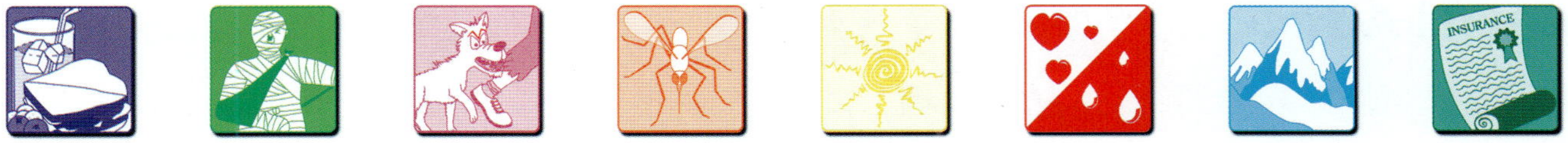

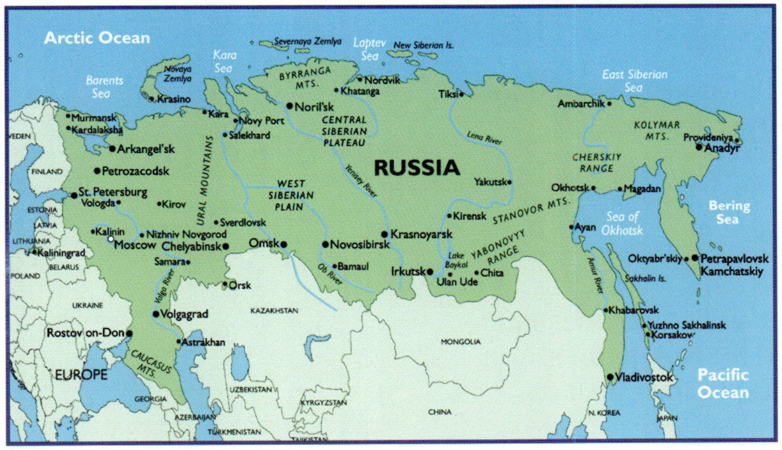

Immunization Advice

- ❑ Immunizations recommended for life should be up to date, especially those for children and boosters of tetanus for adults.
- ❑ Courses or boosters of diphtheria, hepatitis A, and poliomyelitis are usually advised.
- ❑ Vaccines sometimes advised are: BCG, hepatitis B, Japanese encephalitis (only in very far east Siberia close to the Chinese border), rabies, tick-borne encephalitis, typhoid.
- ❑ A yellow fever certificate is required if aged over 9 months old and entering from an infected country.

Malaria Advice

- ❑ Malaria is not normally present.

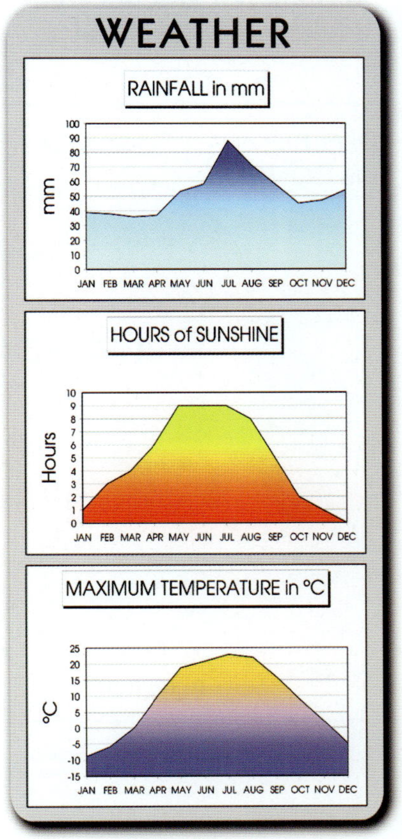

—Weather in Moscow

RWANDA

General Advice

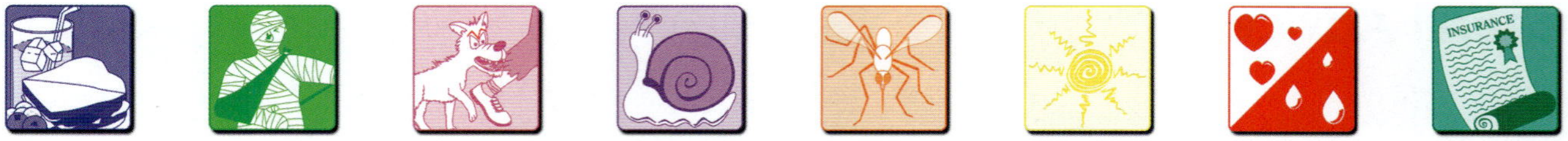

Immunization Advice

- ❑ Immunizations recommended for life should be up to date, especially those for children and boosters of tetanus for adults.

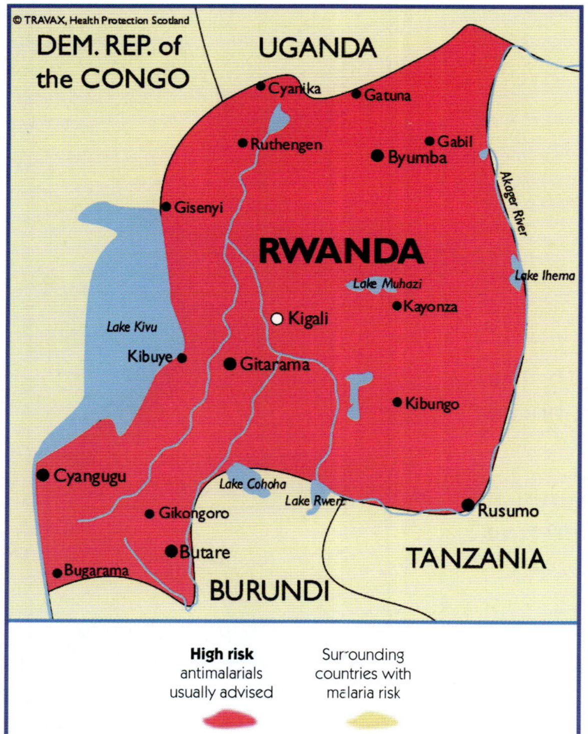

This map is only intended as a guide since mosquitoes do not respect boundaries and the risk areas shown may not be exact. **Reproduced with permission from Fitfortravel, Health Protection Scotland's Travel website www.fitfortravel.nhs.uk.**

- ❑ Courses or boosters of hepatitis A, poliomyelitis, typhoid, and yellow fever are usually advised.
- ❑ Vaccines sometimes advised are: BCG, cholera, hepatitis B, rabies.
- ❑ A yellow fever certificate is required for all travellers aged over 1 year.

Malaria Advice

- ❑ Malaria is a serious and sometimes fatal disease transmitted by mosquitoes. You cannot be vaccinated against malaria.

MALARIA PRECAUTIONS

- ❑ Malaria precautions are essential in all areas all year round. Avoid mosquito bites by covering up with clothing such as long sleeves and long trousers especially after sunset, using insect repellents on exposed skin and, when necessary, sleeping under a mosquito net.
- ❑ Check with your doctor or nurse about suitable antimalarial tablets.
- ❑ Prompt investigation of fever is essential.

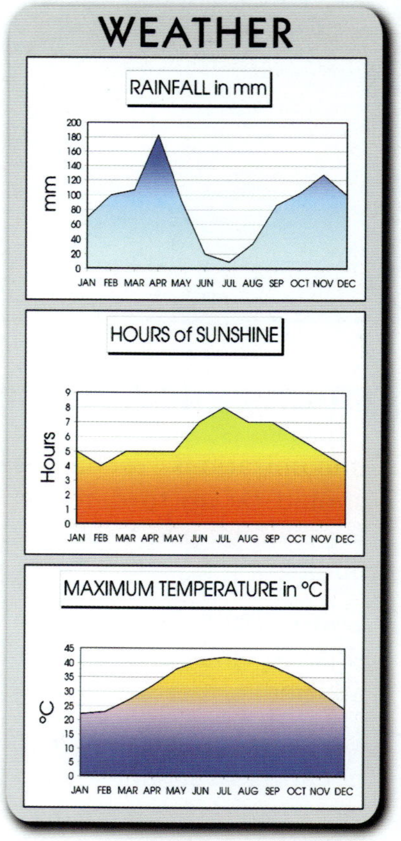

SAINT KITTS and NEVIS

General Advice

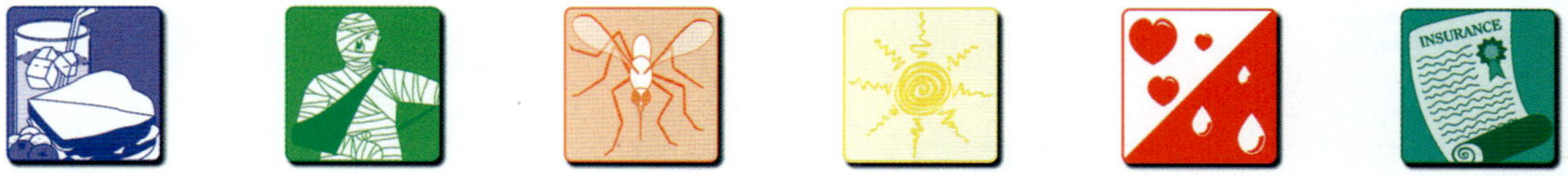

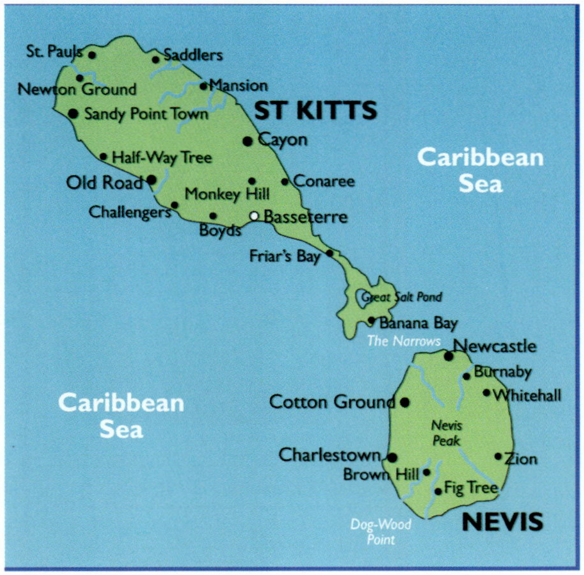

Immunization Advice

- ❑ Immunizations recommended for life should be up to date, especially those for children and boosters of tetanus for adults.
- ❑ Vaccines sometimes advised are: hepatitis A, hepatitis B.
- ❑ A yellow fever certificate is required if aged over 1 year old and entering from an infected country.

Malaria Advice

- ❑ Malaria is not normally present.

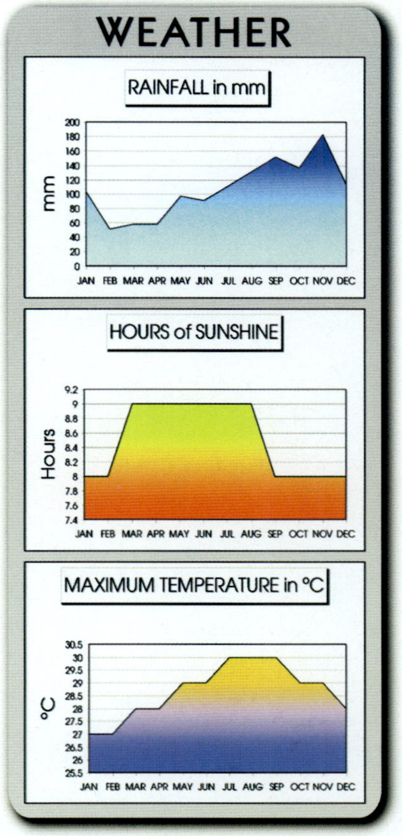

SAINT LUCIA

General Advice

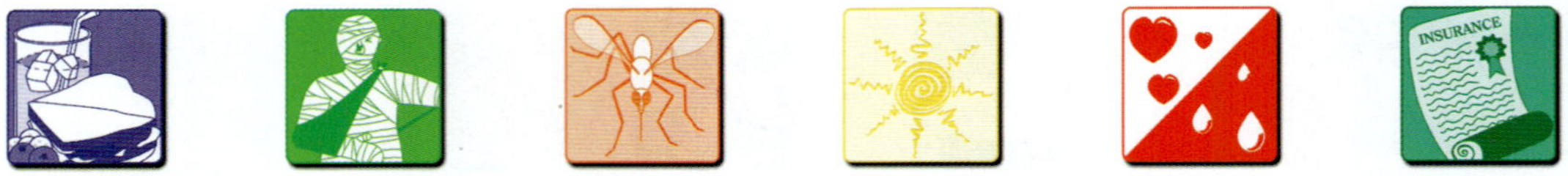

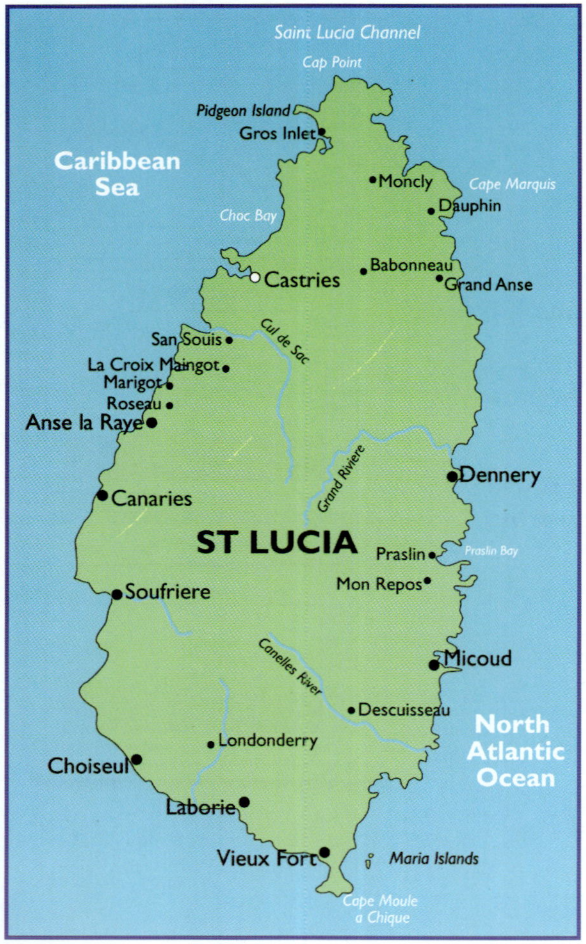

Immunization Advice

- ❑ Immunizations recommended for life should be up to date, especially those for children and boosters of tetanus for adults.
- ❑ Vaccines sometimes advised are: hepatitis A, hepatitis B.
- ❑ A yellow fever certificate is required if aged over 1 year old and entering from an infected country.

Malaria Advice

- ❑ Malaria is not normally present.

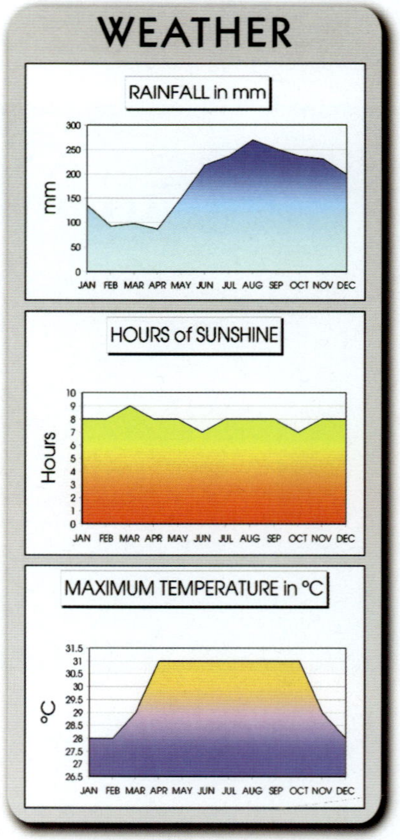

SAUDI ARABIA

General Advice

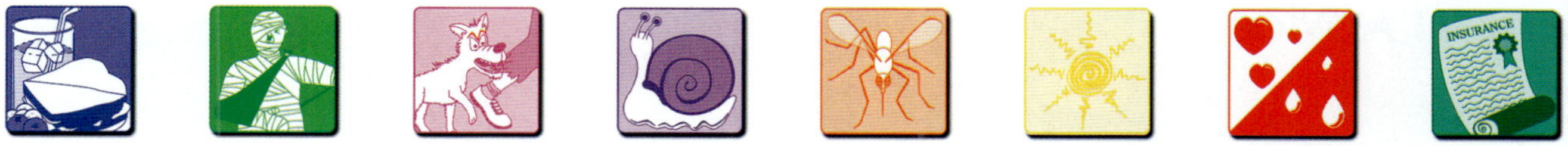

Immunization Advice

❑ Immunizations recommended for life should be up to date, especially those for children and boosters of tetanus for adults.

❑ Courses or boosters of diphtheria and hepatitis A are usually advised.

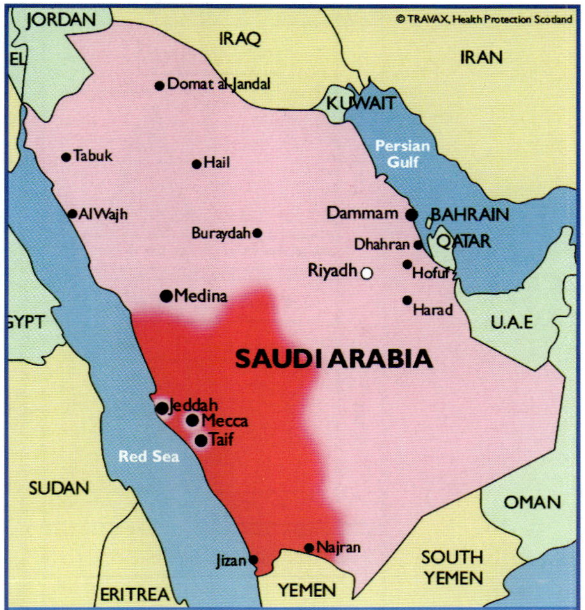

Low to no risk antimalarials not usually advised | **High risk** antimalarials usually advised | Surrounding countries with malaria risk

This map is only intended as a guide since mosquitoes do not respect boundaries and the risk areas shown may not be exact. **Reproduced with permission from Fitfortravel, Health Protection Scotland's Travel website www.fitfortravel.nhs.uk.**

❑ Vaccines sometimes advised are: BCG, hepatitis B, influenza*, meningococcal ACWY†; rabies; typhoid.

*Influenza should be considered for the Hajj especially for those at higher risk of serious complications. The Saudi Arabian Ministry of Health may request proof of vaccination in some circumstances.

†Quadravalent meningococcal (ACWY) vaccine is required by all travellers to the Hajj, or for seasonal work in the Hajj area or arrivals from the African meningitis belt. The Saudi Arabian Ministry of Health will request proof of vaccination.

❑ A yellow fever certificate is required if entering from an infected country.

❑ Check with an online resource for the most up to date advice for travelers to the Hajj.

Malaria Advice

❑ Malaria is a serious and sometimes fatal disease transmitted by mosquitoes. You cannot be vaccinated against malaria.

MALARIA PRECAUTIONS

❑ Malaria precautions are essential in most of the south western region (except in the high altitude areas of Asir Province and the cities of Mecca, Medina, Jeddah, and Taif), all year round. Avoid mosquito bites by covering up with clothing such as long sleeves and long trousers especially after sunset, using insect repellents on exposed skin and, when necessary, sleeping under a mosquito net.

❑ Check with your doctor or nurse about suitable anti-malarial tablets.

❑ Prompt investigation of fever is essential.

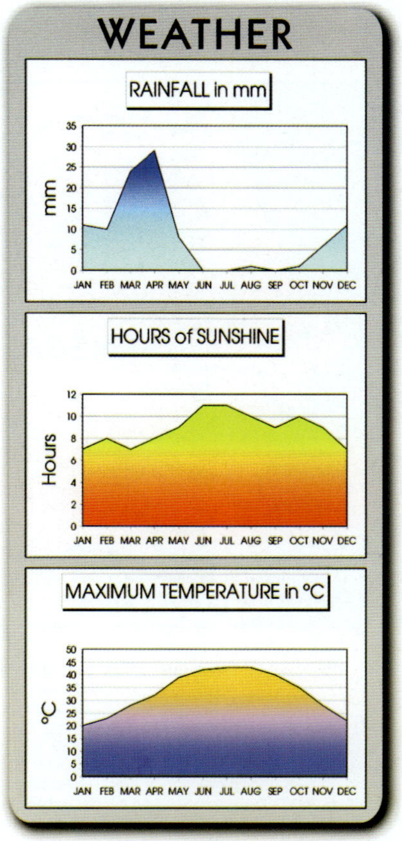

SENEGAL

General Advice

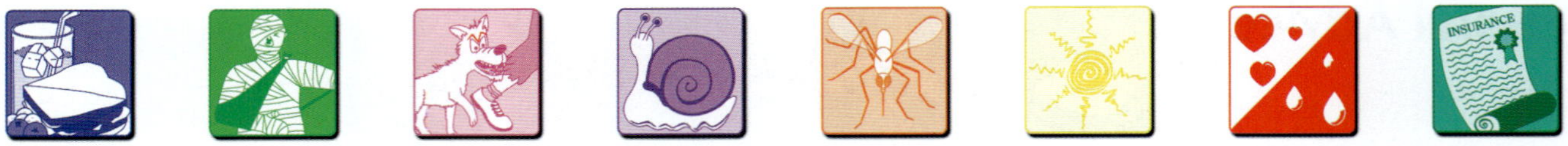

Immunization Advice

- ❑ Immunizations recommended for life should be up to date, especially those for children and boosters of tetanus for adults.

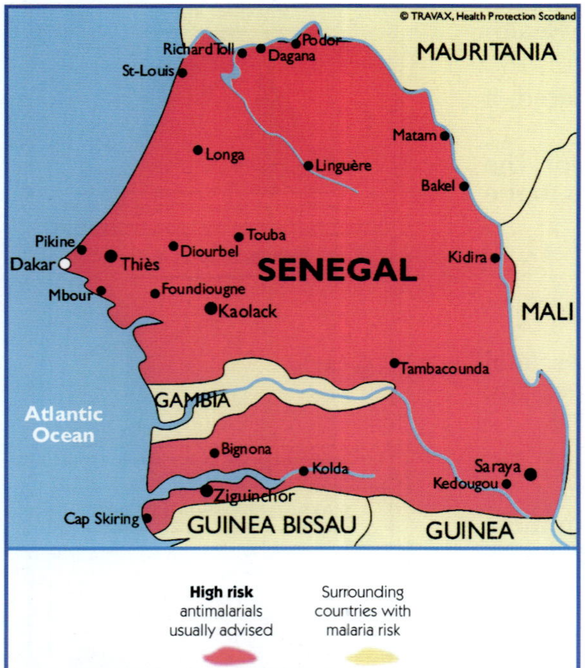

This map is only intended as a guide since mosquitoes do not respect boundaries and the risk areas shown may not be exact. **Reproduced with permission from Fitfortravel, Health Protection Scotland's Travel website www.fitfortravel.nhs.uk.**

- ❑ Courses or boosters of diphtheria, hepatitis A, poliomyelitis, typhoid, and yellow fever are usually advised.
- ❑ Vaccines sometimes advised for: BCG, cholera, hepatitis B, meningococcal A and C, rabies.
- ❑ A yellow fever certificate is required if aged over 9 months old and entering from an infected country.

Malaria Advice

- ❑ Malaria is a serious and sometimes fatal disease transmitted by mosquitoes. You cannot be vaccinated against malaria.

MALARIA PRECAUTIONS

- ❑ Malaria precautions are essential in all areas all year round. Avoid mosquito bites by covering up with clothing such as long sleeves and long trousers especially after sunset, using insect repellents on exposed skin and, when necessary, sleeping under a mosquito net.
- ❑ Check with your doctor or nurse about suitable antimalarial tablets.
- ❑ Prompt investigation of fever is essential.

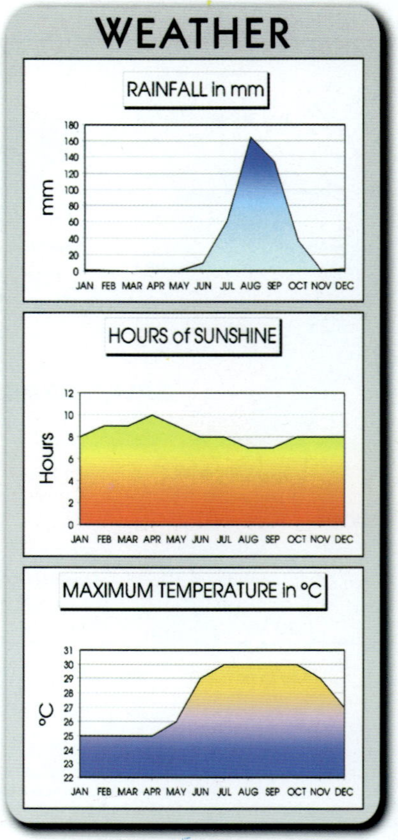

SEYCHELLES

General Advice

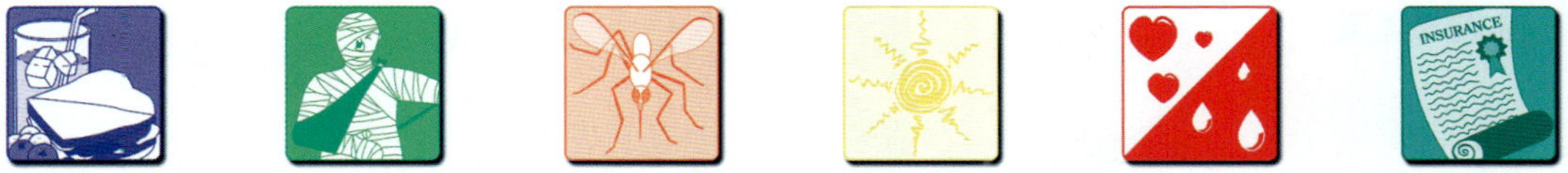

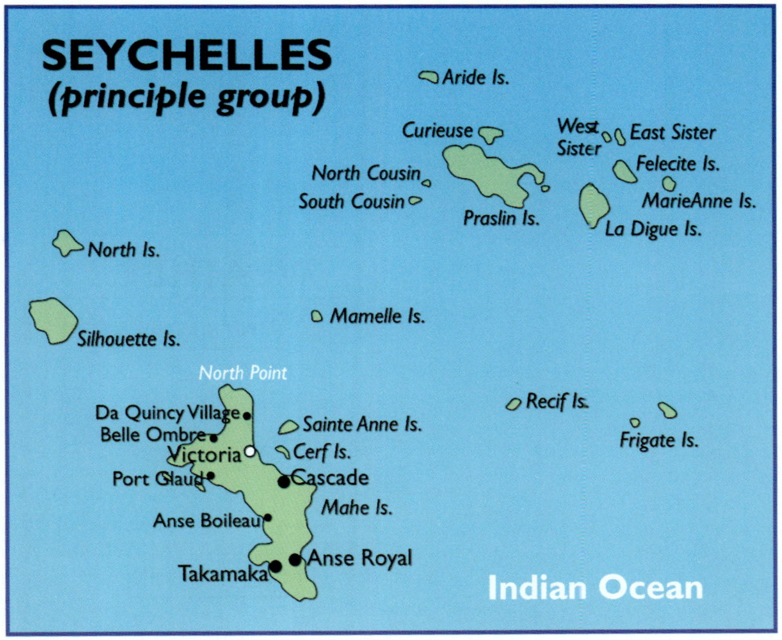

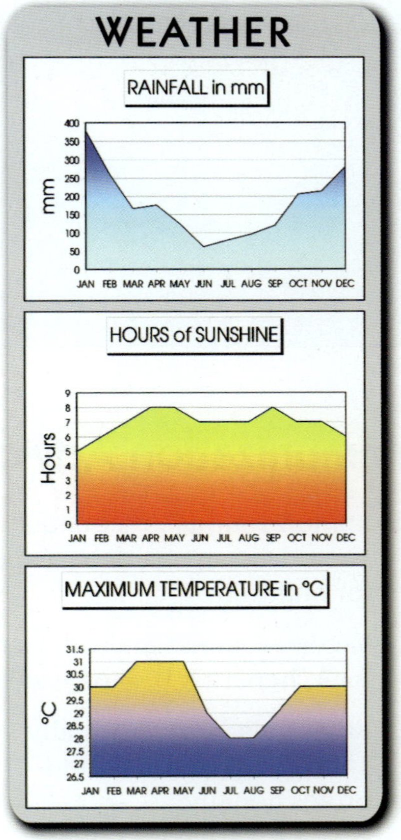

Immunization Advice

- ❑ Immunizations recommended for life should be up to date, especially those for children and boosters of tetanus for adults.
- ❑ Courses or boosters of hepatitis A are usually advised.
- ❑ Vaccines sometimes advised are: BCG, hepatitis B, typhoid.
- ❑ A yellow fever certificate is required if aged over 1 year old and entering from an infected country.

Malaria Advice

- ❑ Malaria is not normally present.

SINGAPORE

General Advice

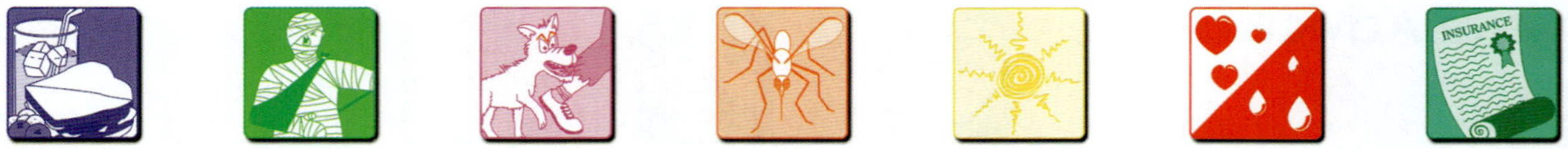

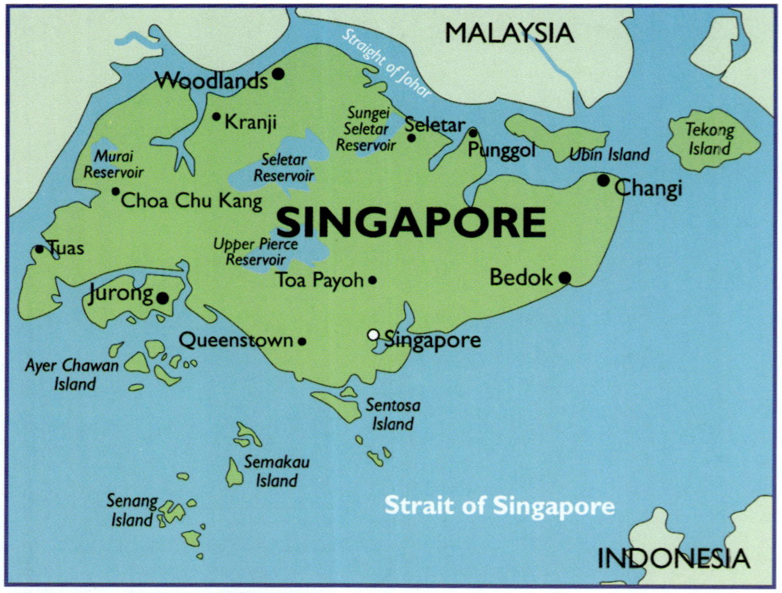

Immunization Advice

- ❑ Immunizations recommended for life should be up to date, especially those for children.
- ❑ Vaccines sometimes advised are: hepatitis A, hepatitis B, Japanese encephalitis.
- ❑ Rabies is not normally present but animal bites should be treated professionally.
- ❑ A yellow fever certificate is required if aged over 1 year old and entering from an infected country or who have been in or passed through any country partly or wholly endemic for yellow fever within the preceding 6 days.

Malaria Advice

- ❑ Malaria is not normally present.

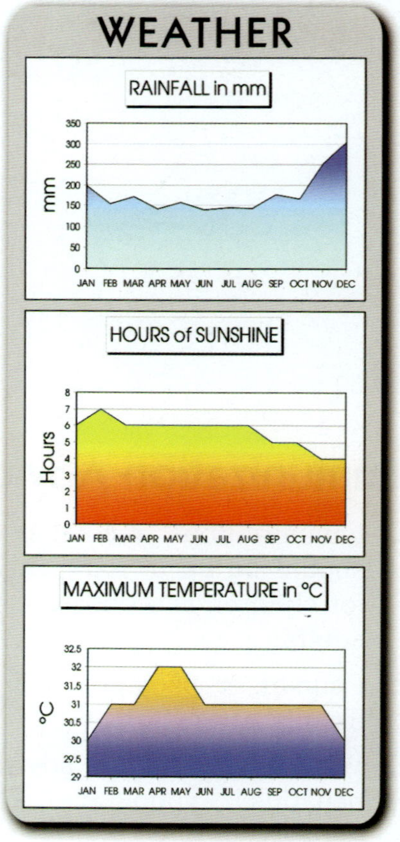

SLOVAKIA

General Advice

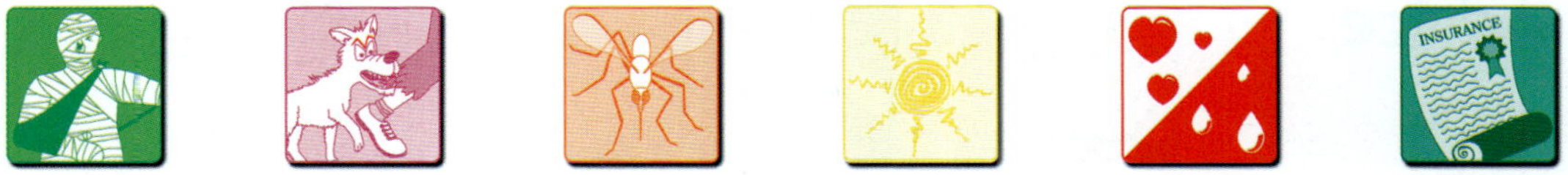

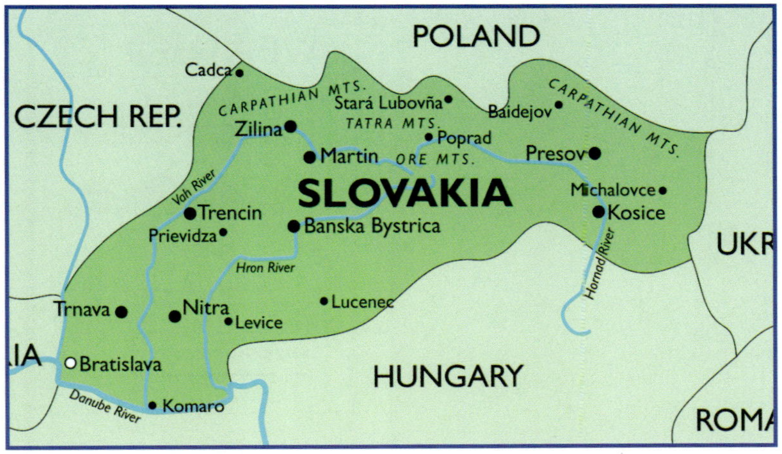

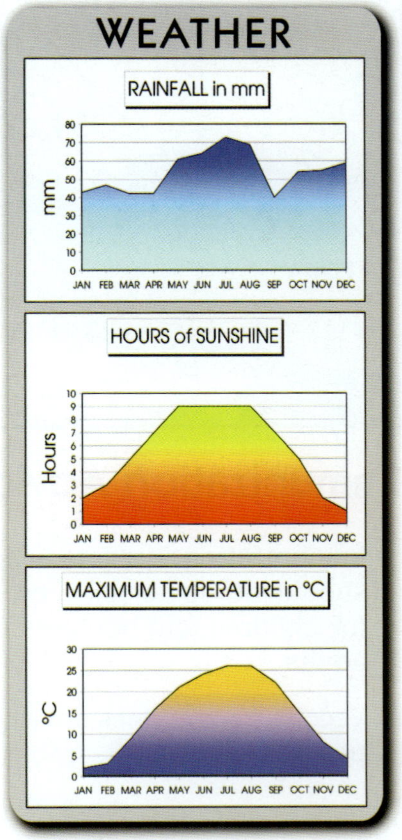

Immunization Advice

- ❑ Immunizations recommended for life should be up to date, especially those for children and boosters of tetanus for adults.
- ❑ Vaccines sometimes advised are: diphtheria, hepatitis A, hepatitis B, rabies, tick-borne encephalitis.
- ❑ No certificate of vaccination for yellow fever is required.

Malaria Advice

- ❑ Malaria is not normally present.

SLOVENIA

General Advice

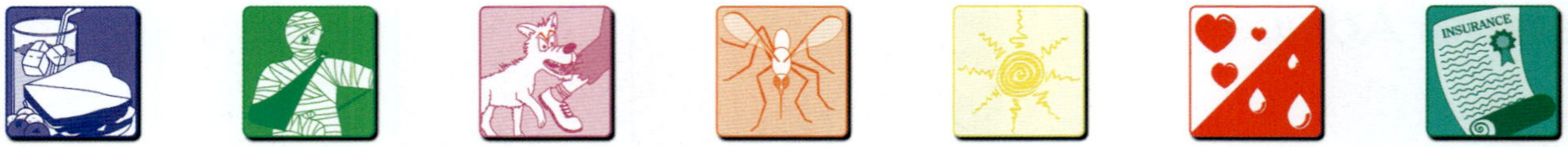

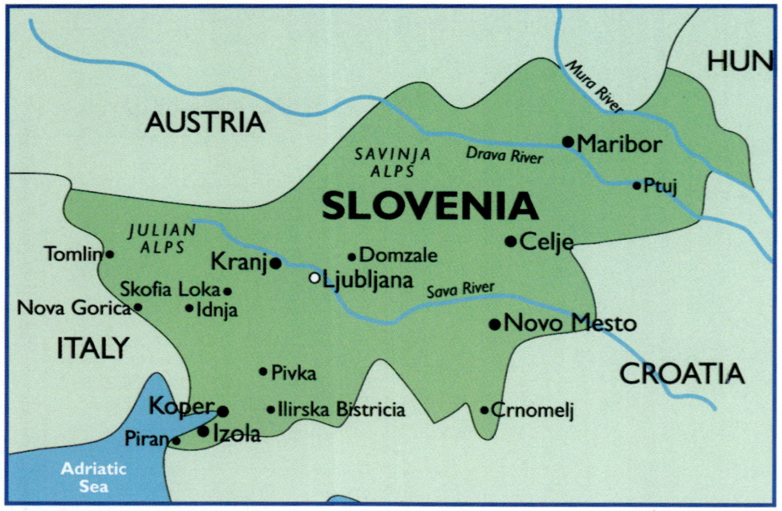

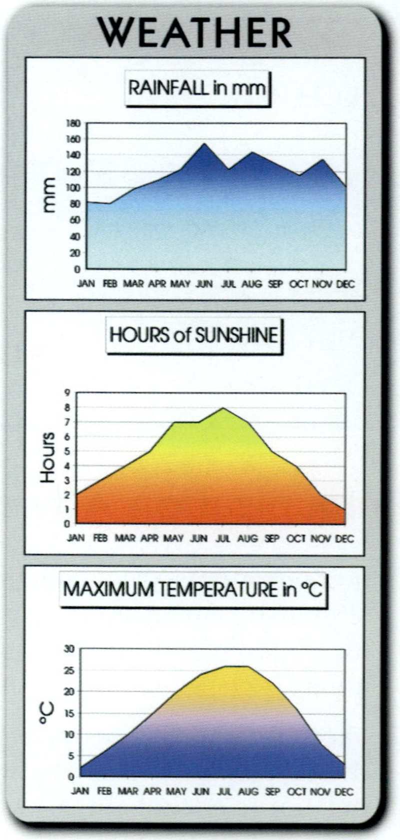

Immunization Advice

- ❑ Immunizations recommended for life should be up to date, especially those for children and boosters of tetanus for adults.
- ❑ Vaccines sometimes advised are: hepatitis A, hepatitis B, rabies, tick-borne encephalitis.
- ❑ No certificate of vaccination for yellow fever is required.

Malaria Advice

- ❑ Malaria is not normally present.

SOMALIA

General Advice

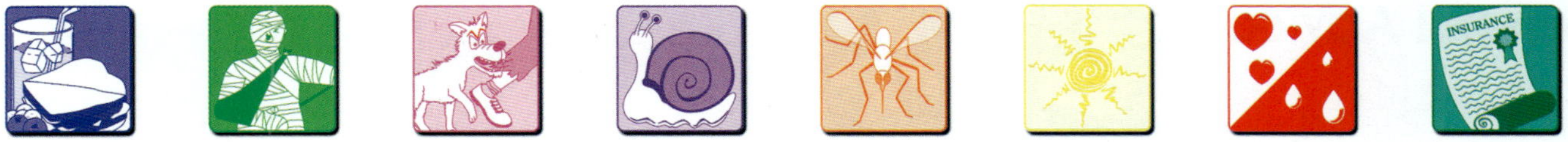

Immunization Advice

- ❑ Immunizations recommended for life should be up to date, especially those for children and boosters of tetanus for adults.
- ❑ Courses or boosters of diphtheria, hepatitis A, and typhoid are usually advised.
- ❑ Vaccines sometimes advised are: BCG, cholera, hepatitis B, rabies, yellow fever (in rare instances; see yellow fever map).
- ❑ A yellow fever certificate is required if entering from an infected country.

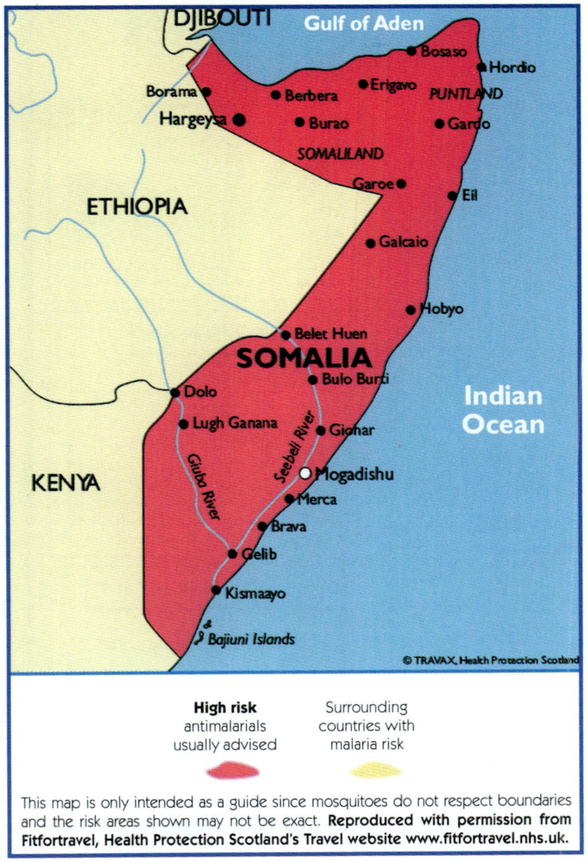

Malaria Advice

- ❑ Malaria is a serious and sometimes fatal disease transmitted by mosquitoes. You cannot be vaccinated against malaria.

MALARIA PRECAUTIONS

- ❑ Malaria precautions are essential in all areas all year round. Avoid mosquito bites by covering up with clothing such as long sleeves and long trousers especially after sunset, using insect repellents on exposed skin and, when necessary, sleeping under a mosquito net.
- ❑ Check with your doctor or nurse about suitable antimalarial tablets.
- ❑ Prompt investigation of fever is essential.

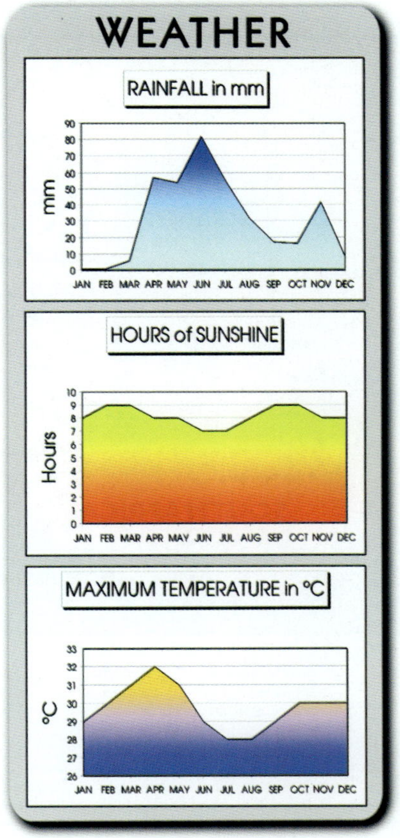

SOUTH AFRICA

General Advice

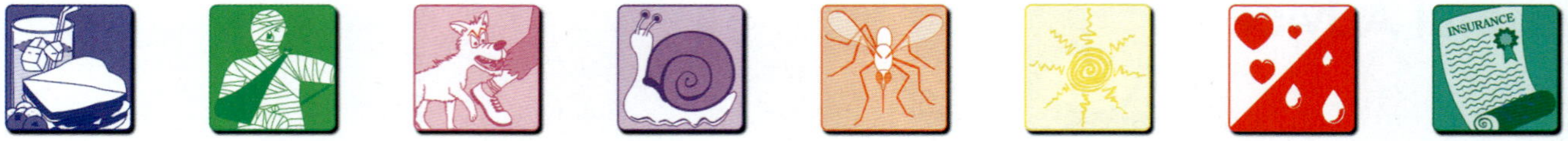

Immunization Advice

- ❑ Immunizations recommended for life should be up to date, especially those for children and boosters of tetanus for adults.
- ❑ Courses or boosters of hepatitis A are usually advised.
- ❑ Vaccines sometimes advised are: BCG, cholera, hepatitis B, rabies, typhoid.
- ❑ A yellow fever certificate is required if aged over 1 year old and entering from an infected country.

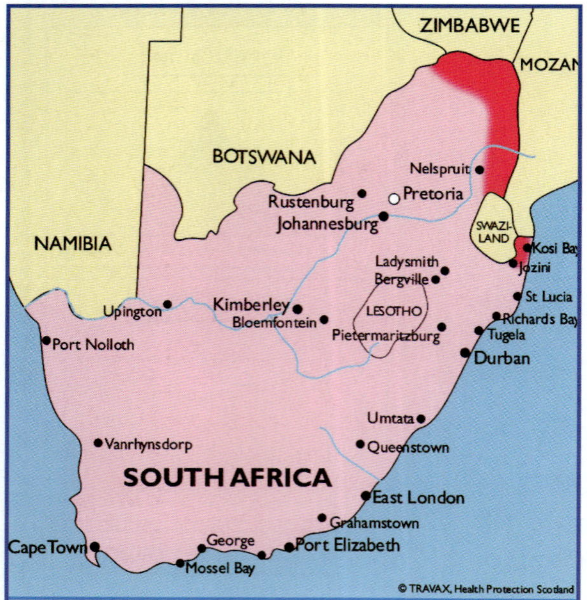

Low to no risk antimalarials not usually advised | **High risk** antimalarials usually advised | Surrounding countries with malaria risk

This map is only intended as a guide since mosquitoes do not respect boundaries and the risk areas shown may not be exact. **Reproduced with permission from Fitfortravel, Health Protection Scotland's Travel website www.fitfortravel.nhs.uk.**

Malaria Advice

- ❑ Malaria is a serious and sometimes fatal disease transmitted by mosquitoes. You cannot be vaccinated against malaria.

MALARIA PRECAUTIONS

- ❑ Malaria precautions are essential in the northeast of the country (Mpumalanga and Limpopo Provinces which border Zimbabwe and Mozambique, and north-eastern KwaZulu-Natal, including Kruger National Park) all year round. Risk is highest in these areas from September to May. Avoid mosquito bites by covering up with clothing such as long sleeves and long trousers especially after sunset, using insect repellents on exposed skin and, when necessary, sleeping under a mosquito net.
- ❑ Check with your doctor or nurse about suitable anti-malarial tablets.
- ❑ Prompt investigation of fever is essential.

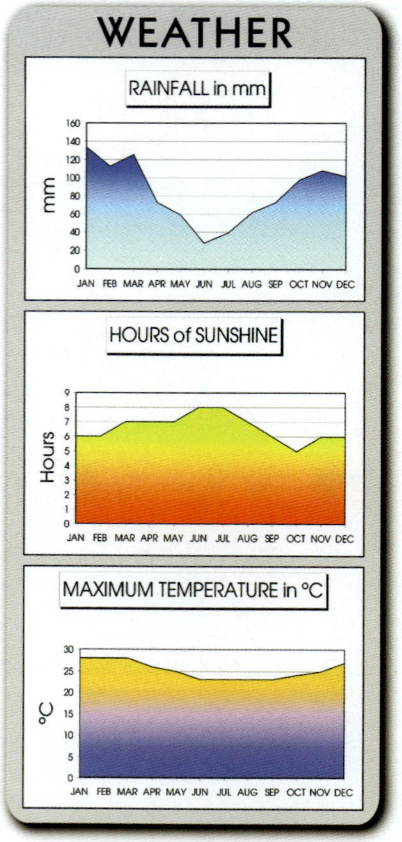

—Weather in Durban—

SPAIN

General Advice

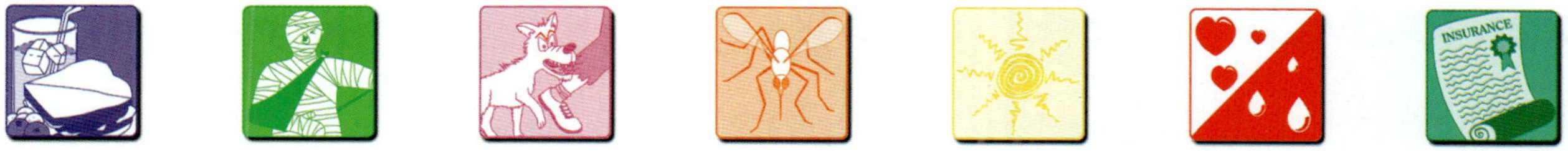

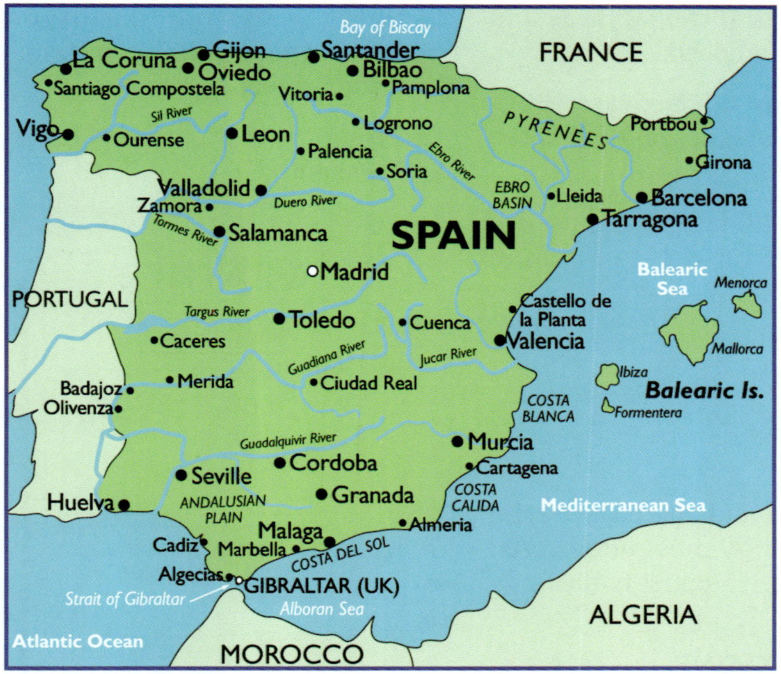

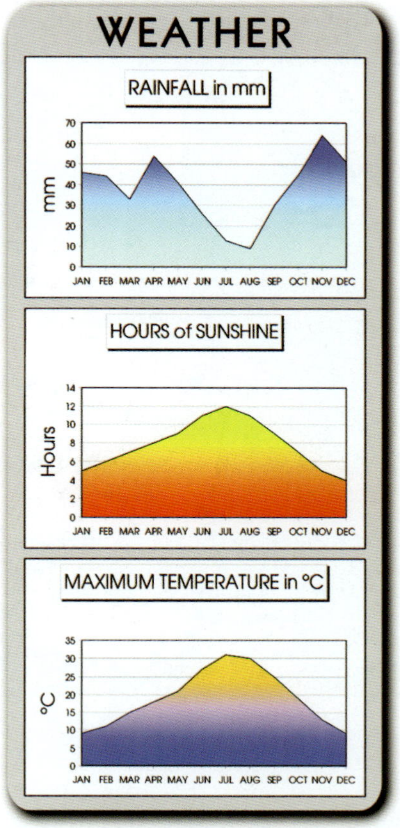

—Weather in Madrid—

Immunization Advice

- ❑ Immunizations recommended for life should be up to date, especially those for children.
- ❑ Vaccines sometimes advised: hepatitis A, hepatitis B.
- ❑ Rabies is not normally present but animal bites should be treated professionally.
- ❑ No certificate of vaccination for yellow fever is required.

Malaria Advice

- ❑ Malaria is not normally present.

SRI LANKA

General Advice

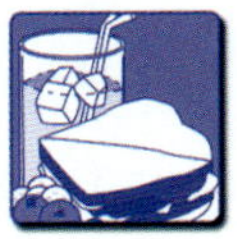

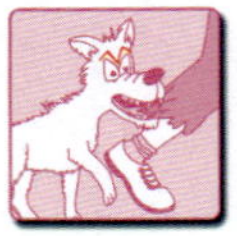
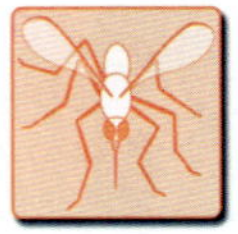

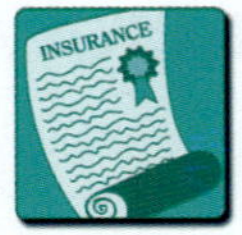

Immunization Advice

- ❑ Immunizations recommended for life should be up to date, especially those for children and boosters of tetanus for adults.
- ❑ Courses or boosters of hepatitis A and typhoid are usually advised.
- ❑ Vaccines sometimes advised are: BCG, hepatitis B, Japanese encephalitis, rabies.
- ❑ A yellow fever certificate is required if aged over 1 year old and entering from an infected country.

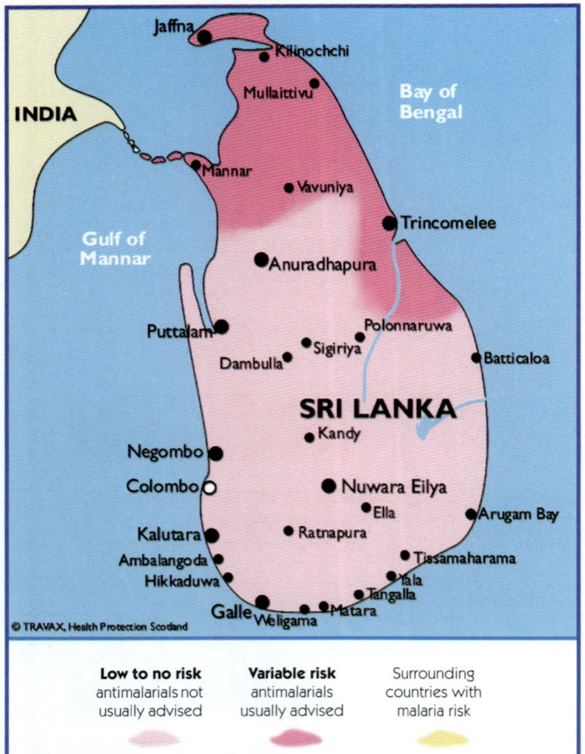

This map is only intended as a guide since mosquitoes do not respect boundaries and the risk areas shown may not be exact. **Reproduced with permission from Fitfortravel, Health Protection Scotland's Travel website www.fitfortravel.nhs.uk.**

Malaria Advice

- ❑ Malaria is a serious and sometimes fatal disease transmitted by mosquitoes. You cannot be vaccinated against malaria.

MALARIA PRECAUTIONS

- ❑ Malaria precautions are essential in most areas all year round. The risk is predominantly in the north. There is low to no risk in Colombo and Kandy. Avoid mosquito bites by covering up with clothing such as long sleeves and long trousers especially after sunset, using insect repellents on exposed skin and, when necessary, sleeping under a mosquito net.
- ❑ Check with your doctor or nurse about suitable antimalarial tablets.
- ❑ Prompt investigation of fever is essential.

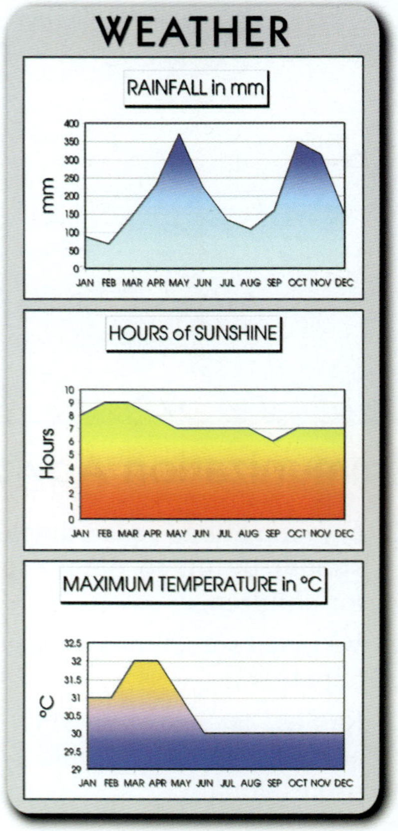

SUDAN

General Advice

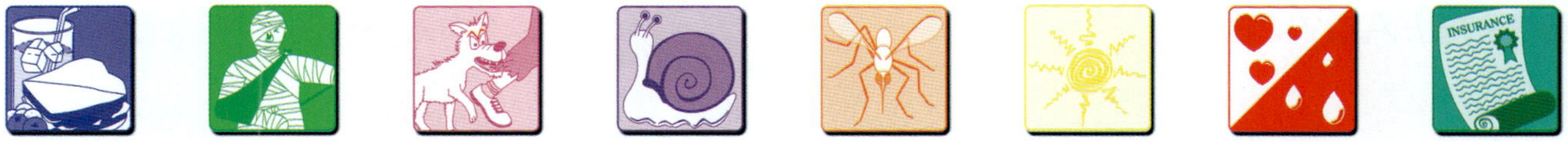

Immunization Advice

- ❑ Immunizations recommended for life should be up to date, especially those for children and boosters of tetanus for adults.
- ❑ Courses or boosters of diphtheria, hepatitis A, and typhoid are usually advised.
- ❑ Vaccines sometimes advised are: BCG, hepatitis B, meningococcal A and C, rabies, yellow fever (see yellow fever map).
- ❑ A yellow fever certificate is required if aged over 9 months old and entering from an infected country. A certificate may be required for travelers leaving Sudan.

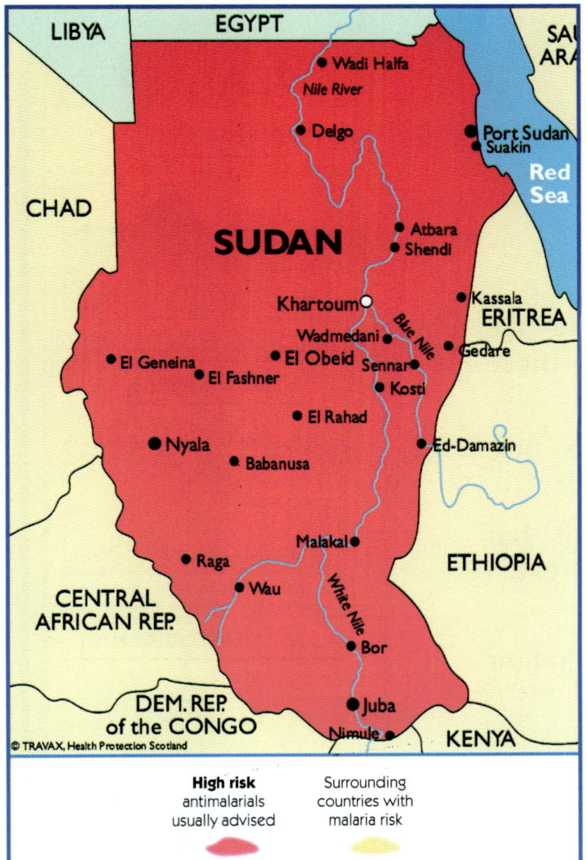

This map is only intended as a guide since mosquitoes do not respect boundaries and the risk areas shown may not be exact. **Reproduced with permission from Fitfortravel, Health Protection Scotland's Travel website www.fitfortravel.nhs.uk.**

Malaria Advice

- ❑ Malaria is a serious and sometimes fatal disease transmitted by mosquitoes. You cannot be vaccinated against malaria.

MALARIA PRECAUTIONS

- ❑ Malaria precautions are essential in all areas all year round. The risk is higher in southern and central areas. Risk is lower and seasonal in the north (April to October). Risk is very low along the Red Sea coast. Avoid mosquito bites by covering up with clothing such as long sleeves and long trousers especially after sunset, using insect repellents on exposed skin and, when necessary, sleeping under a mosquito net.
- ❑ Check with your doctor or nurse about suitable anti-malarial tablets.
- ❑ Prompt investigation of fever is essential.

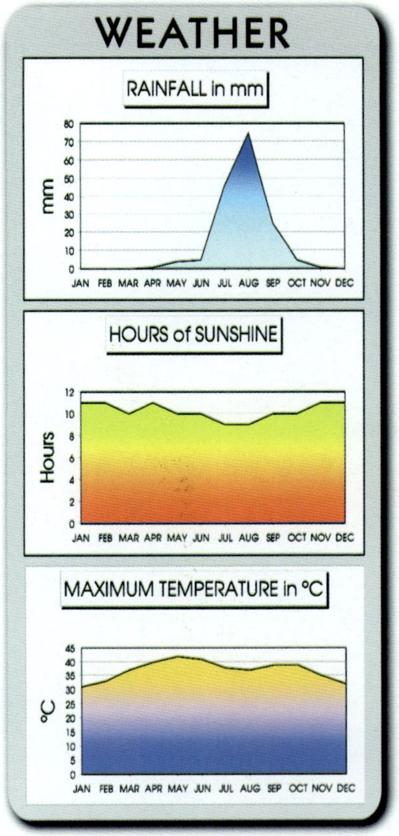

SWEDEN

General Advice

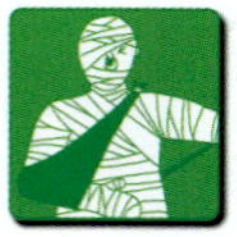

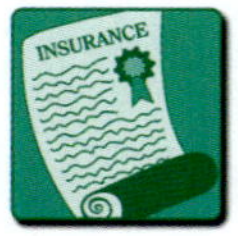

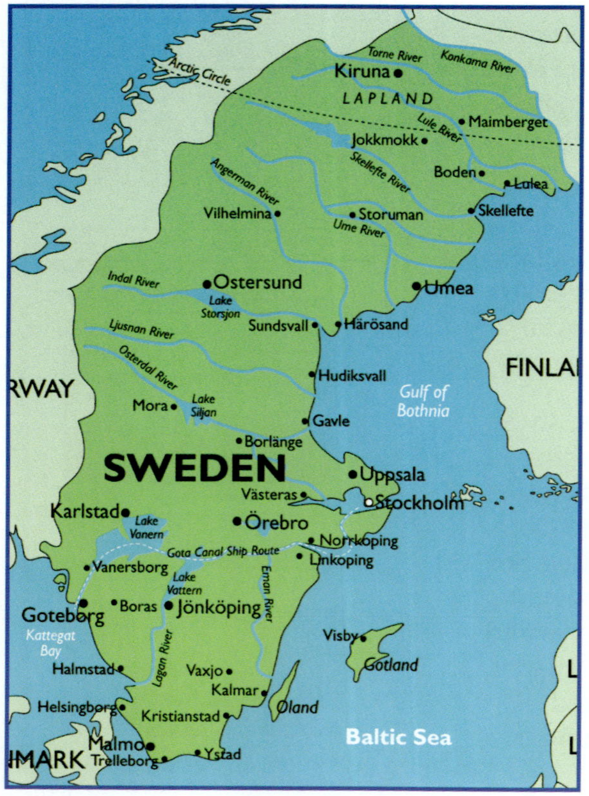

Immunization Advice

- ❑ Immunizations recommended for life should be up to date, especially those for children.
- ❑ Vaccines sometimes advised are: tick-borne encephalitis.
- ❑ Rabies is not normally present but animal bites should be treated professionally.
- ❑ No certificate of vaccination for yellow fever is required.

Malaria Advice

Malaria is not normally present.

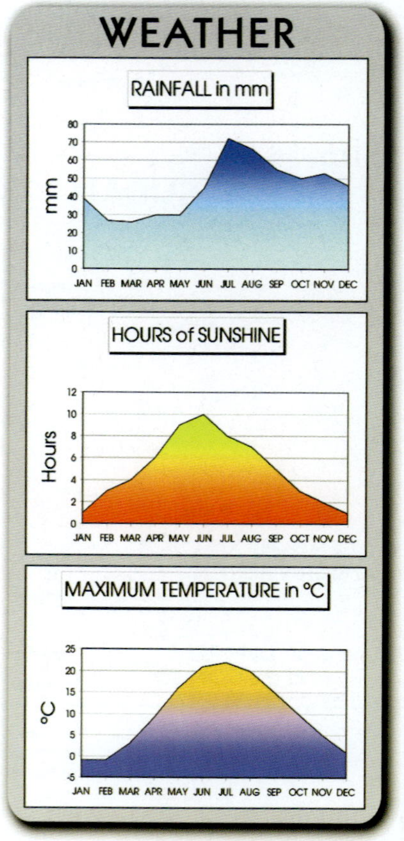

—Weather in Stockholm—

TAJIKISTAN

General Advice

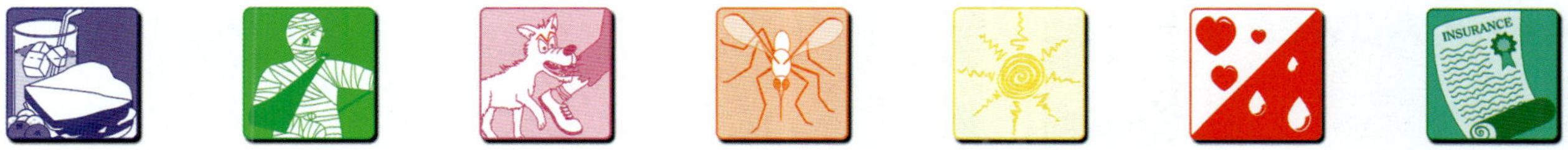

Immunization Advice

❑ Immunizations recommended for life should be up to date, especially those for children and boosters of tetanus for adults.

❑ Courses or boosters of diphtheria, hepatitis A, poliomyelitis, and typhoid are usually advised.

❑ Vaccines sometimes advised are: BCG, cholera, hepatitis B, rabies.

❑ No certificate of vaccination for yellow fever is required.

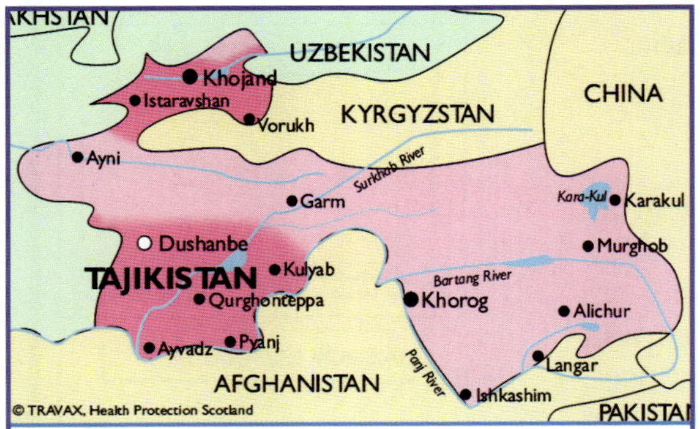

Low to no risk antimalarials not usually advised	**Variable risk** antimalarials usually advised	Surrounding countries with malaria risk

This map is only intended as a guide since mosquitoes do not respect boundaries and the risk areas shown may not be exact. **Reproduced with permission from Fitfortravel, Health Protection Scotland's Travel website www.fitfortravel.nhs.uk.**

Malaria Advice

❑ Malaria is a serious and sometimes fatal disease transmitted by mosquitoes. You cannot be vaccinated against malaria.

MALARIA PRECAUTIONS

❑ Malaria precautions are essential in Khatlon, Dushanbe, Gorno-Badakhshan, and Leninabad, from June to October. Risk is highest in southern areas. Avoid mosquito bites by covering up with clothing such as long sleeves and long trousers especially after sunset, using insect repellents on exposed skin and, when necessary, sleeping under a mosquito net.

❑ Check with your doctor or nurse about suitable antimalarial tablets.

❑ Prompt investigation of fever is essential.

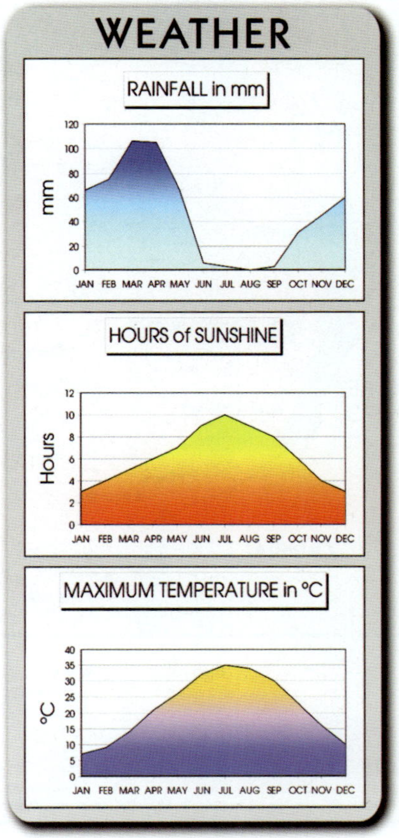

TANZANIA and ZANZIBAR

General Advice

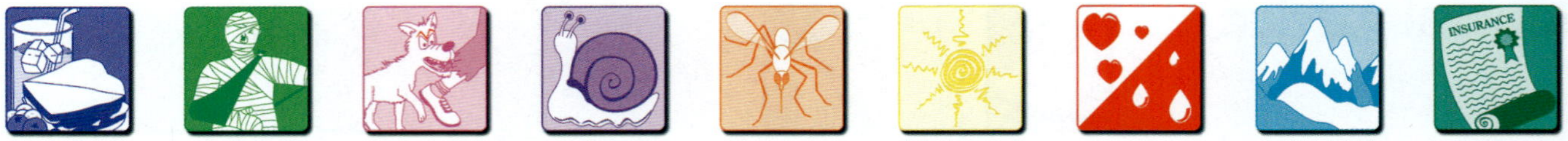

Immunization Advice

- ❑ Immunizations recommended for life should be up to date, especially those for children and boosters of tetanus for adults.
- ❑ Courses or boosters of hepatitis A and typhoid.
- ❑ Vaccines sometimes advised are: BCG, cholera, hepatitis B, rabies, yellow fever (in rare instances; see yellow fever map).
- ❑ A yellow fever certificate is required if aged over 1 year old and entering from an infected country.

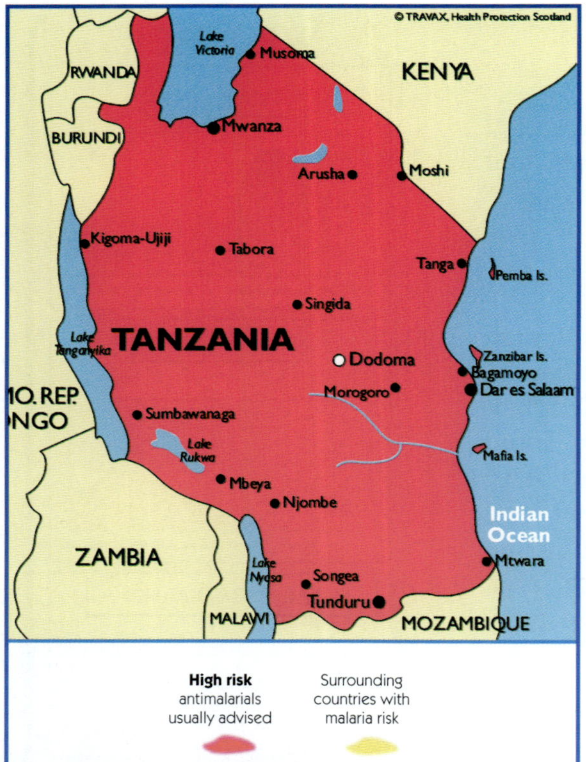

This map is only intended as a guide since mosquitoes do not respect boundaries and the risk areas shown may not be exact. **Reproduced with permission from Fitfortravel, Health Protection Scotland's Travel website www.fitfortravel.nhs.uk.**

Malaria Advice

- ❑ Malaria is a serious and sometimes fatal disease transmitted by mosquitoes. You cannot be vaccinated against malaria.

MALARIA PRECAUTIONS

- ❑ Malaria precautions are essential in all areas below 1800 m all year round. Avoid mosquito bites by covering up with clothing such as long sleeves and long trousers especially after sunset, using insect repellents on exposed skin and, when necessary, sleeping under a mosquito net.
- ❑ Check with your doctor or nurse about suitable antimalarial tablets.
- ❑ Prompt investigation of fever is essential.

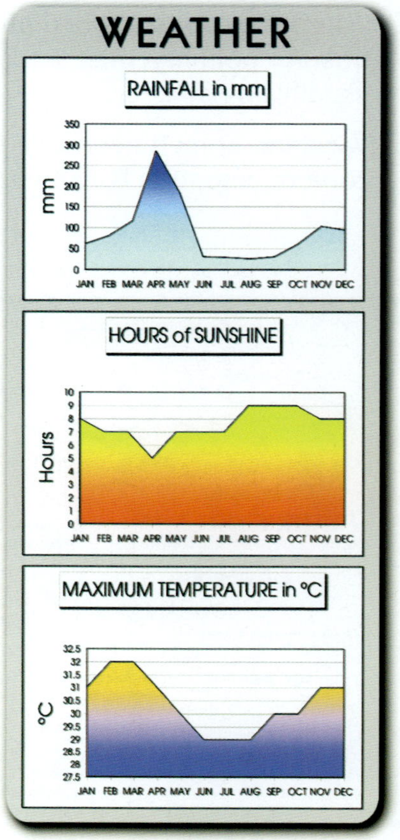

THAILAND

General Advice

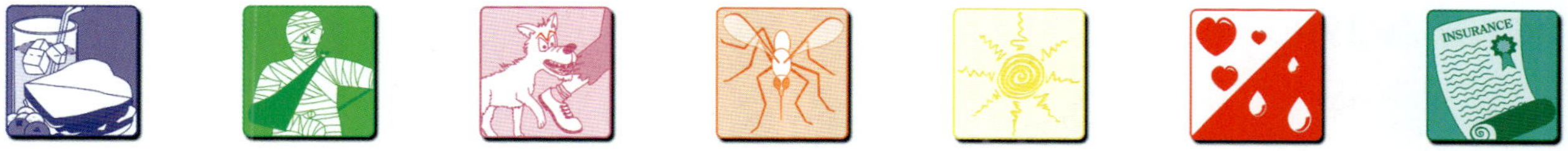

Immunization Advice

❑ Immunizations recommended for life should be up to date, especially those for children and boosters of tetanus for adults.

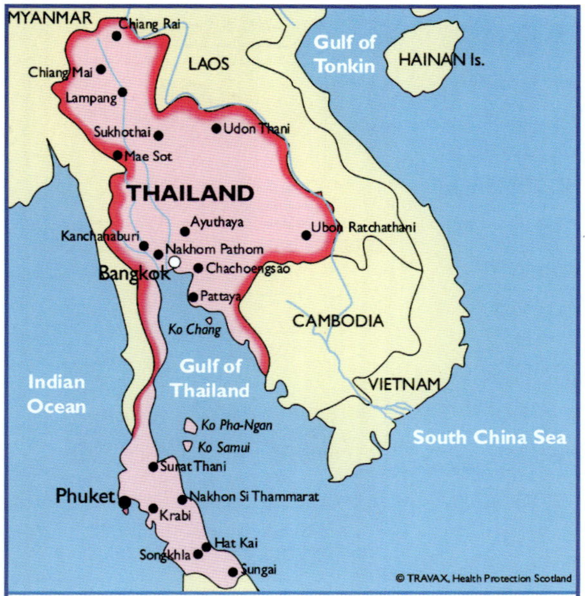

Low to no risk antimalarials not usually advised | **High risk** antimalarials usually advised | Surrounding countries with malaria risk

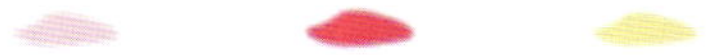

This map is only intended as a guide since mosquitoes do not respect boundaries and the risk areas shown may not be exact. **Reproduced with permission from Fitfortravel, Health Protection Scotland's Travel website www.fitfortravel.nhs.uk.**

❑ Courses or boosters of diphtheria and hepatitis A are usually advised.

❑ Vaccines sometimes advised are: BCG, cholera, hepatitis B, Japanese encephalitis, rabies, typhoid.

❑ A yellow fever certificate is required for all travelers aged over 9 months and entering from an infected country.

Malaria Advice

❑ Malaria is a serious and sometimes fatal disease transmitted by mosquitoes. You cannot be vaccinated against malaria.

MALARIA PRECAUTIONS

❑ Malaria precautions are essential in rural, forested areas near the borders with Myanmar, Laos, and Cambodia, all year round. The risk is minimal in all other areas. Avoid mosquito bites by covering up with clothing such as long sleeves and long trousers especially after sunset, using insect repellents on exposed skin and, when necessary, sleeping under a mosquito net.

❑ Check with your doctor or nurse about suitable anti-malarial tablets.

❑ Prompt investigation of fever is essential.

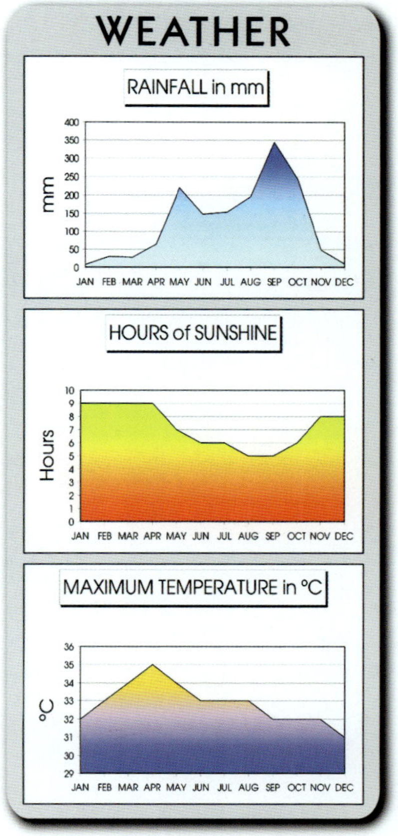

—Weather in Bangkok—

TRINIDAD and TOBAGO

General Advice

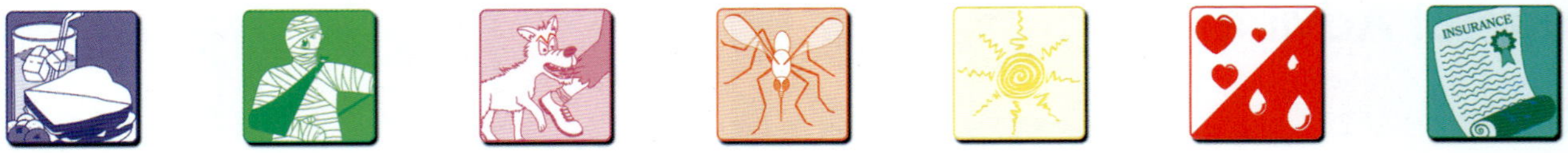

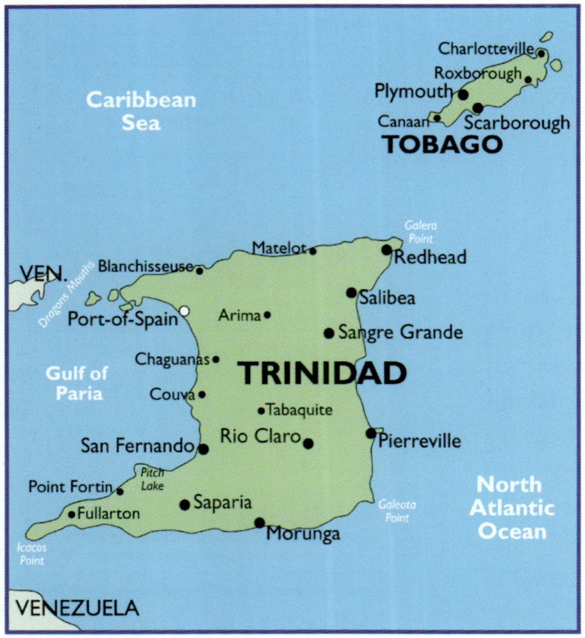

Immunization Advice

- ❑ Immunizations recommended for life should be up to date, especially those for children and adult boosters of tetanus.
- ❑ Vaccines sometimes advised: hepatitis A, hepatitis B, rabies, yellow fever (yellow fever is advised for all travelers aged over 9 months old going to Trinidad; yellow fever vaccination is not recommended if only visiting Tobago).
- ❑ A yellow fever certificate is required if aged over 1 year old and entering from an infected country.

Malaria Advice

- ❑ Malaria is not normally present.

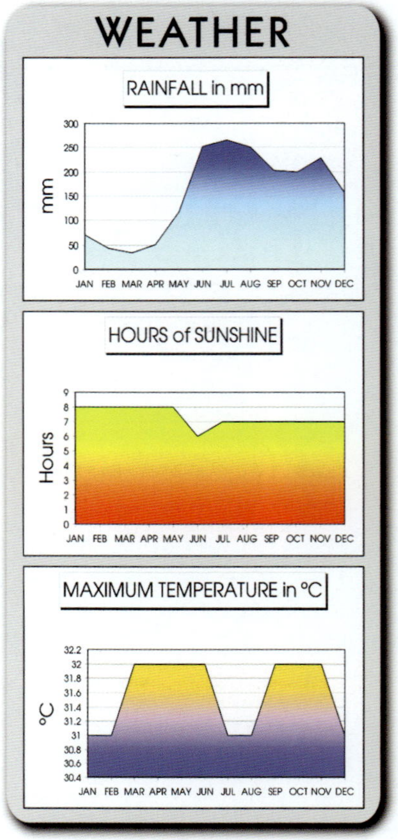

TUNISIA

General Advice

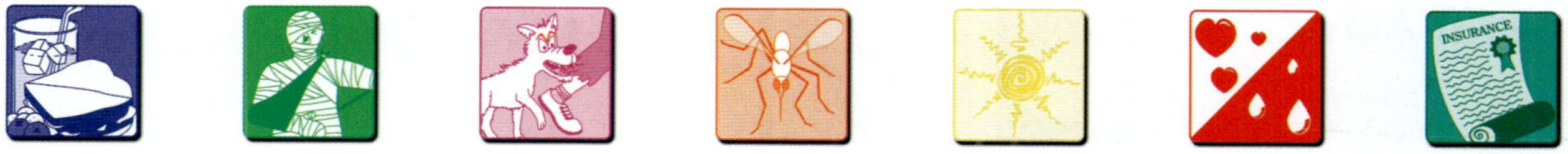

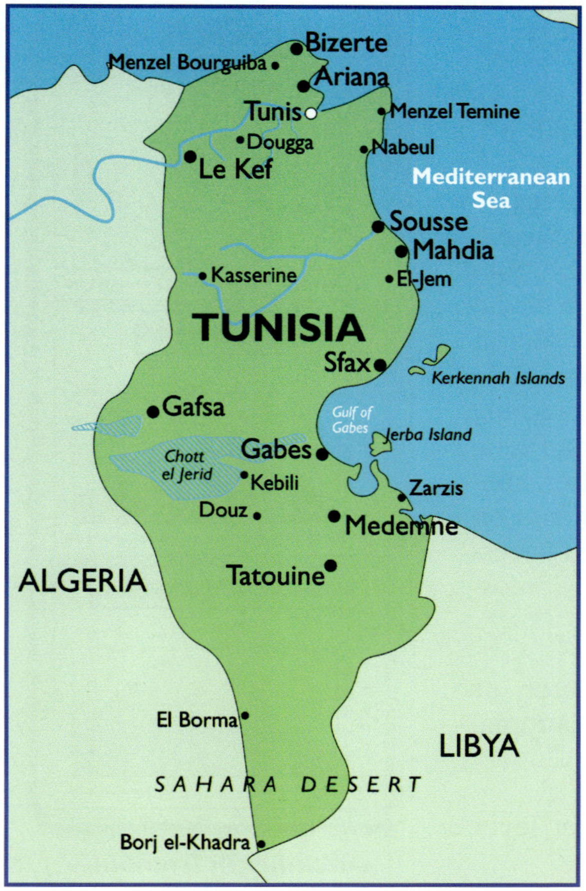

Immunization Advice

- ❑ Immunizations recommended for life should be up to date, especially those for children and boosters of tetanus for adults.
- ❑ Courses or boosters of hepatitis A and typhoid are usually advised.
- ❑ Vaccines sometimes advised are: hepatitis B, rabies.
- ❑ A yellow fever certificate is required if aged over 1 year old and entering from an infected country.

Malaria Advice

- ❑ Malaria is not normally present.

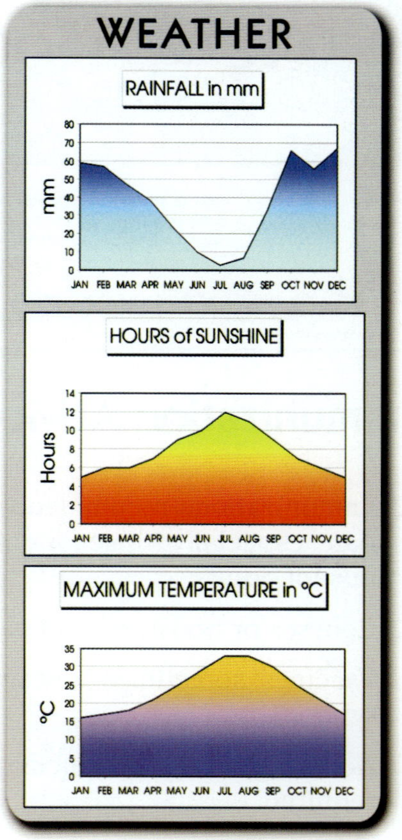

TURKEY

General Advice

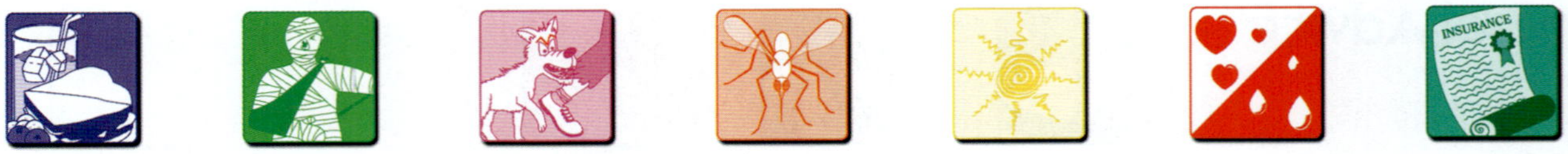

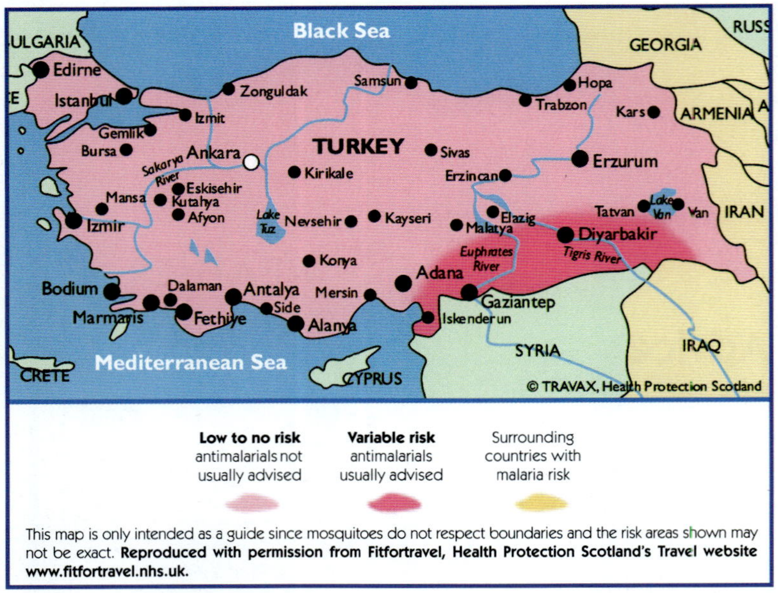

Immunization Advice

- ❑ Immunizations recommended for life should be up to date, especially those for children and boosters of tetanus for adults.
- ❑ Courses or boosters of hepatitis A are usually advised.
- ❑ Vaccines sometimes advised are: hepatitis B, rabies, typhoid.
- ❑ No certificate of vaccination for yellow fever is required.

Malaria Advice

- ❑ Malaria is a serious and sometimes fatal disease transmitted by mosquitoes. You cannot be vaccinated against malaria.

MALARIA PRECAUTIONS

- ❑ Malaria precautions are essential mainly in the southeastern part of the country from May to October. There is no risk in the main tourist resorts. Avoid mosquito bites by covering up with clothing such as long sleeves and long trousers especially after sunset, using insect repellents on exposed skin and, when necessary, sleeping under a mosquito net.
- ❑ Check with your doctor or nurse about suitable antimalarial tablets.
- ❑ Prompt investigation of fever is essential.

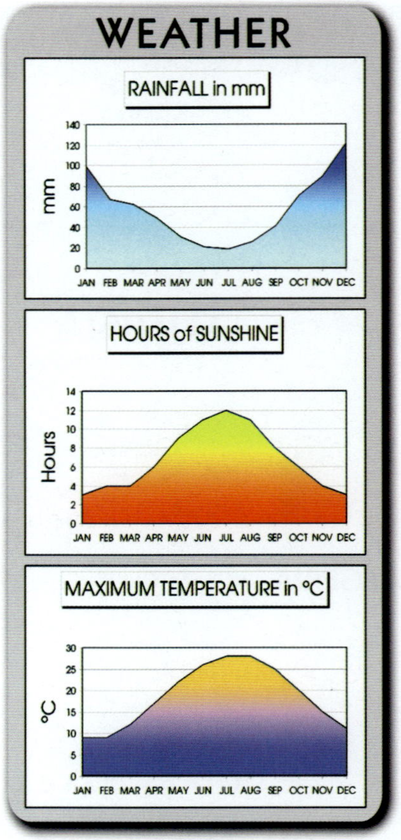

—Weather in Istanbul—

TURKMENISTAN

General Advice

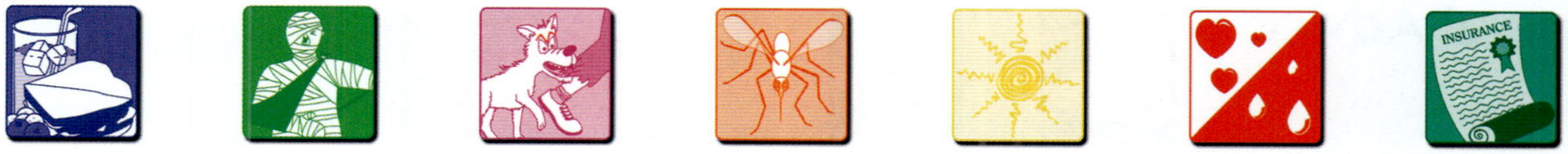

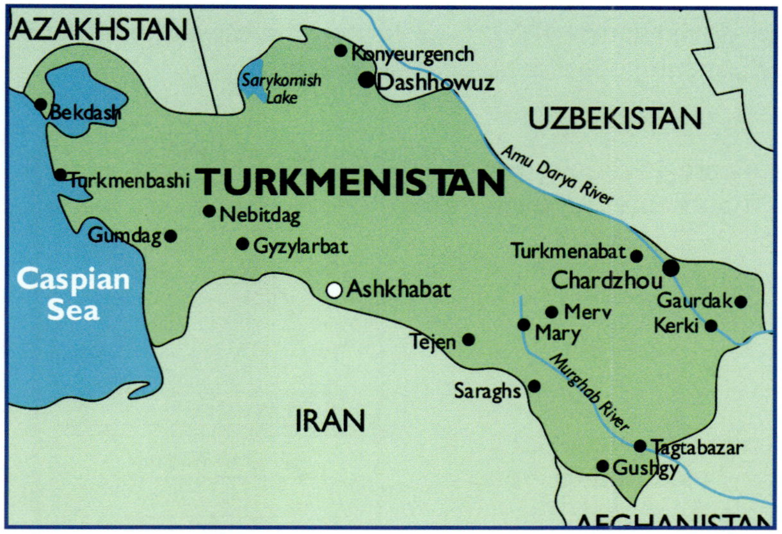

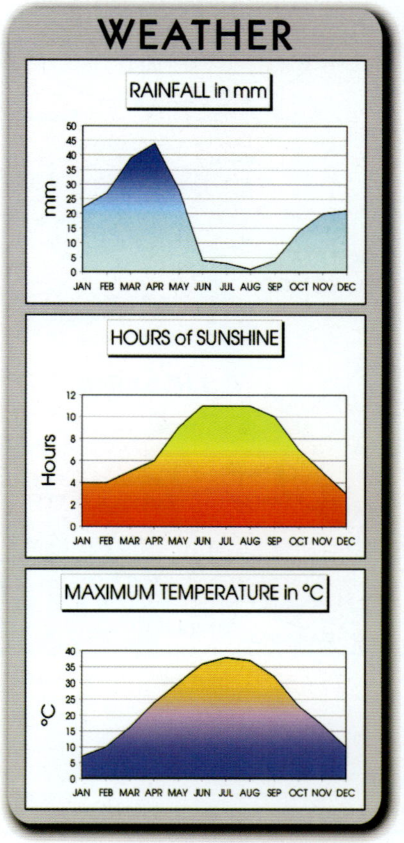

Immunization Advice

- ❑ Immunizations recommended for life should be up to date, especially those for children and boosters of tetanus for adults.
- ❑ Courses or boosters of diphtheria, hepatitis A, and poliomyelitis are usually advised.
- ❑ Vaccines sometimes advised are: BCG, hepatitis B, rabies, typhoid.
- ❑ No certificate of vaccination for yellow fever is required.

Malaria Advice

- ❑ Malaria is not normally present.

UGANDA

General Advice

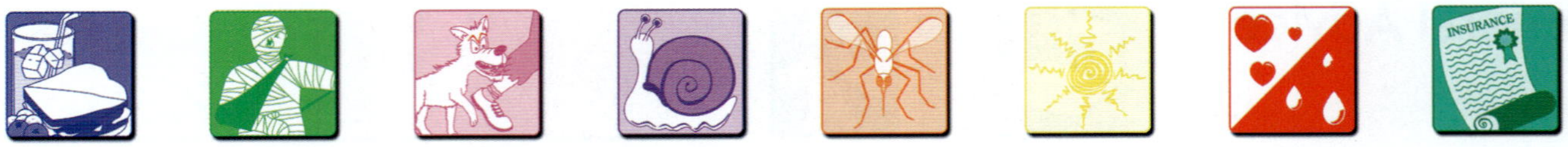

Immunization Advice

❑ Immunizations recommended for life should be up to date, especially those for children and boosters of tetanus for adults.

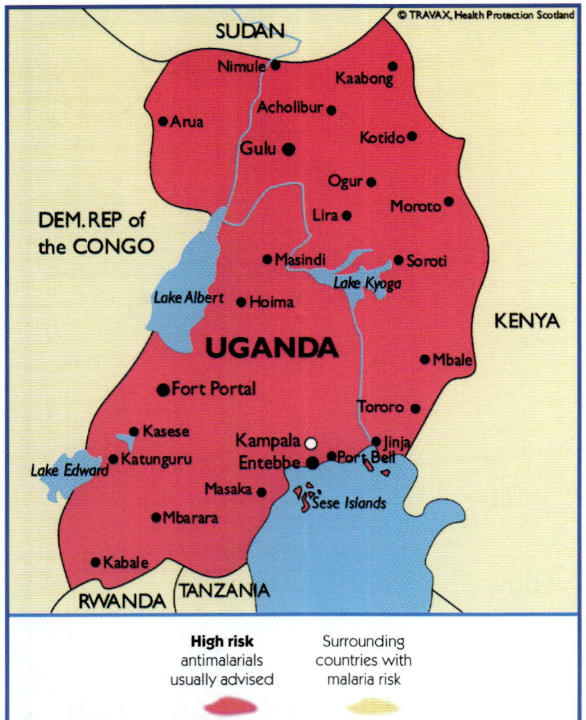

This map is only intended as a guide since mosquitoes do not respect boundaries and the risk areas shown may not be exact. **Reproduced with permission from Fitfortravel, Health Protection Scotland's Travel website www.fitfortravel.nhs.uk.**

❑ Courses or boosters of diphtheria, hepatitis A, poliomyelitis, typhoid, and yellow fever are usually advised.

❑ Vaccines sometimes advised are: BCG, cholera, hepatitis B, meningococcal A and C, rabies.

❑ A yellow fever certificate is required if aged over 1 year old and entering from an infected country.

Malaria Advice

❑ Malaria is a serious and sometimes fatal disease transmitted by mosquitoes. You cannot be vaccinated against malaria.

MALARIA PRECAUTIONS

❑ Malaria precautions are essential in all areas all year round. Avoid mosquito bites by covering up with clothing such as long sleeves and long trousers especially after sunset, using insect repellents on exposed skin and, when necessary, sleeping under a mosquito net.

❑ Check with your doctor or nurse about suitable antimalarial tablets.

❑ Prompt investigation of fever is essential.

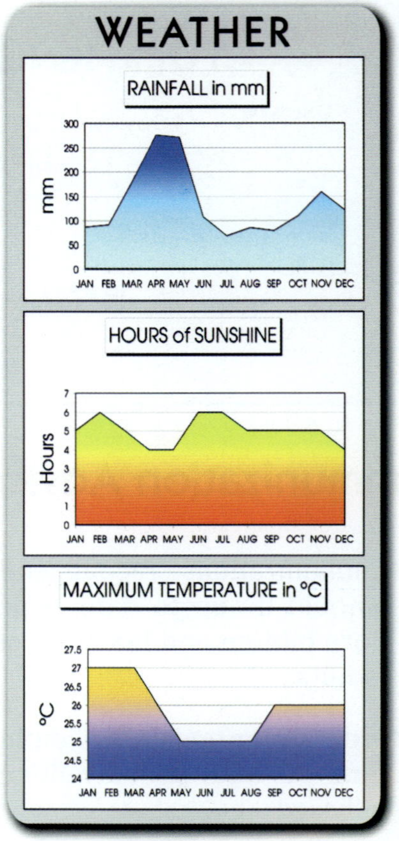

UKRAINE

General Advice

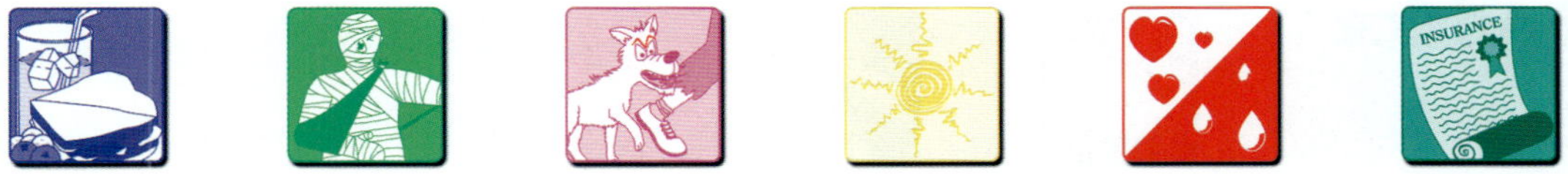

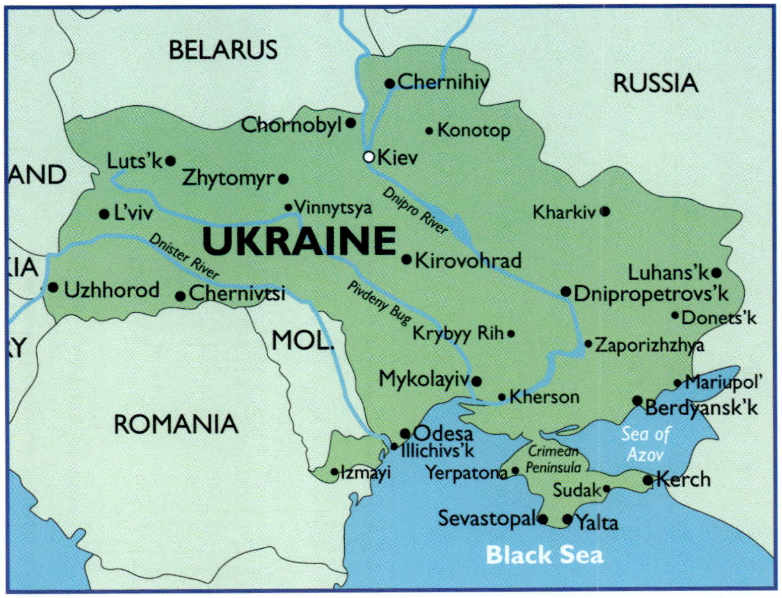

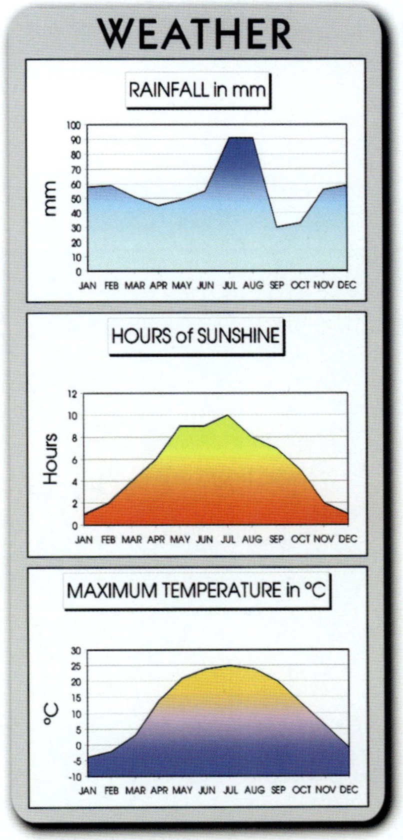

Immunization Advice

- ❑ Immunizations recommended for life should be up to date, especially those for children and boosters of tetanus for adults.
- ❑ Courses or boosters of diphtheria and hepatitis A are usually advised.
- ❑ Vaccines sometimes advised are: BCG, hepatitis B, rabies, tick-borne encephalitis, typhoid.
- ❑ No certificate of vaccination for yellow fever is required.

Malaria Advice

- ❑ Malaria is not normally present.

UNITED ARAB EMIRATES

General Advice

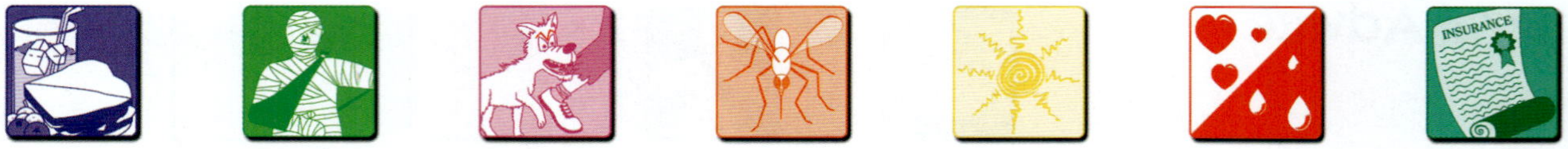

Immunization Advice

- ❑ Immunizations recommended for life should be up to date, especially those for children and boosters of tetanus for adults.
- ❑ Courses or boosters of hepatitis A are usually advised.
- ❑ Vaccines sometimes advised are: hepatitis B, rabies, typhoid.
- ❑ No certificate of vaccination for yellow fever is required.

Malaria Advice

- ❑ Malaria is not normally present.

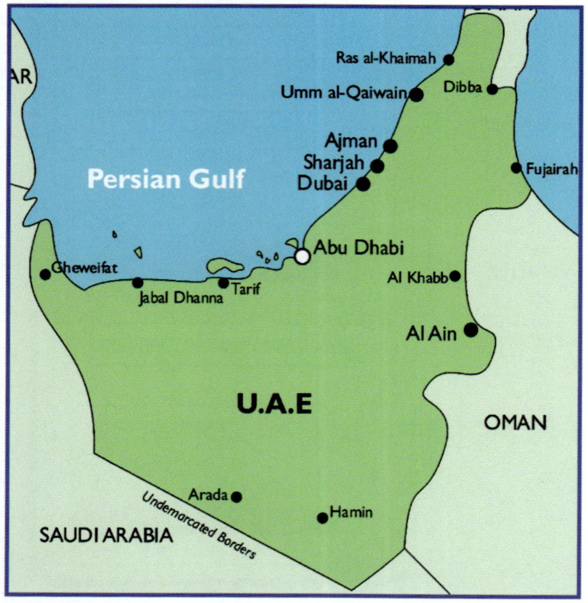

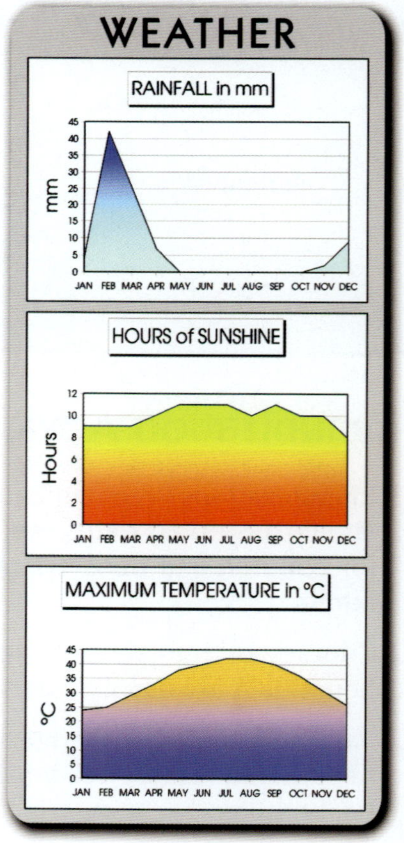

URUGUAY

General Advice

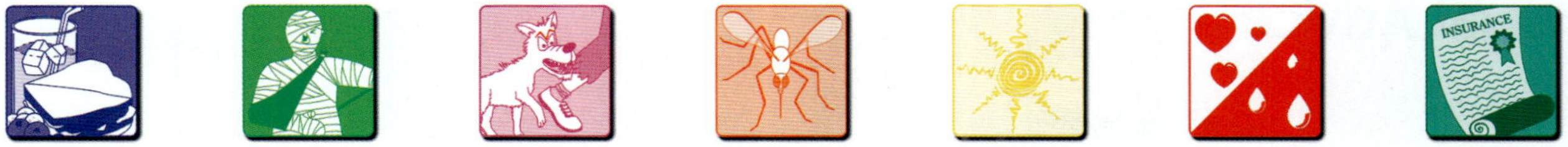

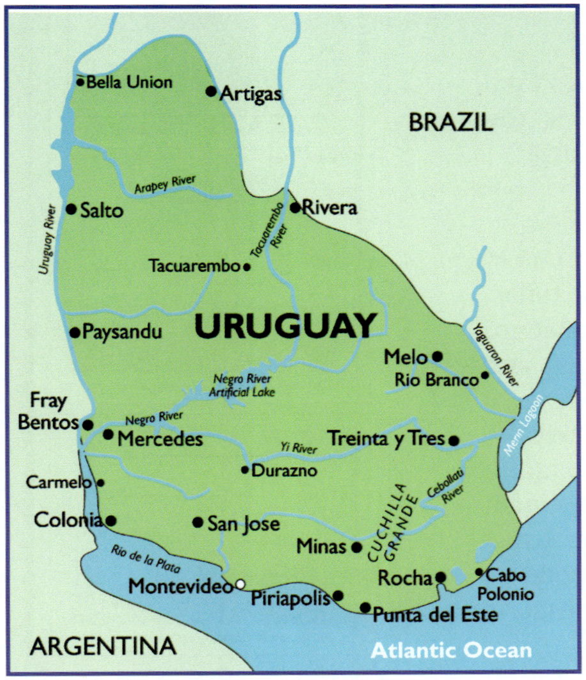

Immunization Advice

- ❑ Immunizations recommended for life should be up to date, especially those for children and boosters of tetanus for adults.
- ❑ Courses or boosters of hepatitis A are usually advised.
- ❑ Vaccines sometimes advised are: diphtheria, hepatitis B, rabies.
- ❑ A yellow fever certificate is required if entering from an infected country.

Malaria Advice

- ❑ Malaria is not normally present.

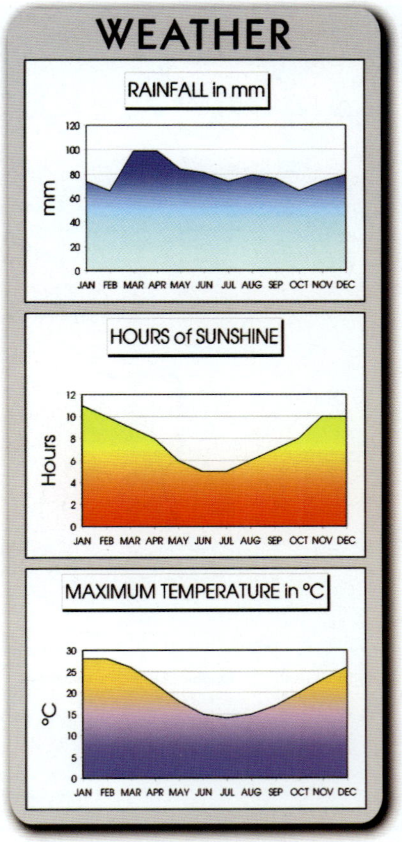

VENEZUELA

General Advice

Immunization Advice

❑ Immunizations recommended for life should be up to date, especially those for children and boosters of tetanus for adults.

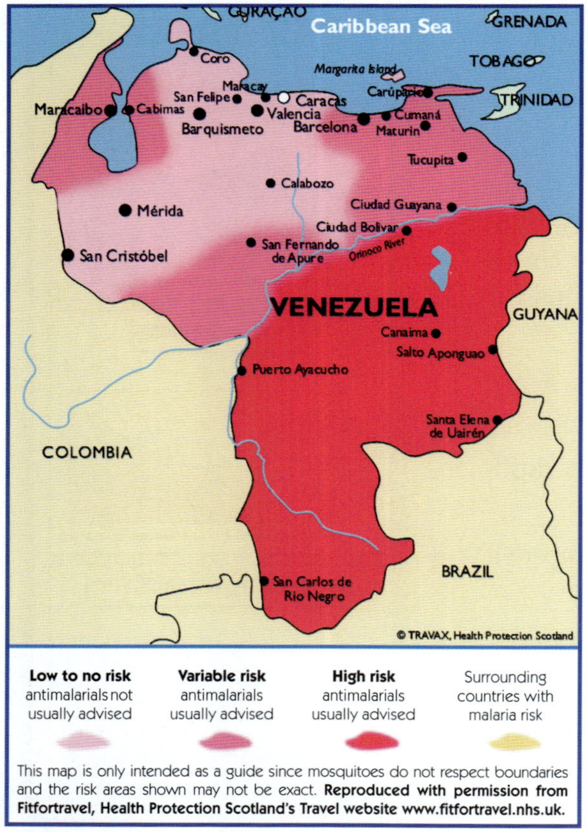

❑ Courses or boosters of hepatitis A and yellow fever are usually advised. Yellow fever is advised for yellow fever areas only. Risk in cities and islands including Margarita is very small; there is a risk at the Angel Falls (see yellow fever map).

❑ Vaccines sometimes advised are: diphtheria, hepatitis B, rabies, typhoid.

❑ No certificate of vaccination for yellow fever is required.

Malaria Advice

❑ Malaria is a serious and sometimes fatal disease transmitted by mosquitoes. You cannot be vaccinated against malaria.

MALARIA PRECAUTIONS

❑ Malaria precautions are essential in most inland rainforest areas of Amazonas, Anzoategui, Bolivar, and Delta Amacuro states. Risk is minimal in Caracas, and Margarita Island (see map). There is a risk at the Angel Falls but this will be small for day trips only. Avoid mosquito bites by covering up with clothing such as long sleeves and long trousers especially after sunset, using insect repellents on exposed skin and, when necessary, sleeping under a mosquito net.

❑ Check with your doctor or nurse about suitable antimalarial tablets.

❑ Prompt investigation of fever is essential.

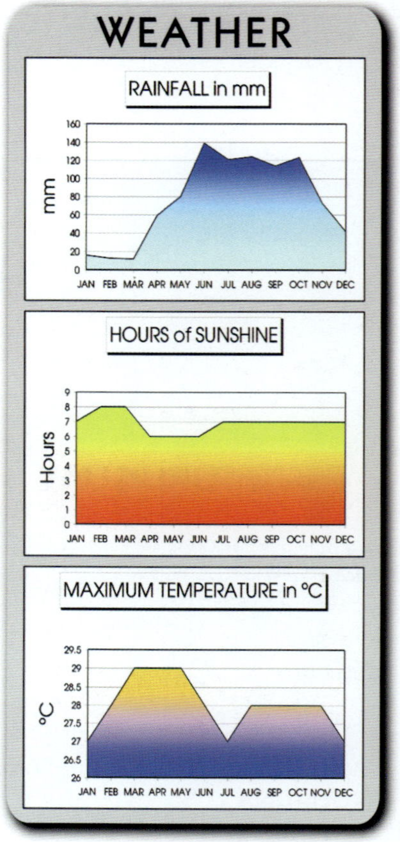

VIETNAM

General Advice

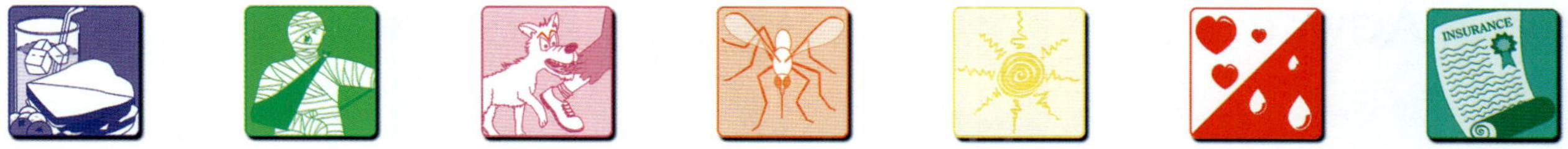

Immunization Advice

- ❑ Immunizations recommended for life should be up to date, especially those for children and boosters of tetanus for adults.
- ❑ Courses or boosters of diphtheria, hepatitis A and typhoid are usually advised.
- ❑ Vaccines sometimes advised: BCG, cholera, hepatitis B, Japanese encephalitis, rabies.
- ❑ A yellow fever certificate is required if aged over 1 year old and entering from an infected country.

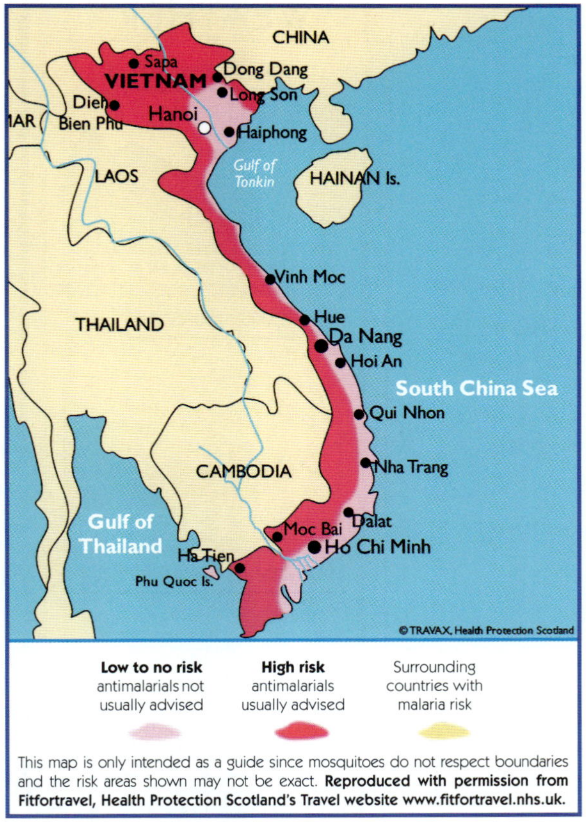

Malaria Advice

- ❑ Malaria is a serious and sometimes fatal disease transmitted by mosquitoes. You cannot be vaccinated against malaria.

MALARIA PRECAUTIONS

- ❑ Malaria precautions are essential in most areas except urban areas such as Ho Chi Min City, Hanoi, the Red River delta and the coastal central plains, all year round. Risk is highest in central highland provinces to the north west of Qui Nhon and provinces south west of Ho Chi Min City. Avoid mosquito bites by covering up with clothing such as long sleeves and long trousers especially after sunset, using insect repellents on exposed skin and, when necessary, sleeping under a mosquito net.
- ❑ Check with your doctor or nurse about suitable antimalarial tablets.
- ❑ Prompt investigation of fever is essential .

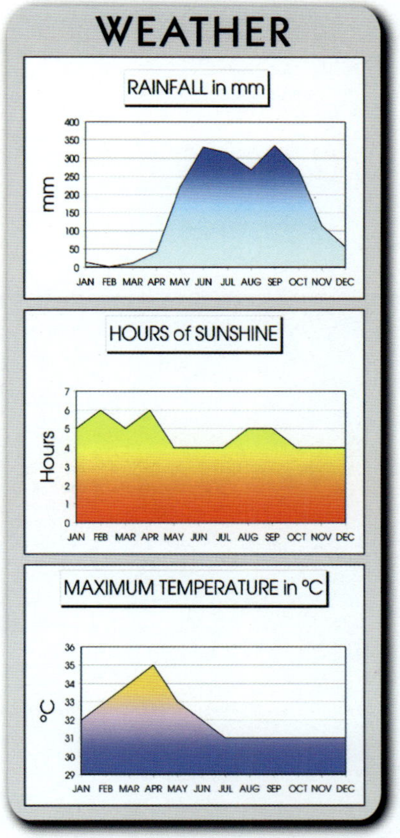

—Weather in Ho Chi Minh City—

VIRGIN ISLANDS

General Advice

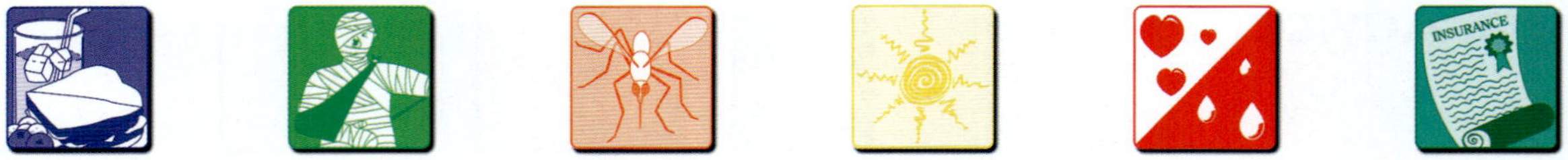

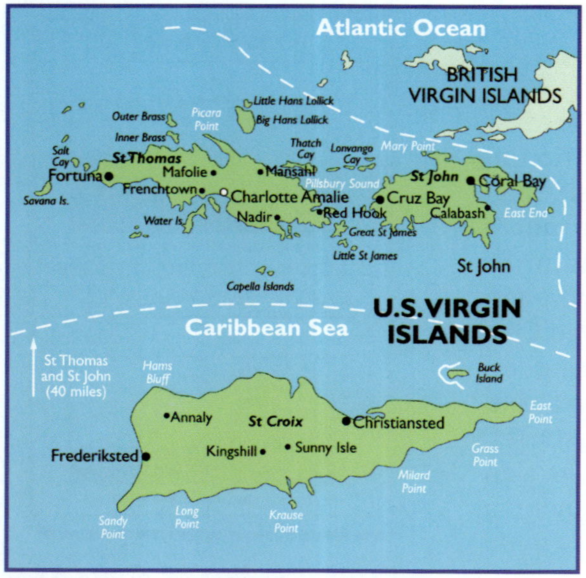

Immunization Advice

- Immunizations recommended for life should be up to date, especially those for children and boosters of tetanus for adults.
- Vaccines sometimes advised: hepatitis A, hepatitis B.
- No certificate of vaccination for yellow fever is required.

Malaria Advice

- Malaria is not normally present.

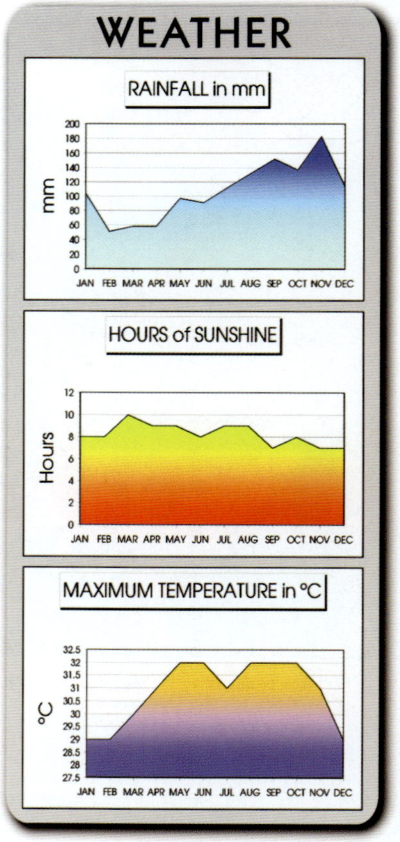

YEMEN

General Advice

Immunization Advice

❑ Immunizations recommended for life should be up to date, especially those for children and boosters of tetanus for adults.

❑ Courses or boosters of diphtheria, hepatitis A, and typhoid are usually advised.

❑ Vaccines sometimes advised are: BCG, hepatitis B, rabies.

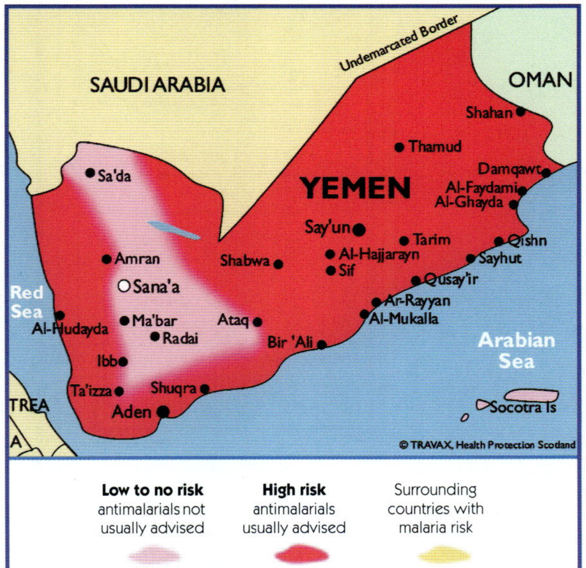

This map is only intended as a guide since mosquitoes do not respect boundaries and the risk areas shown may not be exact. **Reproduced with permission from Fitfortravel, Health Protection Scotland's Travel website www.fitfortravel.nhs.uk.**

❑ A yellow fever certificate is required if aged over 1 year old and entering from an infected country.

Malaria Advice

❑ Malaria is a serious and sometimes fatal disease transmitted by mosquitoes. You cannot be vaccinated against malaria.

MALARIA PRECAUTIONS

❑ Malaria precautions are essential in all areas below 2000 m all year round, but mainly from September to February. There is low to no risk in Socrota Island and no risk in Sanaía City. Avoid mosquito bites by covering up with clothing such as long sleeves and long trousers especially after sunset, using insect repellents on exposed skin and, when necessary, sleeping under a mosquito net.

❑ Check with your doctor or nurse about suitable antimalarial tablets.

❑ Prompt investigation of fever is essential.

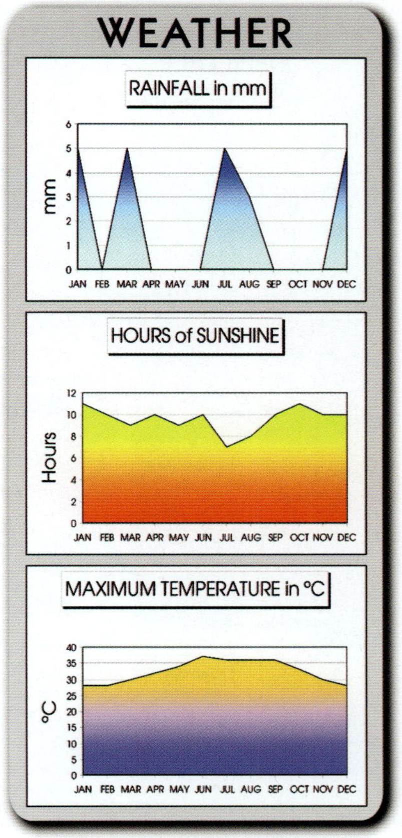

ZAMBIA

General Advice

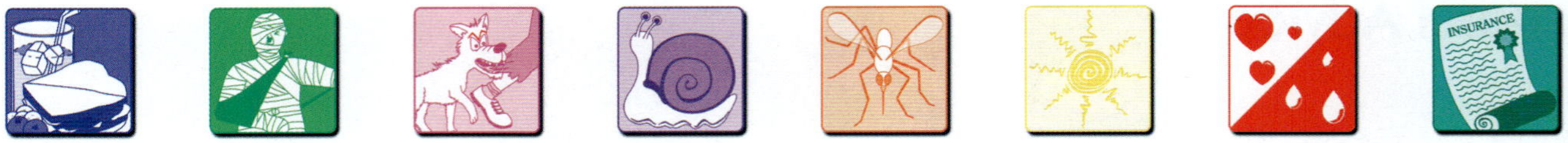

Immunization Advice

- ❑ Immunizations recommended for life should be up to date, especially those for children and boosters of tetanus for adults.

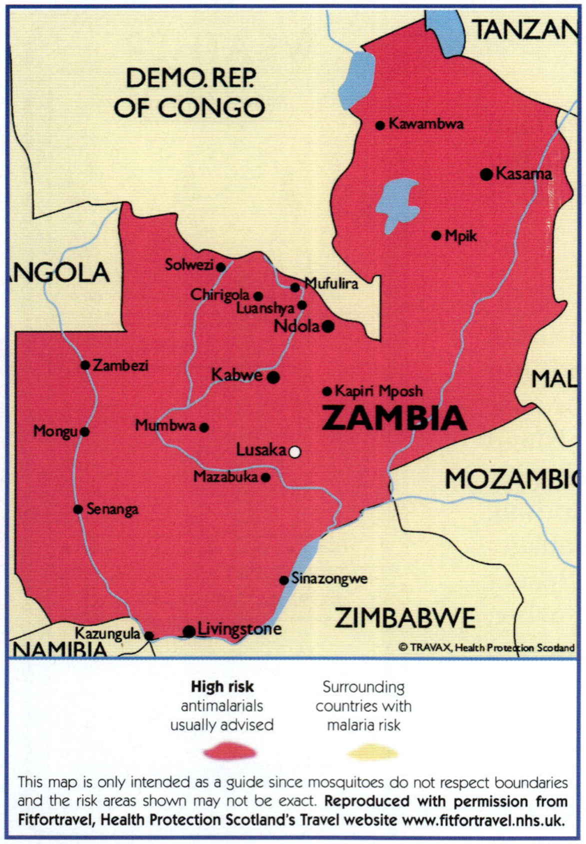

- ❑ Courses or boosters of diphtheria, hepatitis A, and typhoid are usually advised.
- ❑ Vaccines sometimes advised are: BCG, cholera, hepatitis B, rabies, yellow fever (in rare instances; see yellow fever map).
- ❑ No certificate of vaccination for yellow fever is required.

Malaria Advice

- ❑ Malaria is a serious and sometimes fatal disease transmitted by mosquitoes. You cannot be vaccinated against malaria.

MALARIA PRECAUTIONS

- ❑ Malaria precautions are essential in all areas all year round. Risk is highest from November to April. Avoid mosquito bites by covering up with clothing such as long sleeves and long trousers especially after sunset, using insect repellents on exposed skin and, when necessary, sleeping under a mosquito net.
- ❑ Check with your doctor or nurse about suitable antimalarial tablets.
- ❑ Prompt investigation of fever is essential.

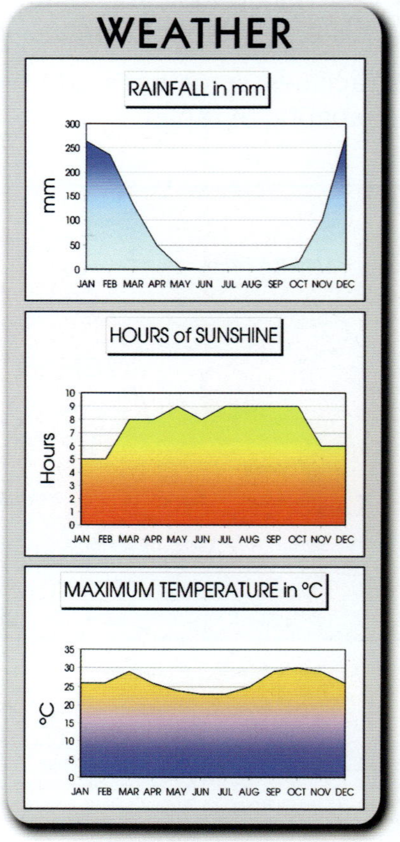

ZIMBABWE

General Advice

Immunization Advice

- ❑ Immunizations recommended for life in Britain should be up to date, especially those for children and adult boosters of tetanus.
- ❑ Courses or boosters of hepatitis A and typhoid are usually advised.
- ❑ Vaccines sometimes advised are: BCG, cholera, hepatitis B, rabies.
- ❑ A yellow fever certificate is required if entering from an infected country.

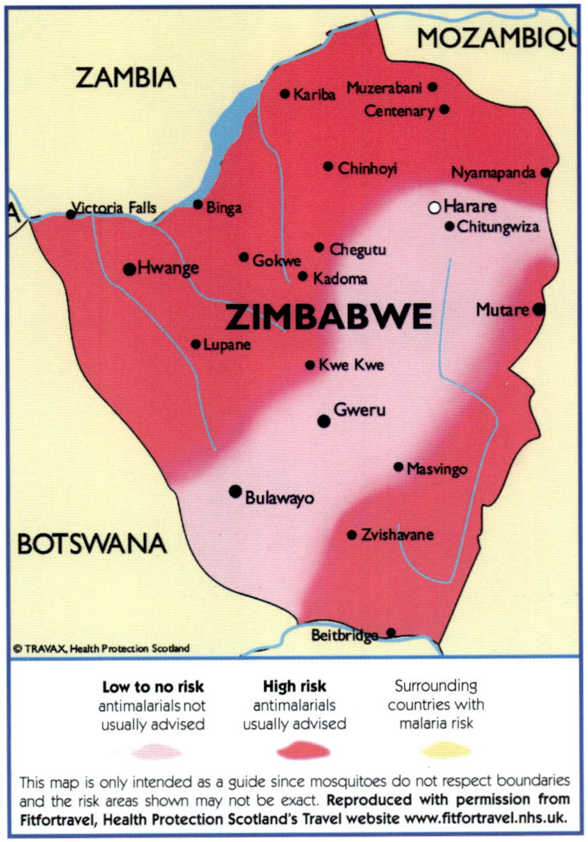

Malaria Advice

- ❑ Malaria is a serious and sometimes fatal disease transmitted by mosquitoes. You cannot be vaccinated against malaria.

MALARIA PRECAUTIONS

- ❑ Malaria precautions are essential in all areas below 1200 m from November to June and all year round in the Zambesi Valley including Victoria Falls. There is minimal risk in Harare and Bulawayo. Avoid mosquito bites by covering up with clothing such as long sleeves and long trousers especially after sunset, using insect repellents on exposed skin and, when necessary, sleeping under a mosquito net.
- ❑ Check with your doctor or nurse about suitable antimalarial tablets.
- ❑ Prompt investigation of fever is essential.

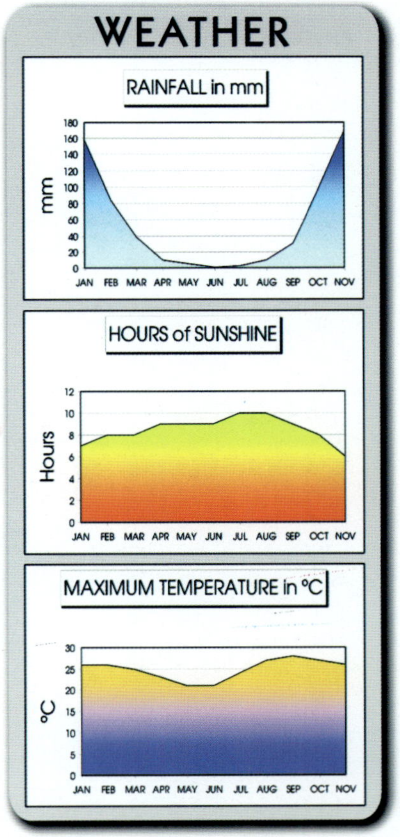

—Weather in Harare—